Dementia and Society

Dementia and Society

An Interdisciplinary Approach

Edited by

Mathieu Vandenbulcke
KU Leuven

Rose-Marie Dröes
Amsterdam University Medical Centers

Erik Schokkaert
KU Leuven

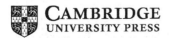
CAMBRIDGE
UNIVERSITY PRESS

CAMBRIDGE
UNIVERSITY PRESS

University Printing House, Cambridge CB2 8BS, United Kingdom

One Liberty Plaza, 20th Floor, New York, NY 10006, USA

477 Williamstown Road, Port Melbourne, VIC 3207, Australia

314–321, 3rd Floor, Plot 3, Splendor Forum, Jasola District Centre, New Delhi – 110025, India

103 Penang Road, #05–06/07, Visioncrest Commercial, Singapore 238467

Cambridge University Press is part of the University of Cambridge.

It furthers the University's mission by disseminating knowledge in the pursuit of education, learning, and research at the highest international levels of excellence.

www.cambridge.org
Information on this title: www.cambridge.org/9781108843508
DOI: 10.1017/9781108918954

First published 2022

A catalogue record for this publication is available from the British Library.

ISBN 978-1-108-84350-8 Hardback

Contents

Contributors

Wilco P. Achterberg, MD, PhD, Department of Public Health and Primary Care, Leiden University Medical Center

Ursula C. Basset, PhD, Center for Research on Family Law, Pontifical Catholic University of Argentina

Dawn Brooker, PhD, Association for Dementia Studies, University of Worcester

Frauke Claes, MSc, Forensic Psychiatry, Psychiatric Centre Sint-Kamillus, Bierbeek

Patrick Cloos, MD, PhD, School of Social Work, Department of Social and Preventive Medicine, School of Public Health, Centre for Public Health Research, University of Montreal

Anja Declercq, PhD, LUCAS – Centre for Care Research and Consultancy and Centre for Sociological Research, KU Leuven

Jan De Lepeleire, MD, PhD, Academic Centre for General Practice, KU Leuven

Laura Dewitte, PhD, Faculty of Psychology and Educational Sciences, KU Leuven

Jessie Dezutter, PhD, Faculty of Psychology and Educational Sciences, KU Leuven

Rudi D'Hooge, PhD, Laboratory of Biological Psychology, and Leuven Brain Institute, KU Leuven

Rose-Marie Dröes, PhD, Department of Psychiatry, Amsterdam University Medical Centers, Location VU Medical Center

Sebastiaan Engelborghs, MD, PhD, Department of Neurology, Universitair Ziekenhuis Brussel; Center for Neurosciences, Vrije Universiteit Brussel; Department of Biomedical Sciences, University of Antwerp

Paul Enzlin, PhD, Centre for Clinical Sexology and Sex Therapy, University Psychiatric Center KU Leuven, and Institute for Family and Sexuality Sciences, KU Leuven

Teake Ettema, PhD, Department of Psychiatry, Amsterdam University Medical Center

Shirley Evans, PhD, Association for Dementia Studies, University of Worcester

Josiane Ezin-Houngbe, MD, Department of Psychiatry, Cotonou, Université Nationale du Bénin

Nelle Frederix, MSc, Aditi vzw

Chris Gastmans, PhD, Centre for Biomedical Ethics and Law, KU Leuven

Debby Gerritsen, PhD, Department of Primary and Community Care, Radboud university medical center Nijmegen

Peter Hacker, DPhil, Emeritus Research Fellow, St John's College, Oxford University

Gørill Haugan, PhD, Department of Public Health and Nursing, NTNU Norwegian University of Science and Technology; Faculty of Nursing and Health Science, Nord University

Ann Heylighen, PhD, Research[x]Design, Department of Architecture, KU Leuven

John Keady, PhD, Division of Nursing, Midwifery and Social Work, University of Manchester

Martin Knapp, PhD, Care Policy and Evaluation Centre, Department of Health Policy, London School of Economics and Political Science

Ruslan Leontjevas, PhD, Faculty of Psychology, Open University of The Netherlands

Catarina Lundberg, PhD, Traffic Medicine Centre and Medical Unit Medical Psychology, Karolinska University Hospital

Jeroen Luyten, PhD, Leuven Institute for Healthcare Policy, KU Leuven

Constantine G. Lyketsos, MD, MHS, Johns Hopkins Bayview, Johns Hopkins Medicine

Mary S. Mittelman, DrPH, Department of Psychiatry, NYU Grossman School of Medicine

Tim Opgenhaffen, PhD, Institute for Social Law KU Leuven; Centre for Government and Law, Hasselt University

Bart Pattyn, PhD, Institute of Philosophy, KU Leuven

Marleen Prins, MSc, Department on Aging, Netherlands Institute of Mental Health and Addiction (Trimbos Institute)

Johan Put, PhD, Institute for Social Law and Leuven Institute of Criminology, KU Leuven

Dorota Religa, MD, PhD, Traffic Medicine Centre, Karolinska University Hospital; Department of Neurobiology, Care Sciences and Society, Karolinska Institutet

Martin Rossor, MD, PhD, Dementia Research Centre, Institute of Neurology, University College, London

Erik Schokkaert, PhD, Department of Economics, KU Leuven

Aline Sevenants, PhD, LUCAS – Centre for Care Research and Consultancy, KU Leuven

Cheng Shi, PhD, Department of Social Work and Social Administration, The University of Hong Kong

Peter Simonsen, PhD, Department for the Study of Culture, University of Southern Denmark

Mythily Subramaniam, MD, PhD, Institute of Mental Health, Singapore and Saw Swee Hock School of Public Health, National University of Singapore

Aagje Swinnen, PhD, Department of Literature and Art, Faculty of Arts and Social Sciences, Maastricht University

Jos Tournoy, MD, PhD, Gerontology and Geriatrics, Department of Public Health and Primary Care, KU Leuven

Lies Van Assche, PhD, Geriatric Psychiatry, University Psychiatric Center KU Leuven

Chantal Van Audenhove, PhD, LUCAS – Centre for Care Research and Consultancy, and Department of Public Health and Primary Care, KU Leuven

Maarten J. A. Van Den Bossche, MD, PhD, Geriatric Psychiatry, University Psychiatric Center, KU Leuven, and Leuven Brain Institute, KU Leuven

Mathieu Vandenbulcke, MD, PhD, Geriatric Psychiatry, University Psychiatric Center, KU Leuven, and Leuven Brain Institute, KU Leuven

Ann Van der Jeugd, PhD, Laboratory of Biological Psychology, and Leuven Brain Institute, KU Leuven

Henriëtte G. van der Roest, PhD, Department on Aging, Netherlands Institute of Mental Health and Addiction (Trimbos Institute)

Jenny T. van der Steen, PhD, FGSA, Department of Public Health and Primary Care, Leiden University Medical Center; Department of Primary and Community Care, Radboud university medical center

Baldwin Van Gorp, PhD, Institute for Media Studies, KU Leuven

Iris Van Steenwinkel, PhD, Department of Architecture, KU Leuven

Pieter Vermeulen, PhD, Department of Literary Studies, KU Leuven

Frans Boch Waldorff, MD, PhD, Research Unit and Section of General Practice, Department of Public Health, University of Copenhagen

Perla Werner, PhD, Department of Community Mental Health, University of Haifa

Introductory chapter illustrations and cover art
© Luisa Jung

Preface

As the population grows older, dementia becomes more noticeable in our society. Most of us sooner or later have to deal with dementia in our close environment or personally. Although there are some promising reports of decreasing incidence, prevalence is on the rise, especially in low- and middle-income countries. Surveys tell us that cognitive decline is the biggest concern among older adults. Both the unfamiliar realm of dementia and the prospect of losing one's cognitive abilities are terrifying. Most people fear to lose themselves and their dignity. People are afraid of not being taken seriously anymore, of being pushed aside in society. Such feelings express the imminent degradation of the very essence that a society stands for. The word 'society' comes from the Latin word *societas*, which is derived from the noun *socius*, meaning ally or friend, and describes a bond between people. Society is about living together as prosperously as possible. Of course, by the nature of their condition, persons with dementia are at higher risk of losing connection with the community they belong to and vice versa. To mitigate the risk of alienation and to safeguard the well-being of humans with cognitive impairment and their caregivers, society must consider how its policy and organization can best be tailored to the needs of people with dementia. This requires deep reflection on a range of topics: What defines dementia? Does the meaning of dementia depend on the perspective taken? How is dementia perceived in our society? Do portrayals of dementia affect persons living with dementia? How is dementia experienced and how does it affect relationships with others? What determines quality of life for persons with dementia? Can people with dementia still have a meaningful life? How to create a supportive and safe environment, when to decide on future care decisions and how to organize and finance care? Obviously these questions can only be answered by bringing together expertise from different disciplines, which was the set-up of this book.

Metaforum

This book is part of an initiative of the University of Leuven (KU Leuven) called Metaforum. Metaforum is an interdisciplinary think tank that brings together Leuven academics and international colleagues to reflect on societal themes. Its mission is to make the wealth of scientific and scholarly expertise on pressing societal issues available to policymakers and the general public. In 2018, a working group on dementia was launched, assembling KU Leuven scholars and international experts with an interest in dementia from different fields, including medicine, biology, psychogeriatrics, epidemiology, nursing, social law, economics, social psychology, human movement sciences, moral philosophy, architecture and literary studies. This initiative was sponsored by Opening the Future, a philanthropic campaign at KU Leuven targeting neurodegenerative diseases. The gathering led to a series of animated interdisciplinary discussions and lectures on various topics related to societal aspects of dementia. The fellows consented to share their ideas in the form of a book that reflects Metaforum's way of working – that is, offering different perspectives on themes raised by the experts rather than aspiring to an exhaustive account on the consequences of dementia for the community. In general, choices were based on a common interest of scholars from different disciplines who participated in the discussions, the feeling that the topic required an interdisciplinary approach, and consensus among the fellows that the topic was timely and of interest to a broad audience eager to learn about societal aspects of dementia. Accordingly, most of the chapters are the result of intensive crosstalk between a group of authors of different disciplines and include different points of view.

Audience

The book targets a broad audience of professionals working in the field of dementia, academics, students and lay readers with an interest in dementia, as well as policy advisors and representatives from politics who want to learn more about the impact of dementia on society and its citizens and good ways to deal with it.

Flow

All chapters stand on their own and can be read separately depending on the interest of the reader. For the reader new to the field of dementia, or with a more general interest in the topic, we ordered the chapters so that the reader's view on dementia gradually broadens as the book progresses. Although most chapters focus on a specific topic or perspective, they also contribute to the understanding of other topics or perspectives on dementia.

A clustering principle that we loosely kept in mind after introducing the origins of the concept and public perception of dementia (Chapters 1 and 2) was moving from the micro level – that is, the person with dementia (Chapters 3–5) – to the meso level – that is, close environment (Chapters 6 and 7) – and the macro level, corresponding with society and public policy (Chapters 8–14).

Brief Outline

To familiarize the reader with the concept of dementia, we describe in Chapter 1 the history and current definition of dementia and give an overview of perspectives on dementia beyond the biomedical approach. We discuss several psychosocial models as well as anthropological, societal and political views on dementia. In Chapter 2, complementary to Chapter 1, we offer a sociocultural perspective on dementia and explore the history and meaning of the stigma of dementia as well as how dementia is portrayed in language, media and literature. In the three following chapters, we discuss how dementia affects the person living with it. In Chapter 3, we discuss from a philosophical perspective how the dignity of persons with dementia can be respected, even if dementia affects identity, autonomy and personhood, and we confront this philosophical analysis with juridical and clinical reflections. In Chapter 4, we argue that meaning in life matters

for persons with dementia and is an important determinant of well-being. In Chapter 5, we examine what quality of life, as the main outcome of care intervention, represents, how different measures reflect different conceptions of well-being and how these cover what people with dementia find important in life. In the next two chapters, we discuss how dementia affects relationships and informal carers as well as the support provided to deal with it. Chapter 6 focusses on partner relationships, from the perspectives of both the person with dementia and the partner. We examine how dementia affects relational roles, intimacy and sexuality. In Chapter 7, we describe the characteristics of informal care and evidence-based interventions to support caregivers. Next, in Chapter 8, we discuss psychosocial interventions that could mitigate the risk of developing dementia, followed by a description of the principles of an empowering environment for persons with dementia and several operationalizations in Chapter 9. The COVID-19 crisis uncovered some serious shortcomings in the way care is organized for people with dementia, which are addressed in Chapter 10. In Chapter 11, we discuss participation and inclusion of persons with dementia, both from a human rights and ethical perspective, and in Chapter 12, the specific issue of end-of-life decisions. In Chapter 13, we turn theory into practice by discussing the specific case of driving in dementia, illustrating the delicate balance between individual freedom, social inclusion and public safety. Finally, in Chapter 14, we discuss the economic consequences of inclusive policies and care initiatives that improve quality of life of people with dementia.

Cross-links

There are many connections between the different chapters, leading to complementary insights on various topics. Let us illustrate this point by focussing on one of the book's central themes – namely, *social inclusion* as a means to improve the quality of life of persons with dementia. In Chapter 1, we introduce the person-centred care model, which is about knowing the person through interpersonal relationships and actively involving persons with dementia in social life, searching for sources of fulfilment or meaning, and being aware of disempowering communication strategies in social interactions with broad negative effects. The latter includes discriminatory attributions of the general public, called public stigma, that hamper integration of persons with dementia, which we discuss in Chapter 2. In Chapter 4, we argue that experiencing meaning in life, which is frequently related to having social connections, strongly contributes to well-being in dementia, and that people with dementia are still able to indicate what the sources of meaning are in their life, even in advanced stages. However, creating togetherness and finding shared meaning in relationships and activities is challenged by dementia and also dependent on the well-being of caregivers, as discussed in Chapters 6 and 7 respectively. In Chapter 9, we discuss how the organization of both the physical and social environment can maximize social inclusion and quality of life, and in Chapter 10, what detrimental effects disruption of this empowering environment can have, which became dramatically clear during the COVID-19 crisis. Although the effects of loneliness and lack of social engagement on well-being and cognitive outcome have been well known to the field for many years, the COVID-19 crisis clearly exposed the negative consequences of social isolation and demonstrated the necessity of good psychosocial care for people with dementia. The presence of such negative psychosocial factors may even increase the risk of developing dementia, as discussed in Chapter 8. Finally, Chapter 14 shows that there is a clear association between some of the factors that negatively impact social inclusion and socio-economic status, leading to inequality in health at old age. Thus,

throughout the book, different perspectives complement each other, creating a multifaceted view on social inclusion and on other themes that are important for living well with dementia.

Rational scientific language is not adequate to capture all the different dimensions of the experience of persons with dementia and of the persons interacting with them. That is why we have included in the book some selected poems that have the power to touch more directly our emotions.

Clearly, we took advantage of the many interactions between the experts during the meetings organized by Metaforum. We also believe that many authors were inspired by the interdisciplinary discussion during the writing process. Nevertheless, despite the high interrelatedness of the contributions, we found it challenging to bridge the gaps between theory and practice and to really integrate the viewpoints of the different disciplines. We strongly feel that this book is not an end point, but rather an attempt to find a common language between various disciplines which is an indispensable first step to address a complex problem such as dementia. We hope that this book will be a source of inspiration for an integrative policy that aims for a better life for people with dementia. We also hope that it becomes increasingly clear to the reader, as it became to us, that improving the lives of people with dementia is a collective responsibility.

Mathieu Vandenbulcke, Erik Schokkaert and Rose-Marie Dröes

Then it was autumn.

Carol Frost

Each morning she would rise and dress
and walk out the back door where orange rounds
hung from boughs – breasts, big acorns, eggs, jewelry bags?
She waited, she told me, for the right word
to come back to her. Maybe she stood on the patio a few minutes
or hours. The closing click of the door behind her
made her look back, and she stepped inside.
I don't think I believed her then. The weeks passed,
the months, then her forgetfulness blended with angers,
as if red wild bees were knocked from large red blossoms
by witches. When she began her wandering
along cracking pavement, by blank billboards, toward lights
that in the distance must have seemed mythic (or she slept,
intent on making time go away, like a vagrant),
then I felt hushing in her before, by dark severance,
flesh no longer could feed the sweetest mind.
Honeycomb, goddess, death, fate, and the human heart,
they lived in her until too many of her words
flew like birds of the muses away, so few at first
that their disappearance didn't much matter.

Different Perspectives on Dementia

Lies Van Assche, Martin Rossor, Constantine Lyketsos, John Keady and Mathieu Vandenbulcke

1 A Brief History of the Concept of Dementia

1.1 Earliest Historical Traces of Dementia

The earliest references to dementia were discovered in an ancient Egyptian text written in the twenty-fourth century BCE. Even though it is not a medical record, the text describes clearly in hieroglyphs the situation of Ptah-Hotep, who was a vizier during the Fifth Dynasty of Egypt. According to the text, Ptah-Hotep spent every night becoming more 'childish'. His inability to remember yesterday was also noted. Progressive behavioural changes as well as memory decline suggested that Ptah-Hotep was developing a dementia syndrome [1]. Ironically, he was highly esteemed for writing maxims, early Egyptian 'wisdom' literature, that instructed young men on appropriate behaviour and promoted self-control instead of childishness. The next identified reference to dementia or mental decline in old age was in the writings of classical authors.

1.2 Transition from Age-Related Senility to Dementia

Papavramidou [2] studied ancient Greek and Byzantine writings from the seventh century

BCE up to the fourteenth century CE in order to examine how people viewed ageing, senility or dementia in the classical era. She studied literary texts as well as scientific manuscripts and concluded that the history of dementia may be divided into two periods distinguishing between different types of ontologies associated with mental decline, the period before and after Posidonius in the late second to the early first century BCE (see Figure 1.1).

In the first period, authors mainly refer to dementia or senility as a condition brought forward by age. Indeed, already in the seventh century BCE, Pythagoras proposed that old age came with mental derangement. Specifically, a regression of mental faculties began at age 60 and by the age of 80 one would have reached a state of 'imbecility' or 'infancy'. Two centuries later, Hippocrates referred to a similar phenomenon using the term 'morosis' (*becoming a child*) as a decline in the intelligence associated with ageing. Plato and Aristotle explained this decline as a result of bilious 'humours' or excessive black bile that was trapped in the body in old age and hence led to forgetfulness and reasoning problems.

However, in the second period, starting with Posidonius in the late second to the early first century BCE, there was a differentiation of the medical ontologies relating to dementia.

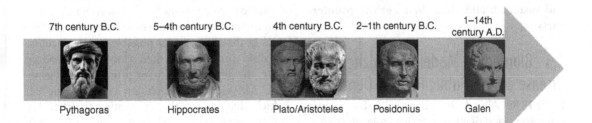

7th century B.C.	5–4th century B.C.	4th century B.C.	2–1th century B.C.	1–14th century A.D.
Pythagoras	Hippocrates	Plato/Aristoteles	Posidonius	Galen

Figure 1.1 Scholars addressing senility and dementia in the Greco-Roman period

Posidonius was the first to separate dementia due to old age ('leros') from dementia due to other causes ('morosis'). In a similar vein, Cicero – second century BCE – noticed that not all older people developed 'senile imbecility', only the 'weak'. According to him, an active mental life could offer the possibility of postponing senility. In the centuries that followed, many causes for dementia were described. Galen in the late first to the early second century CE clarified that a little humidity adding to cold in the brain was the main reason for morosis, as this mixture leads to inertia of the brain. Aretaeus in the second century CE referred to morosis occurring when melancholia aggravates. Psellus in the eleventh century and Actuarius in the thirteenth to fourteenth century CE wrote that cold and humidity specifically affect the ventricles of the brain, thus causing morosis. These concepts and ideas were maintained for several centuries as during the 'dark' Middle Ages, advances in understanding of dementia halted abruptly. Even though people were undeniably afflicted by dementia in this period, no relevant written sources are known.

According to Berchtold and Cotman [3], the next notable step in understanding dementia after the classical period was taken in the early 1600s during the Enlightenment. The English philosopher Francis Bacon wrote a book entitled *Methods of Preventing the Appearance of Senility* in which he noted that old age is the home of forgetfulness. In the second part of the seventeenth century, different types of dementia were characterized by Thomas Willis (1621–75), who was the personal doctor of Charles II. In his book *Practice of Physick*, he suggested that dementia might result from: (1) congenital factors, (2) age, (3) head injury, (4) disease or (5) prolonged epilepsy.

Only in the eighteenth century was 'senile' dementia considered distinct from usual ageing since the emerging new science of post-mortem study had shown that people with this condition had smaller brains than their healthy counterparts [4].

1.3 Biomedical Model with Alzheimer's Disease as the Public Face of Dementia

In the 1890s, Alois Alzheimer and Otto Binswanger extensively described the critical role of atherosclerosis in the development of brain atrophy and coincident senile dementia. A decade later,

Alzheimer was the first to discover specific changes in the brain that might be associated with symptoms of dementia. He studied a relatively young woman, Auguste Deter, who displayed progressive personality changes, confusion, suspiciousness towards her husband and hallucinations. Afterwards, pronounced memory problems occurred [5]. After her death at age 56, Alzheimer investigated changes in her brain post-mortem and found senile plaques that had been observed before only in older people, and first described neurofibrillary tangles. He reported on this in a case study entitled 'About a Peculiar Disease of the Cerebral Cortex' in 1907 and gave a lecture that received little attention.

For most of the twentieth century, Alzheimer's disease (AD) was considered a rare condition that affected mainly younger people and caused 'presenile' dementia. Hardening of the blood vessels, on the other hand, was considered a major contributor to cognitive decline in late life. Moreover, the causes for hardening of the blood vessels were sought in the organization of society that forced seniors to become inactive and isolated. According to Rothschild and many other psychiatrists, reduced stimulation of the brain was believed to result in cognitive deterioration [4].

A shift occurred in the early 1970s when studies of large numbers of post-mortem brains of older individuals observed extensive senile plaque loads that correlated with the clinical occurrence of dementia [6]. This shifted the field to attributing senile dementia to 'Alzheimer' pathology as opposed to vascular pathology and brought forward the term 'senile dementia of the Alzheimer's type', later to be replaced by AD irrespective of age, although early-onset (i.e. before the age of 65) and late-onset AD do have some different clinical features.

While recognition that senile plaques contain an amyloid protein was first proposed by Bielschowsky [7], the insoluble nature of the deposited protein made biochemical characterization difficult. With advances in molecular techniques in the 1980s, it was possible to sequence the amyloid protein and then clone the encoding gene, the amyloid precursor protein (APP) gene. The APP gene is located on chromosome 21, which aligned with the observation that trisomy 21 (Down's syndrome) individuals universally develop AD pathology by their early 40s with most also developing dementia. Subsequently, mutations in the APP gene were identified in autosomal dominant early-onset AD and soon after in presenilin genes that influence APP processing. This led to the formulation of the amyloid cascade hypothesis that postulated that the primary pathology is in amyloid deposition, which then leads to neurofibrillary tangles, synaptic dysfunction, neuronal loss and symptoms. Alzheimer's disease thereafter remained the 'face' of dementia for a long period. However, increasingly, it has become clear that there are many 'faces' of dementia and many degenerative illnesses that trigger cognitive decline or behavioural changes and subsequent dementia.

1.4 The Current Definition of Dementia

Dementia is a condition that may be caused by a wide range of diseases. Specifically, dementia is defined as a clinical syndrome of global cognitive decline affecting one or more cognitive domains, including complex attention, learning and memory, language, executive function, perceptual motor function and social cognition. The cognitive decline is severe enough to cause loss of independence by impairing the capacity to perform instrumental and/or basic activities of daily living. Individuals with dementia may experience difficulties that are so pronounced that they cannot live independently and over time become fully dependent on others.

Alzheimer's disease is the most common form of dementia, accounting for approximately 60% of all dementia diagnoses either alone or in combination [8]. However, many diseases are associated with dementia. The most recent (fifth) edition of the *Diagnostic and Statistical Manual* (DSM-5) replaces the term 'dementia' with 'major neurocognitive disorder' (NCD) and also distinguishes between acquired and developmental NCD, although many of the conceptual challenges are common to both [9].

1.5 The Spectrum of Cognitive Decline

In older people, dementia can be conceptualized as a syndrome encompassing advanced cognitive and functional decline, representing one end of a loose continuum ranging from 'usual' ageing to subjective cognitive impairment, mild cognitive impairment and finally dementia [10].

Usual – as opposed to 'normal' – cognitive ageing is characterized by reduced mental speed and less working memory capacity, leading to difficulties in spontaneous recall, less ability to multitask, slower organization and the appearance of greater indecision. These changes typically do not interfere with the level of functioning in an individual and do not cause distress. Subjective cognitive decline (SCD), on the other hand, refers to an experience of cognitive failing that is distressing to the individual. Subjective cognitive decline is not a universal aspect of ageing, and it should be noted that many individuals with dementia do not perceive and are not distressed by their cognitive impairment. There are several possible causes of SCD. For some individuals, the experience of deteriorating cognitive skills might be a first signal of a pathological process that has not yet been detected in neuropsychological testing or brain imaging. For others, these distressing subjective changes may not reflect brain pathology, but rather result from a tendency to be introspective or to value cognitive functioning more than other domains of functioning. For yet others, this might reflect experiences resulting from depression, sleep impairments or alcohol use.

Mild cognitive impairment (MCI) is different from SCD because cognitive decline, beyond what might be expected from usual ageing, is present but does not impair functioning enough to be dementia. These alterations are detected in neuropsychological testing and others also notice a change in functioning [11]. Still, a person with an MCI can function at a high level and continue to live independently. Clinicians distinguish single-domain and multiple-domain MCI, as well as amnestic and non-amnestic MCI. These all have different prognoses, although with enough time most individuals with MCI develop different types of dementia, which is why MCI is often referred to as a dementia 'prodrome' [12, 13]. For instance, an amnestic, multiple-domain MCI may result in Alzheimer's dementia more often than a non-amnestic, single-domain MCI [14]. In contrast, non-amnestic MCI appears more likely to be a prodrome for non-Alzheimer's dementia.

Dementia, finally, represents the most severe form of decline, in which a person is no longer able to function independently, with the term 'de-mentia' referring to the loss of mind. As is common in this 'medical' discourse, the most important discriminator of dementia from MCI or usual ageing is in the functional and social domain, referring to the possibility to function day to day independently or need support from others.

While there have been considerable scientific advances in understanding the pathogenesis of the several dementia aetiologies, many challenges remain. First, the distinction between a disease, referring to the underlying pathology, and a syndrome, referring to the impact a disease has on the experience and functioning of an individual, often remains troublesome to clinicians as well as to patients and their families. As a result, people are unsure concerning the prognosis of a condition, or which types of symptoms can be understood as a part of the disease and which symptoms might represent a psychological reaction to disease symptoms. Another issue is the current focus on early detection of diseases, even in the presymptomatic phases. Often, to people in whom a vulnerability to develop a certain disease has been detected, such a vulnerability is implicitly considered a first stage in the disease process [15]. Even to clinicians or researchers, this distinction is not always clear. This may cause unnecessary distress, even more so as there is currently not yet a cure for the neurodegenerative causes underlying dementia.

To add to the confusion that sometimes arises from the different names that exist for a condition characterized by progressive cognitive decline, the latest version of the DSM-5 has utilized an alternative categorizing system to refer to cognitive impairment [9]. As mentioned earlier, the manual distinguishes between mild and major neurocognitive disorders corresponding with MCI and dementia, respectively. Indeed, dementia was considered as a stigmatizing label that needed to be replaced by a more neutral reference to the symptoms that are observed [16, 17]. However, there was no clear consensus on the use of the terms 'major' and 'mild' neurocognitive disorder [17, 18].

2 Broader Models of Dementia

2.1 Challenges to the Traditional Medical Model

The development of a biomedical model has certainly advanced the approach to dementia. In previous centuries, largely devoid of scientific medical knowledge, individuals with symptoms of dementia such as disorientation or hallucinations were at risk of being persecuted for witchcraft; they were stigmatized and often isolated. Also, old age was often unconditionally associated with senility.

Fortunately, biomedical research has enlightened some of the pathogenic mechanisms behind dementia, hence making it an identifiable disease that does not warrant punishment or exorcism. Instead a treatment is required whereby the primary focus is on reversing impairments by means of 'medical-somatic' therapy or pharmacotherapy. Still, the application of a bygone biomedical model aimed at curing impairments caused by an illness has been limited as there is no cure for many of the neurodegenerative causes of dementia and quite often there are few effective pharmacological treatments of burdensome disease symptoms such as memory loss and disorientation [19]. Finally, neurobiological changes can explain only some of the considerable variety that is observed in individuals with dementia, with little conformity to any predetermined stage-like progression.

Hence, an excessively narrow application of the medical model risks minimizing the psychological and social sequelae of the disease, especially its effects on a person's experience of and reaction to certain symptoms. It also carries the risk of limiting the therapeutic potential of interventions focussing on the social environment by underappreciating the role of caregiving in patient outcomes.

Fortunately, in the 1970s, treatments were also starting to focus on the consequences of dementia, concentrating on how to deal with impairment, the reorganization of the living environment and social environments. Also, psychosocial care gradually gained importance, defined as the treatment of psychological and behavioural symptoms that occur when an individual tries to cope with or adapt to the limitations caused by dementia (see Figure 1.2) [20–21]. This treatment aims to support the person with dementia and their family and thus increase well-being.

2.2 Biopsychosocial Models of Dementia

A treatment that encompasses all three perspectives and that considers interventions focussed on cure, rehabilitation and support as complementary is the biopsychosocial model, which was

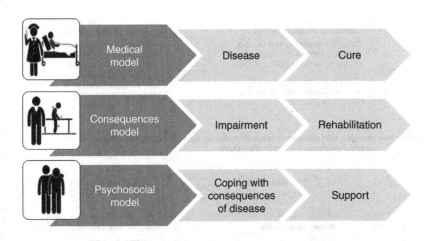

Figure 1.2 Different perspectives in the treatment of dementia [19]

introduced in 1977 by the internist and psychiatrist George Engel at Rochester University Medical Center in the USA [22]. He stated that to understand the full impact of an illness and treat it adequately, one should not just consider biological factors, but also personal and social factors of the individual with the illness.

In the 1980s and 1990s, many researchers developed biopsychosocial models that focus specifically on psychogeriatric care and dementia. A review by Finnema et al. [21] describes among others the dynamic systems analysis (DSA) model, utilizing a system-theory perspective in which complex interactions are emphasized instead of 'simple' and linear relationships. Hence, treatment of symptoms coinciding with dementia is based on the understanding of symptoms as the result of an interaction between somatic disease, cognition, personality, communication, the social environment and life history. Changes in any of these factors may have a therapeutic effect by altering the interaction.

Many practical applications exist of such biopsychosocial models. For instance, a major success in the USA is the person-centred, individualized Maximizing Independence at Home (MIND at Home) approach, which was developed in 2006 at Johns Hopkins University; it derives from an assessment of the individual needs of persons with dementia living at home, along with those of their caregivers [23–24]. It accounts for psychosocial determinants of health and behaviour and appreciates the importance of individual psychology in the development of illness and the central role of non-pharmacological therapies in improving clinical outcomes and quality of life. The assessment leads to a tailored set of interventions to address these needs using continuously evolving, evidence-based protocols. The MIND approach has been shown to delay transition from home to a nursing home, improve life quality and reduce care burden and healthcare costs.

Similarly, in the UK, Spector and Orrell [25] have developed a biopsychosocial approach which can be used as a tool for understanding individual cases (see Figure 1.3).

In this illustration, a 75-year-old person with Alzheimer's dementia is admitted to hospital as a result of increased anxiety and the need to constantly be with the partner, who reports a great care burden. Psychologically, there are events in the past that cannot be changed. The man lost his mother at an early age. Additionally, his father was unable to be responsive and care for his son, as he was experiencing a complicated grief process himself. Biologically, AD causes disorientation and memory problems. Therefore the environment is often unfamiliar, which causes anxiety, and the man seeks reassurance through proximity of carers. At home, this is usually the partner. Finally, sensory deficits increase feelings of being isolated and alone. Interventions can be aimed at reducing this feeling of loneliness and hence decreasing levels of anxiety. Specifically, proximity to others may be promoted, and sensory function may be ameliorated. Feelings of anxiety may hence be reduced. In some cases, however, when other interventions appear insufficient, pharmacological treatment can be indispensable to alleviate symptoms. The biopsychosocial model illustrated summarizes the disease process (using a timeline), fixed and changeable psychological or

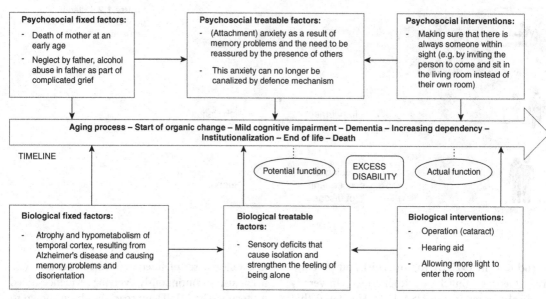

Figure 1.3 Case illustrating the biopsychosocial approach of Spector and Orrell [25]

biological factors. It encourages that dementia is recognized as something which is flexible, allowing for change, adaptation and improvement. The discrepancy between potential and actual function can be diminished, leading to less 'excess' disability. In some cases, this can postpone institutionalization and promote well-being. Preliminary research has already shown the benefits of applying such a model as this leads to a greater understanding of individuals with dementia and an improvement in caregivers' abilities to develop interventions. Caregivers also report feeling more knowledgeable [26].

Obviously, many more approaches in Europe and worldwide have proven their value as interventions that successfully concentrate on the well-being of the individual with dementia and their caregivers by focussing on disease symptoms, consequences and psychosocial factors. Interestingly, there are also different psychosocial models used in dementia care, derived from more general theoretical frames, such as the attachment theory, psychodynamic models or crisis and coping models. The majority of the research on biopsychosocial models in dementia, however, involves the person-centred approach, originally introduced by Kitwood [27]. We first discuss the

person-centred approach to dementia care and then briefly describe some of the other psychosocial models that have been developed.

2.3 Person-Centred Models of Dementia

I had become the guardian not only of George's medical history but also of the story of his life, a story that was increasingly difficult for him to articulate and of which it seemed that I alone knew many of the facts. Experiences, feelings, all kinds of memories from six decades of lived life, somehow all this had come into my keeping.

Hadas [28], p. 14

Kitwood [29] proposed an integrative and dialectical framework for dementia. In order to visualize the model, he used a simple equation:

$$D = P + B + H + NI + SP$$

In the equation, D stands for dementia, P for personality, B for biography, H for physical health, NI for neurological impairment and SP for social psychology.

There is a primary focus on the experience of an individual with dementia. In particular, person-centred models aim to understand how identity is formed and how it can be maintained in individuals with dementia. Kitwood and Bredin [30] believe the psychological 'self' has the potential to survive long into the illness. Hence, they looked at what a person with dementia needs and suggest that it is (1) *love*, (2) *comfort* and *trust* that comes from others, (3) *attachment* and a sense of familiarity when individuals with dementia so often feel as though they are in a strange place, (4) to be *included* in care and in the lives of others, (5) to be involved in the processes of normal life and have sources of *fulfilment* and, finally, (6) to have an *identity* related to personal history and preferences that distinguish them from another person and make them unique [27, 31].

According to Sabat and Harré's [32] social constructionist view, there is a personal singularity, a private self, that remains intact throughout the illness despite the debilitating effects of dementia (see Chapter 3). However, there is also a 'public' self or selves that can be lost indirectly as a result of the illness. In particular, negative social interactions can bring forth a detrimental effect on the sense of identity and well-being of a person with dementia. Kitwood [27] also delineated 17 types of 'malignant' social interactions which can lead to a diminished sense of self and self-worth (see Table 1.1).

Snyder [33] illustrated how negative social interactions may impact the well-being and 'personhood' of individuals with dementia. She describes how patients experienced being informed about their diagnosis by a neurologist and found that many had the impression that there was no compassion, no regard for or interest in the feelings of the individual who received a diagnosis, leading to an experience of being depersonalized by the healthcare professionals rather than feeling cared for. Snyder [33] speculated that perhaps these healthcare professionals were not uncaring, but they might have been inclined to position the person with dementia wrongly as someone who, because of the illness, cannot engage in a discussion about what the diagnosis means to him or her.

Table 1.1 'Malignant' social psychology developed by Kitwood [27]

Type	Definition
Treachery	Use of deception to distract or manipulate
Disempowerment	Not allowing someone to use abilities that one still has
Infantilization	Treating someone like a child
Intimidation	Causing someone to feel frightened as a result of verbal threat or physical power
Labelling	Referring to people inappropriately by using a term that describes and classifies them (associated with concepts of self-fulfilling prophecy or stereotyping)
Stigmatization	Treating someone as if they were an outcast
Outpacing	Providing information or asking questions/offering choices too quickly so information becomes difficult to understand or questions become impossible to respond to adequately
Invalidation	Not acknowledging the reality or experience of a person
Banishment	Excluding someone physically and/or emotionally
Objectification	Treating someone as an object (e.g. during washing, clothing etc.)
Ignoring	Talking about someone in their presence as though they are not there
Imposition	Forcing someone to do something
Withholding	Failing to provide attention or to fulfil an obvious need
Accusation	Blaming someone for their inability or misunderstanding
Disruption	Suddenly disturbing a person and interrupting their activity, speech or thought
Mockery	Making fun or joking at the expense of someone
Disparagement	Telling someone that they are worthless

Case

DOCTOR: How are you today?

PERSON WITH DEMENTIA: I am alright, but I need to get home. My children need to be picked up from school. Can someone show me the way out?

DOCTOR: There's no need for that. Your children are at home. You are in hospital. We will take care of you.

PERSON WITH DEMENTIA: I don't need to be taken care of. It's my children that need taking care of! Who can let me out? [Walks impatiently towards the exit and then towards the nursing station.]

DOCTOR: Has she been agitated all afternoon?

NURSE: Yes, we've tried to distract her, but she doesn't want any coffee ...

This conversation illustrates how individuals with dementia are sometimes subtly and involuntarily excluded from conversations, not taken seriously, and hence isolated in their experience. In some cases, this means that activities are taken over unnecessarily and decisions are made for the person with dementia without involving him or her. Specifically, in this example, the doctor addresses a nurse when the person with dementia is still present and talks about her behaviour as though she was not there. She is treated as someone who needs help from others rather than as a concerned mother who wants to take care of her children. She feels misunderstood. This interaction causes further distress rather than being reassuring.

The opposite of malignant social psychology, according to Kitwood, is positive person work [27]. It consists of 12 different types of behaviours and may lead to improvement of the condition, referred to as 'rementia' (see Table 1.2) [27, 34].

One example of positive person work is recognition, which occurs when someone thanks a person with dementia, affirms his or her views or greets him or her with his or her preferred name. Another form of positive person work is play – for instance, when individuals with dementia can undertake activities that engender spontaneity, self-expression, giving and enjoyment, such as a gardening session in which they can explain to the therapist how to tend to a plant.

In line with the effect that Kitwood [29], predicted Macrae [35] found no loss of self or personhood in a small group of Canadian individuals with AD who were surrounded by supportive caregivers, with little evidence of negative social interactions. Individuals led meaningful lives and they were not concerned with the loss of their identity. Hence, indirectly, this study could support the hypothesis of how the absence of malignant social psychology and the presence of positive person work may reduce threat to the 'self' or 'selves' and promote well-being [29].

Other researchers have also looked at possibilities for strengthening a person's sense of self-worth and identity. Harrison [36], for instance, suggested that caregivers try to look at the individual with dementia within the context of this person's life, which may help strengthen a feeling of continuity and hence preserve personhood. A recent systematic review found that reminiscence and life story work – which is not restricted to the recollection of memories, but also concerns an evaluation and reappraisal of the life course – are important interventions in trying to understand a person's biography and in stimulating a sense of identity [37].

However, there are some criticisms of the personhood notion proposed by Kitwood [29] and Sabat and Harré [32]. In particular, Kontos [38] states that the body should be given an active and agential role in the constitution and manifestation of selfhood as it is a substantive means

Table 1.2 Positive person work as developed by Kitwood [27]

	Type	Definition
Social interactions	Recognition	Being recognized as a person with unique thoughts, feelings or preferences
	Negotiation	Consulting with someone about their preferences and if possible involving them in decision-making
	Collaboration	Promoting partnership between the healthcare professional and the person with dementia in carrying out an activity
	Play	Providing activities that stimulate self-expression and enjoyment
	Timalation/ stimulation	A form of interaction that stimulates the senses (e.g. massage or aromatherapy)
	Celebration	Celebrating special occasions such as an anniversary or an achievement
	Relaxation	Offering a low-level intensity of stimulation and providing personal comfort
Psychotherapeutic interactions	Validation	Acknowledging someone's emotions and feelings and responding to them
	Holding	Creating a safe psychological space by containing distress and allowing self-revelation
	Facilitation	Enabling a person to do what he or she would otherwise be unable to do; stimulating the use of remaining abilities rather than pointing out errors
People with dementia can take a leading role in	Giving	Person with dementia presents him or herself in a positive, helpful way
	Creation	Individual is stimulated to be creative and offer something to the interaction spontaneously

by which individuals with dementia engage in the world and in which agency is not derived from a cognitive form of knowledge. She refers to an 'embodied selfhood' that has the potential to improve dementia care when it is better understood, and hence needs to be explored further in empirical research. In a similar vein, Fazio and Mitchell [39] studied the persistence of 'self' in AD using visual recognition of the body. Even though individuals did not remember a photographic session that occurred a couple minutes earlier, there was an unimpaired self-recognition of themselves on the pictures taken, suggesting that the body is an essential element in the maintenance of a sense of 'identity' [39].

Irrespective of the definition of personhood and self, the person-centred approach to dementia has been broadly applied and it has evolved over the years – for example, the Values-Individualized approach-Perspective taking-Social environment or 'VIPS' framework developed by Dawn Brooker [40] and applied by Rosvik et al. [41]. There have been several literature reviews looking at commonalities in the models and practices derived from the concept of 'person-centred care', leading to a general conclusion that personal choice and autonomy are of great importance [42]. In the most recent review, Fazio, Pace, Flinner and Kallmyer [43] concluded that, even though there is no consistent and clear statistical proof of the impact of person-centred care, there is sufficient evidence to warrant six recommendations. First of all, it is important to know the person living with dementia as a unique person who supersedes his or her diagnosis. Second, it is important to accept the person's reality, thereby promoting effective and emphatic communication. Third, it is important to identify and support ongoing opportunities for meaningful engagement, related to earlier or new interests and preferences, and to stimulate the experience of joy and purpose in life. Fourth, it is important to build and nurture authentic, caring relationships. People with dementia need to be connected and treated with dignity and respect. Also, it is important to create a supportive community for individuals, family and staff. This allows for comfort and creates opportunities to celebrate accomplishments. Finally, care practices need to be evaluated regularly and changed if necessary.

2.4 Psychological Adaptation-Based Models of Dementia

When models focus on individual psychology and specifically on coping of the person with dementia in order to explain behaviour or mood symptoms, they may be referred to as 'psychological adaptation-focussed' models of dementia.

In the psychodynamically inspired model of Hagberg [44], for instance, personality-related symptoms are considered one of the most sensitive indicators of the onset of dementia. In particular, the development of defence mechanisms is hypothesized to depend on cognitive maturation. Defence mechanisms are conceptualized as 'mediators' in conflicts between the individual's needs and environmental requirements. Rather than immediately showing feelings of frustration or anxiety, as they age, individuals become more efficient in channelling conflicts between their own needs and limitations in fulfilling these needs that are induced by the environment. Cognitive development and maturity is thought to solidify these strategies and, given intact cognition, the 'solutions' are believed to become more and more sophisticated. As dementia primarily affects cognition, defence mechanisms will change or become inefficient. This, in turn, can become evident in behavioural changes in a person with dementia. Changes are twofold, according to Hagberg [44], as the author suggests that there may be regressive behaviour on one hand and a shift in the dynamics from a conflict-free sphere to a conflict area on the other. Lack of defence strategies could uncover anxieties that are overwhelming for the individual with dementia and have to be dealt with by family or healthcare professionals. Hence, the kind of behaviour that becomes evident as a result of failing defence mechanisms may feel childlike to the social environment.

Another model that is in essence an interactive psychodynamic model is the adaptation-coping model. This model is also concerned with understanding the person's adaptation to the consequences of living with dementia and the influence the relationship with the social and physical environment can have on this process, in addition to personal history and disease-related factors. According to the adaptation-coping model [21, 45], which was based on the coping theory of Lazarus and Folkman and the crisis model of Moos and Tsu, living with dementia demands fulfilling certain adaptive tasks, such as dealing with increasing disabilities, developing an adequate care relationship with caregivers, preserving an emotional balance and positive self-image, maintaining social relationships and coping with an uncertain future. When the coping is less adequate, behavioural and mood symptoms can develop. Also, when the person is unable to cope with one or more adaptive tasks, he or she can even end up in a crisis. Support is therefore based on an individual psychosocial diagnosis which indicates the tasks and context in which the person experiences difficulties or distress, as shown by behaviour and mood disruptions and the defence and coping strategies he or she uses to maintain emotional balance. The three strategies to support the cognitive/practical, social and emotional adaptation are reactivation, resocialization and optimizing the emotional functioning, respectively. The subsequent concrete action plan consists of relevant psychosocial interventions, varying from cognitive stimulation activities, music therapy, art therapy and psychomotor therapy to reminiscence, and depends on the personal preferences and cognitive and functional abilities of the person.

A final model concerning the understanding of behaviour of people with dementia as an expression of their needs and as a manner in which they hope to fulfil these needs has been inspired specifically by a combination of ethology, psychodynamic theory and psychiatry. Attachment theory, originally conceived of by the psychiatrist John Bowlby [46] in the context of behaviour displayed by children towards their parents, was used as an explanatory model in understanding 'parent fixation' in individuals with dementia [47]. Attachment behaviour consists of all efforts to gain proximity to a primary caregiver or attachment figure in order to experience feelings of safety, warmth and security. It is especially prominent in stressful situations. Based on his clinical experience and behavioural experiments, Miesen [47] found that almost every older adult with dementia, at some point in the disease process, develops the conviction that his or her parents are still alive and some also experience the desire to find them (referred to as 'parent fixation'), leading to 'wandering' or emotionality. He interprets this behaviour as a need for security while being confronted with the many losses, disorientation

and anxiety that are the result of the disease. Interestingly, empirical research showed that a staff training in attachment theory resulted in an increased awareness of emotional needs of residents and at the same time in a reduction of anxiety and distress in these residents [48]. More in general, a homelike, familiar and secure environment seems crucial to promote well-being in individuals with dementia.

2.5 Environmental Adjustment-Focussed Models of Dementia

When the focus lies specifically on adjustment of the social or living environment to the needs of a person with dementia, models may be referred to as 'environmental adjustment focussed'. Hall and Buckwalter [49], for example, developed the progressively lowered stress threshold (PLST) model. According to them, it is important that the environment of individuals with dementia is adjusted to their cognitive as well as their functional abilities. The model distinguishes four stages in AD, each associated with different levels of stress tolerance further reducing throughout the day, and warranting a different organization of the physical and social environment. Factors that can increase distress throughout the day are fatigue, demands that exceed the capacities of the person with dementia, exposure to overwhelming or conflicting stimuli, emotional reactions to losses, physical stressors and, finally, changes regarding the caregiver, environment or routine.

Similarly, Souren and Franssen [50] emphasize that there are four different stages in AD, originally conceptualized by Reisberg et al. [51], and postulate that each stage warrants a specific approach and environment. In the first phase, there is a loss of planning and initiative, and therefore encouragement is needed. When insight, judgement and motivation reduce in the second phase of the illness, the caregivers need to intervene more actively in order to ensure safety and well-being. The third phase encompasses a loss of learned routine activities and speech, necessitating a partial taking over of activities. In the final phase, with complete loss of spontaneous motor movement, there is a complete taking over of activity.

2.6 Relationship-Centred Care in Nursing Homes

A final framework focusses on relationship-centred care. This approach supersedes the idea of adjusting the living and social environment to the needs of the person with dementia. Instead, in the development of relationship-centred care in nursing homes, Nolan and his colleagues [52] highlighted the importance of staff, carer and the person with dementia all working together. The Senses Framework addressed a sense of security, continuity, belonging, purpose, achievement and significance with the goal of attaining/reaching an enriched environment of care for the person with dementia and for the caregiver [52]. Table 1.3 provides a little more detail on the Senses Framework.

Importantly, the Senses Framework emphasizes interpersonal processes and experiences from a range of stakeholders, ensuring that a balanced approach to care and decision-making is taken whenever possible.

It is clear that there are many different models focussing on the treatment of dementia and derived from several (psycho)social theories. These models are not mutually exclusive, but are best used alongside each other as they can broaden our perspective

and allow us to better tailor our interventions to each person and caregiver individually. Still, there are limitations to the models discussed.

2.7 Limitations and Possible Routes for Further Development of a Biopsychosocial Model of Dementia

First of all, the development of biopsychosocial models have tended to use AD as the exemplar, mainly amnestic AD as the most common type of dementia. The combination of biological and psychosocial models is best understood in this context, and provides powerful approaches to management. Atypical AD and the other dementias, specifically the behavioural variant and semantic variants of frontotemporal lobar degeneration, have been less explored and create particular challenges. For example, in biparietal AD and cortical basal degeneration, the prominent parietal damage can mean that touch becomes unpleasant and individuals may demonstrate rejection behaviour [53]. This can negate the advice of Kitwood [27] to use massage. The behavioural changes in the behavioural variant of frontotemporal degeneration (bvFTD) and a number of individuals with semantic dementia present

Table 1.3 The six senses [52]

Sense	Definition
Sense of security = to feel safe within relationships	
For person with dementia: For staff:	Attention to essential emotional and physiological needs to promote a sense of safety Have secure conditions of employment, the emotional demand of work recognized, work within supportive culture
Sense of continuity = to experience consistency	
For person with dementia: For staff:	Recognition and valuing of personal biography Positive experience of work with older people from an early stage of career, positive role models
Sense of belonging = to feel part of things	
For person with dementia: For staff:	Opportunity to form meaningful relationships Feel part of a team
Sense of purpose = to have personally valuable goals	
For person with dementia: For staff:	Pursue personally relevant goals on a day-to-day base Have a sense of therapeutic direction, a clear set of goals
Sense of achievement = to make progress towards a desired goal	
For person with dementia: For staff:	Ability to engage in meaningful and satisfactory activity Be able to provide good care, feel satisfied with one's efforts
Sense of significance = to feel that you matter	
For person with dementia: For staff:	Feel recognized and valued as a person Feel that gerontological practice is valued and important, that work efforts 'matter'

another unique challenge for the application of psychosocial models developed for AD. In contrast to the preservation of the psychological self until late in AD as described by Kitwood and Bredin [30], personality in FTD can be the first change preceding deficits in cognitive domains. Moreover, nosognosia (lack of illness insight) can present a particular challenge in management. Nosognosia is well described in survivors of stroke – for example, Anton syndrome with cortical blindness and lack of awareness of a left hemiparesis, referring to the weakness or the inability to move on one side of the body in right hemisphere strokes in right-handed people. Nosognosia of cognitive deficits also occurs in the dementias – for example, the memory deficit in AD. It appears distinct from denial of cognitive failure that might reflect psychological defence mechanisms, but rather seems related to damage to the neural network that can compute awareness of the deficit. Future biopsychosocial models will need to accommodate not only the rich variety of psychological and social factors, but also variability in the pattern of neurodegeneration.

Still, irrespective of these limitations, as is the case in psychotherapeutic practice in general, an important guideline seems to be that the basis of warm and genuine contact, time and attention, and respecting autonomy and individuality seems necessary in professional dementia care [54].

3 Anthropological Perspectives on Dementia

It is a mistake to assume that Western classifications, explanations and subsequent decisions concerning treatment of disease are self-evident across the world [55]. There is relatively little knowledge about how disorders of old age are experienced and understood in non-Western settings [56]. Yet anthropology emphasizes that knowledge and behaviour are usually logical but highly dependent on a person's context [57]. Hence, in order to fully comprehend the impact of dementia, it is important to gain an idea of the different contexts in which individuals with dementia reside, even more so as social and cultural factors predict recognition of symptoms, help-seeking strategies and caregiving behaviours. Researchers have looked at different types of societies in different areas of the world, such as

the USA, Hawaii, Africa, UK, China, India and Japan.

One major difference in perspective that has become evident concerns the level of *material well-being* and the development of a healthcare system, which was for a long time associated with industrialization. Even though there are differences in levels of 'acculturation' as a result of increased migration [58], in most underdeveloped nations across the world, knowledge of dementia remains limited [59, 60]. Memory problems or other cognitive symptoms are usually still interpreted as a natural result of ageing. As older people are often highly respected in less developed countries because of the wisdom they can share with younger members of society, people with memory problems are well cared for at home. When the prestige of being an elder decreases, often alongside the level of industrialization or development, neglect becomes more apparent. For instance, in more urbanized regions of sub-Saharan Africa, older adults with dementia are neglected more often than in rural areas because they cannot be productive and provide income [61–62]. Behavioural issues associated with dementia are often more problematic. In some African regions, it is believed that an individual with behavioural problems may be possessed by a demon or affected by a curse, or this person might be suspected of willingly committing a criminal offence [62]. Hence, people are sometimes put through exorcist rituals or they may be incarcerated for several years, instead of receiving the medical or psychosocial aid they need (see Box 1).

In Indian American societies, some behavioural or psychological symptoms that coincide with dementia are considered a supernatural gift. Specifically, hallucinations are regarded as communications with the dead ('those we cannot see', rather than 'those who are not there') [63–65]. This interpretation is consistent with the context, as Indian American tribes are convinced that older individuals who are closer to death may have more contact with the deceased.

In 'developed' countries such as the USA, UK or China, people are often aware that dementia is an illness that requires medical and psychosocial treatment and that it may be characterized by cognitive as well as psychological and behavioural symptoms. However, there are still differences in the way people with dementia are viewed and

---

Box 1 Sociocultural representations of dementia in Benin

Benin, like other sub-Saharan African countries, is faced with an ageing population. Approximately 4.4% of the population is currently older than 60 years. As a result, the prevalence of old age diseases such as dementia is also rising. Specifically, there is a prevalence rate of 2.3% in the rural areas of Benin and up to 3.7% in urban areas. Hence, people are increasingly confronted with dementia and it is therefore interesting to see how the disease is experienced and conceptualized.

A qualitative study conducted by Josiane Ezin-Houngbe in a few large communities in southern Benin (Porto-Novo, Allada, Comé, Lokossa) included the responses of 30 individuals, and it showed that there was not a *single* word that refers to dementia. Instead, there were several terms referring to dementia:

- 'the spirit has gone into childhood' or 'the person has returned to childhood' (Ayi-yikpè)
- 'the disease of old age' (Kpeykpozon)
- 'the person who says things that have no coherence or meaning' (Numalémalé)
- 'the person who speaks to say nothing' (Gblo-no)
- 'a person who forgets, a person whose thinking is unstable' (Ayifena-No)

Interestingly, dementia was not always considered a disease. Sometimes it was conceptualized as a normal part of ageing. A man is born as a child, grows up and ends up again as a child. Other non-medical causes for dementia were witchcraft or punishment for previous crimes. Indeed, it is believed that a person who has done much harm to innocent souls may be haunted by them in the 'evening of his or her life'.

Caregiving is mostly done by women, partners or children of the person who is ill. If family members refuse to take on this role, they risk being isolated, scorned and even cursed for it. Whereas female members of the family are usually involved in caregiving, male family members are often responsible for financial contributions to the household. When a parent becomes ill, a woman is expected to leave her own home and take care of her mother or father, which may lead to marital conflicts. Many children solve this problem by taking on a housekeeper.

Josiane Ezin-Houngbe

---

treated. One study demonstrated that American society may be more instrumentalist, emphasizing the disability and need for institutionalization associated with dementia, whereas the UK tends to focus more on emotional aspects of the disease. In China, dementia care was usually provided by family, most often the eldest son. However, cultural values are changing, partly as a result of the 'one child' policy and the subsequent shift in the demographic reality. Many children are unable to care for ageing parents and meet other demands in life at the same time. In a recent study by Calia, Johnson and Cristea, [66] a task that requires people to associate freely to the word 'dementia' illustrates how dementia has become more of an 'inconvenience' to Chinese individuals (see Figure 1.4).

Another difference in the way people are viewed and treated when they display symptoms of dementia across the world is related to the findings displayed in Figure 1.4 and refers to the more *individualistic versus more sociocentric* orientation of a society [61, 67]. Japanese culture is typically described as sociocentric, whereas American culture is often regarded as more individualistic. Some authors argue that these orientations are mutually dependent and dynamically constituting the experiences of one individual within a specific culture [68]. One may conclude that, even though there is no clear-cut difference, some cultures have a more individualistic or a more sociocentric orientation and people with dementia appear to be treated differently, in line with the most dominant orientation in one culture. For instance, behavioural problems or increased dependency on others are considered 'shameful' in Japan. People have not been able to care for themselves and prevent the development of cognitive decline through exercise. Hence, they become a burden to others. In India, there is a taboo as well. However, this is related to the belief that dementia may be caused by a 'neglectful family'. Cohen [69], for instance, describes a situation of a woman who is thought to have become forgetful and disorientated as a result of intergenerational conflict. In particular, her son marrying a foreigner is considered the direct cause of her illness. Behavioural problems are interpreted as the result of neglect, memory loss as the consequence of shock and sorrow. Many

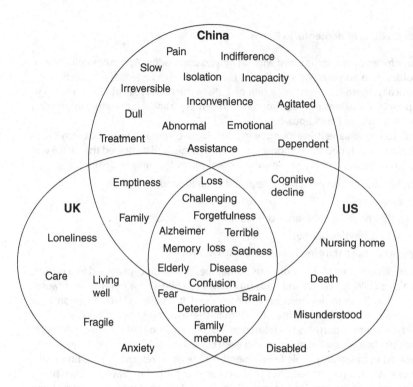

Figure 1.4 Results from a free association task with 'dementia' as a stimulus across the USA, UK and China, based on results from the study by Calia et al. [66]

doctors view medical treatment as ineffective. Rather, changes in the family might procure improvement in functioning.

In most sociocentric countries, care is provided by the family. Usually female members of the family are responsible for older people who display symptoms of dementia. However, there is one exception. A study that researched caregiving for older people with dementia in Hawaii found that care for older people with dementia is provided by the person the family thinks could care best. This may be a male or female member of the family. He or she receives control over and becomes the 'coordinator' of the care. Medical care is only sought when the doctor is a friend or someone the family knows well [62]. However, the only study on caregiving for a relative with dementia in Hawaii was conducted in 1998, which may mean that the findings do not take into account changes that have taken place in the social structure in Hawaii in the past decades.

Finally, irrespective of the level of development and the individualistic or more sociocentric orientation of society, dementia is seen as a condition that may lead to dehumanization globally. In Japan, for instance, to become a burden without ever being able to reciprocate

the care offered may procure the loss of one's basic humanity [64]. In Western cultures, on the other hand, cognitive changes that impact autonomy and personal control may result in a similar experience of not being a full human being. Hence, across cultures it seems important to seek out ways in which people with dementia might retain a continued sense of identity and purpose by contributing to society [70]. The importance of 'empowering' individuals with dementia, making them feel in control of their life, as well as valued as a person with a history, cannot be underestimated. The following paragraphs summarize the first steps that have been taken in order to promote empowerment in people with dementia, a feeling of control and safety, primarily looking at the history of dementia care in the UK, where the movement towards social inclusion of individuals with dementia knew an early start and has shown much progress.

4 Societal Perspectives on Dementia: A Movement towards Social Inclusion

We first outline how people with dementia moved from being positioned as those who were considered not to have a 'self' into today's citizens with growing peer-to-peer self-advocacy opportunities. Indeed, it is people with dementia who are now taking forward their own campaign for civil liberties under the banner of human rights and they are supported in this endeavour by the Alzheimer organizations and the World Health Organization in their (2017–25) global action plan on the public health response to dementia [71]. It is this movement and momentum towards social inclusion in society that we now trace, but to do that we must first turn back the clock to view a previous landscape of (in)formal care and organizational language that negatively framed the lived experience of dementia (see also Chapter 2).

4.1 Times Past

In the early 1980s, Brice Pitt's text *Psychogeriatrics* [72] explored the clinical characteristics of dementia, diagnostic considerations and procedures that needed to be followed during the person with dementia's inevitable downward trajectory towards double incontinence, faecal smearing and death. As Pitt [72] himself indicated, dementia was a 'tragic disorder' whereby:

> Sometimes it seems as if the true self dies long before the body's death, and in the intervening years a smudged caricature disintegrates noisily and without dignity into chaos. *(p. 39)*

Chaos and faeces – hardly an enticing introduction to the field. At this time, as it had been for many decades beforehand, it was not uncommon for people with dementia to be admitted to single-sex psychogeriatric wards – for example, at one of the (many) Victorian asylums spread across the UK – once care had broken down at home [73]. Such asylum-based care was provided free by the National Health Service and it is safe to say that most people with dementia admitted to such ward environments lived and died there hidden away from the public, their families and the gaze of the outside world. Looking at the (limited) literature from this time [73], it is difficult to find any positive language, imagery or affirmations about living with dementia and a rationale as why anyone would want to take on a caring role in such circumstances, either as a family member or as a member of a profession such as social work or mental health nursing.

However, amongst this societal neglect, the seeds of change were beginning to be sown. In the UK, one of the few policy reports in the 1980s that addressed the needs of people with dementia and their carers – a 1982 Health Advisory Service report called 'The Rising Tide' [74] – set out the components of a service for people with dementia and recommended that 'the role in providing support, advice and relief at times of special difficulty to families and primary health and social services is an essential ingredient in a successful comprehensive service' (p. 17). Such an overt commitment to carers and people with dementia was later reinforced by the King's Fund Centre [75] in a far-sighted project paper published two years later that detailed the principles of good service practice. By astutely avoiding sharing any exemplars of good practice in the report, the authors were able to set out a challenge to service providers and national policymakers. This was achieved by providing five key principles that outlined philosophical and practical beliefs about personal empowerment for people with dementia. These five key principles [75] (pp. 7–8 abridged) called for an acknowledgement that:

1. People with dementia have the same human value as anyone else irrespective of their degree of disability or dependence.
2. People with dementia have the same varied human needs as anyone else.
3. People with dementia have the same rights as other citizens.
4. Every person with dementia is an individual.
5. People with dementia have the right to forms of support which do not exploit family and friends.

Nearly 40 years on, these five key principles still speak a truth. However, in 1984, society and the caring professions were not quite ready to listen to these empowering values or, perhaps more important, to act on them.

As a consequence, in the research literature of the 1980s, people with dementia were predominantly positioned as a 'burden' and the direct cause of the caregiver stress and coping so widely reported at the time [76–77]. As an illustration, a significant contribution to advancing understanding about the meaning of care from the experiences of carers of people with dementia emerged from a study conducted in the USA by Miriam Hirschfield [78–79]. In this study, the author interviewed 30 carers of people with dementia (the sample also included unstructured interviews with seven people with mild cognitive impairment, but those data were not reported), and developed the concept of 'mutuality' as 'the most important variable' ([79] p. 26) to explain the social relationship between families and the person with dementia. In outlining the properties of 'mutuality', Hirschfield [79] suggested that:

> It grew out of the caregiver's ability to find gratification in the relationship with the impaired person and meaning from the caregiving situation. Another important component to mutuality was the caregiver's ability to perceive the impaired person as reciprocating by virtue of his/her existence.　　　　*(p. 26)*

Accordingly, mutuality was about carers' ability to find meaning, gratification and reciprocity in their caregiving role and relationship to 'the impaired person' (i.e. the person with dementia). Hirschfield [79] also reported that 'mutuality' was seen to exist within four parameters:

1. High mutuality from within the relationship (internally reinforced mutuality).
2. High mutuality due to circumstances (externally reinforced mutuality).
3. Low mutuality.
4. No mutuality survived.

Feelings of low mutuality were synonymous with poor adjustment within the family and negative feelings towards the person with dementia. This negative adjustment was as likely to be present in those caring for a person with mild dementia as those caring for a person living through its later stages. Hirschfield [79] outlined three other variables which influenced the planned continuation of home care: (1) management ability, (2) morale and (3) tension. Interestingly, the operational definition of tension included the feeling of 'being tied down', and this was conceptualized as the carer's restricted opportunity for free time and lack of individual privacy. Indeed, it was the combination of low/no mutuality survived coupled with 'severe tension' that Hirschfield believed to be the driving force for carers to consider admission into care for the person with dementia, thus predicting the breakdown of care at home. Hirschfield [79] illustrated the existence of this phenomenon via the following case example of 'no mutuality existing':

> I used to love my father; I used to love to see him come through the door. Now when he comes I hate it. It is like my emotions have changed. I hate to think that I hate my father now, but I just hate the disease he has. It's like I consider him dead three or four years ago ... some people say 'that's your father' but when you hear a door banging all night long you can't sleep.　　*(p. 28)*

With the son's description of the father being considered dead 'three or four years ago' Hirschfield's case illustration also identified another significant concept in the literature at the time – namely, anticipatory grief and social death [80–81]. Such imagery and negative language were later used to define the experience of living with AD as 'coping with a living death' [82], an identity marker that left little room for hope or well-being. A new broom was necessary to sweep away such negative and troubling representations, however well intentioned the overarching messages and the underpinning social science.

4.2　Time for a Change

Starting with the work on personhood and person-centred care by Tom Kitwood and members of the Bradford Dementia Group in the UK in the late 1980s [83, 84], and later built upon by others (see paragraph 2.3), new conceptual theories and standpoints about the lived experience of dementia began to emerge. This new wave of studies put the person with dementia's experience front and centre. As Kitwood wrote as the suffix to the title of his seminal book *Dementia Reconsidered*, published in 1997, and shortly before his untimely death, 'the person comes first' [84]. Such an open acknowledgement of the value attached to the experience of living with dementia helped create the space for the social inclusion and social citizenship to emerge: a relational dynamic for people with dementia that continues to the present day.

Whilst academic insights are important, they are not the final word. Indeed, it could be argued that the words and communicated life experiences of people who live with dementia both say so much and do so much to promote social change and social awareness. Stemming from the USA, two books published four years apart kick-started this new insight into the lived experience of dementia based upon individual testimonies. The first publication (in the world) emerged at the time of Kitwood's early writings in the late 1980s and was published in 1989. This was a relatively short book entitled *My Journey into Alzheimer's Disease* written by the Reverend Robert Davis [85], who was aged 54 at the time of the onset of (undiagnosed) AD. Underpinned by his Christian faith, pages 21–82 of this publication were written by the Reverend Davis and articulated a seven-month transition and adjustment to the onset of AD. The remainder of the publication was an interpretation of the later experience of dementia written by Reverend Davis' wife. This moving account portrayed the fear and uncertainty which accompanied Reverend Davis' journey into AD:

> I can no longer speak in public, and I shatter psychologically in any pressure situation. Mental and emotional fatigue leave me exhausted and confused. Mental alertness comes now only in waves at random hours of either the day or night.
> *(p. 24)*

The book also revealed that the couple's close marital relationship held them together during the onset and progression of dementia, particularly during the early months when Reverend Davis was struggling to make sense of his accumulating losses. Despite his best efforts, his inability to correct the situation was personally devastating to him as he had 'read a book a day from seventh grade on' (p. 29). Indeed, it was his inability to resolve this situation that eventually led Reverend Davis and his wife to seek medical help, although their diagnostic quest would prove to be a traumatic experience. In the book, Reverend Davis [85] continually cites his reliance on existential coping techniques to make sense of this experience with the dementia, 'part of God's plan' (p. 80) to test his faith, reconcile his past and affirm the durability of his marital relationship. There was also the belief, expressed both during his account and later by his wife, that AD had brought the couple closer together and that they were able to 'work through it' as a partnership once there was an awareness of the name and prognosis of the condition. It was this overriding combination of Christian belief, love and partnership that best summarized Reverend Davis' journey into AD and one that appeared to continue until the time of his death.

Four years later, another younger person with dementia living in the USA, Diana Friel McGowin, also wrote an influential book/testimony that provided a lucid account of being 'dragged' into AD

[86]. McGowin described the emotional, physical, social and sexual turmoil this process had upon her life and that of her family. However, in contrast to the account provided by Reverend Davis and his wife, for McGowin, the early transition into AD was marked by the denial of events by her husband and his reticence to acknowledge that she was failing in any way, as this extract from the book highlighted:

> The electric bill was higher than usual because my clothes dryer was not shutting off automatically. I frequently forgot to remove the clothes from the dryer and there were many days when the laundry load tumble-dried all day. Jack was furious, emphasising how much current the clothes drier used. All I had to do was remember to take the clothes out, he said. *(p. 82)*

For McGowin, such an exchange placed an additional layer of stress upon an already difficult situation, a process that led to ever-increasing cycles of blame and recrimination. Indeed, McGowin revealed that her husband continued to deny the reality of events for several years, which placed responsibility for responding to the symptoms directly with her and led to 'severe tension' in their marital relationship – a descriptive marker that directly echoes the earlier work of Miriam Hirschfield outlined in this section [78–79]. However, this time, it was McGowin, as the person with dementia, who was communicating the relationship challenges she was facing and proving, at a stroke of a pen, that care was not a unidirectional process (i.e. carer to person with dementia) and instead consisted of complex interrelational dynamics.

The importance of these two pioneering personal testimonies should not be overlooked. In their own ways, both books enabled people with dementia to voice their own lives and to remind the public and society as a whole that people with dementia were not simply objects to be studied and reported upon, but human beings who had much to give, share and communicate. It was, after all, their condition and not the exclusive property of others.

4.3 Time for New Horizons

Fast forward to the present day and people with dementia are now intertwined in the fabric of many procedures and practices in dementia care, be that service planning, research, policy, education, disseminations or design. Global, national and local forums have been established to enable the voices of people with dementia to be heard, with examples including:

- Dementia Alliance International (www.dementiaallianceinternational.org)
- European Working Group of People with Dementia (www.alzheimer-europe.org/Alzheimer-Europe/Who-we-are/European-Working-Group-of-People-with-Dementia)
- DEEP network (www.dementiavoices.org.uk)
- Scottish Dementia Working Group (www.alzscot.org/our-work/campaigning-for-change/have-your-say/scottish-dementia-working-group).
- 3 Nations Dementia Working Group (www.alzheimers.org.uk/get-involved/engagement-participation/three-nations-dementia-working-group)

Many of these initiatives are supported by public donations and/or dedicated charitable organizations such as Alzheimer Europe (www.alzheimer-europe.org) and the Alzheimer's Society (www.alzheimers.org.uk). Over the past 20 years or so, the pace of change has been rapid. However, it should not be forgotten, that in the UK at least, it was not until 2012 that people living with dementia were called 'citizens' in influential policy and strategy reporting and ascribed a status that was first set out in the five key principles of the 1984 King's Fund Centre report [75].

Developing this point, Bartlett and O'Connor [87] have put forward ideas around social citizenship to describe the ways in which people with dementia could remain socially included and active citizens. The authors underpinned social citizenship with an ongoing rights-based approach, as seen in their definition of social citizenship:

> Social citizenship can be defined as a relationship, practice or status, in which a person with dementia is entitled to experience freedom from discrimination, and to have opportunities to grow and participate in life to the fullest extent possible. It involves justice, recognition of social positions, rights and a fluid degree of responsibility for shaping events at a personal and societal level.
> (p. 37)

Constructing a theory of dementia through a rights-based approach has also been picked up and articulated by people with dementia

themselves and adopted by the World Health Organization in its (2017–25) global action plan on the public health response to dementia [71]. As a further illustration of this movement and momentum, in England, the Dementia Action Alliance has outlined five 'Dementia Statements' that people with dementia believe are essential to upholding their everyday quality of life:

- We have the right to be recognized as who we are, to make choices about our lives including taking risks, and to contribute to society. Our diagnosis should not define us, nor should we be ashamed of it.
- We have the right to continue with day-to-day and family life, without discrimination or unfair cost, to be accepted and included in our communities and not live in isolation or loneliness.
- We have the right to an early and accurate diagnosis, and to receive evidence based, appropriate, compassionate and properly funded care and treatment, from trained people who understand us and how dementia affects us. This must meet our needs, wherever we live.
- We have the right to be respected, and recognized as partners in care, provided with education, support, services and training which enables us to plan and make decisions about the future.
- We have the right to know about and decide if we want to be involved in research that looks at cause, cure and care for dementia and be supported to take part.[1]

As current policy and practice strategies develop to take account of the everyday lives of people with dementia, a rights-based approach to social citizenship that embodies such relational qualities may well be a foundation on which to build lasting change for people with dementia.

Finally, as we have highlighted throughout this section, sensitive language use is very important to the positive positioning of people with dementia and to enabling social inclusion. As a recent example of such work, in a co-produced study conducted alongside people with dementia, and with people with dementia as part of the authorship team, Caroline Swarbrick and her

---

[1] For further information, see www.dementiaaction.org.uk/news/23236_news_launching_the_dementia_statements, accessed 12 July 2020.

Table 1.4 Language guidance for use in any dementia-related outputs or publications

When writing about 'dementia'
Terms to use:
• Dementia • Symptoms of dementia • Younger onset dementia
Terms to avoid:
• Senile/senility • Slang expressions of dementia • Early onset dementia • Disease
When writing about 'people'
Terms to use:
• Person with dementia • Person living with dementia • Person supporting someone living with dementia • Living with/caring for/supporting a person who has dementia • Effect/impact of supporting someone with dementia
Terms to avoid:
• Demented/dementing • Sufferer/suffering • Subject • Patient (unless in a clinical context) • Service user • Client • Victim • Abbreviations, such as PWD • Carer burden

Adapted from Swarbrick et al. [88]

colleagues in the UK [88] provided language guidance for use in any dementia-related outputs or publications. Some of the main outcomes of this work are highlighted in Table 1.4.

Socially inclusive practices for people with dementia also extend to the environments where everyday life is played out. This can be seen in the rise of the dementia-friendly community movement [89] and in better understanding how people living with dementia age in place [90]. On this latter issue, Clark et al. [91] have recently undertaken a major mixed-methods study looking at how people with dementia connect to the spaces, places and people in their neighbourhood. The authors suggested that 'small acts of kindness' displayed by neighbours and friends helped people with dementia remain both socially connected and positively positioned in a relational network. The transcending message here is that it is sometimes not only major public health and dementia awareness initiatives that are required, but also a recognition that micro interpersonal practices in the neighbourhood help maintain the social identity and inclusivity of people with dementia. And in many ways, all of us have a civic obligation to play our part in both undertaking and maintaining such actions.

5 Political Perspectives on Dementia

In line with this, there is also an increased political interest in dementia, which results in part from the demographic reality that populations globally are ageing and hence the number of individuals with dementia is rising, which leads to rapidly increasing healthcare costs. The World Health Organization estimated that 47 million people worldwide had dementia, which results in a total cost of more than $1 trillion (USD) in 2019 [92]. Moreover, the number of individuals with dementia will increase to 75.6 million by 2030, leading to even greater costs in the near future (see also Chapter.14).

In 2013, the world's first G8 summit on dementia was organized. Ministers from the G8 countries, researchers, pharmaceutical companies and charities gathered in order to discuss the way in which prevention of dementia as well as treatment of the condition can improve [93]. The main resolutions involved the development of a coordinated research plan with international collaboration, the call for greater innovation in order to improve the quality of life for people with dementia and their carers while reducing emotional and financial burden, the development of cross-sector partnerships (research, industry, society at large etc.). Finally, there was an aspiration to increase awareness of the disease and its societal implications, and to continue global efforts to reduce stigma, exclusion and fear. These ambitions were confirmed during a second summit in 2015.

Also, as a part of the Access to Timely Formal Care (ActifCare) project, expert interviews were conducted in eight different European countries with political decision makers or representatives of relevant institutions in order to clarify their views on treatment of individuals with dementia. The results showed that there appears to be a need for a coordinating role in the organization of care, which should be person-centred, tailored to individual needs and in part formal and multi-disciplinary. According to the experts, there should also be an increased awareness of the impact of the condition [94]. Additionally, several politicians have argued that society as a whole should become more dementia friendly in order to allow individuals to continue to fulfil their responsibilities in life and contribute to society rather than being considered merely a 'burden' [93]. Hampson and Morris [93] discuss that a different societal view on dementia may further reduce the 'disability' caused by dementia and enable those affected to live well in spite of their cognitive impairment.

6 Conclusions

Dementia is a chronic condition that potentially affects several domains of functioning and hence impacts the sense of identity. Indeed, not only are cognitive deficits evident, but in some individuals with dementia, behavioural changes and difficulties in sensing other people's state of mind also occur, which leads to problematic social functioning. Also, many individuals with dementia suffer from psychological symptoms such as anxiety or depression, and personality changes are described by the family or partner.

The pervasive and complex nature of these changes requires a diversified response or treatment. In Western countries, scientific evolution has advanced medical thinking and has allowed for pharmacotherapy as a means to reduce burden in individuals with dementia or their caregivers. Without denying the beneficial effects of medical interventions, research has also suggested that it is important to support and empower persons living with dementia and their caregivers and value personhood through psychosocial interventions. Many individuals with dementia at some point in the disease process tend to feel identified with their diagnosis ('Not everything I do can be explained by the Parkinson's disease!'). In line with what Cloos [95] writes, medicalization might be seen as a reductionist process if it does not consider personal, family or social issues. When describing experiences with his own mother who was diagnosed with AD, he remarks that 'for the medical staff, the disease explained everything' (p. 65) [95], and he attempts to illustrate the importance of circumstances and biographical elements to explain a situation. Rather than

denying the disease, Cloos looks for a 'complete' view encompassing the awareness that AD is also a social construction and in that respect certainly heterogeneous and more dynamic than a 'narrow' medical approach might suggest. Therefore, it is important to be aware of possibilities for social inclusion and continue to explore these.

In summary, it is necessary to integrate valuable insights from different views on dementia and in that way allow for good care. Still, individuals with dementia should not just be recipients of care. One of the future societal challenges may be to further explore ways to allow individuals with dementia to continue to contribute to society and hence stimulate meaningful activity and a sense of purpose, leading to higher quality of life.

References

1. Smith M, Atkin A, Cutler C. An age old problem? Estimating the impact of dementia on past human populations. *J Aging Health* 2017; **29**: 68–98.

2. Papavramidou N. The ancient history of dementia. *Neurol Sci* 2018; **39**: 2011–16.

3. Berchtold NC, Cotman CW. Evolution in the conceptualization of dementia and Alzheimer's disease: Greco-Roman period to the 1960s. *Neurobiol Aging* 1998; **19**: 173–89.

4. Fotuhi M, Hachinski V, Whitehouse PJ. Changing perspectives regarding late-life dementia. *Nat Rev Neurol* 2009; **5**: 649–58.

5. Cipriani G, Danti S, Carlesi C. Three men in a (same) boat: Alzheimer, Pick, Lewy. Historical notes. *Eur Geriatr Med* 2016; **7**: 526–30.

6. Blessed G, Tomlinson BE, Roth M. The association between quantitative measures of dementia and of senile change in the cerebral grey matter of elderly subjects. *Br J Psychiatry* 1968; **114**: 797–811.

7. Bielschowsky M. Zur Kenntnis der Alzheimerschen krankheit (präsenilen Demenz mit Herdsymptomen). *J Psychol Neurol* 1911; **18**: 1–20.

8. Schachter AS, Davis KL. Alzheimer's disease. *Dialogues Clin Neurosci* 2000; **2**: 91–100.

9. *Diagnostic and Statistical Manual of Mental Disorders* (5th ed.). Washington, DC, American Psychiatric Association, 2013.

10. Knopman DS, Beiser A, Machulda MM, Fields J, Roberts RO, Pankratz VS, ... Petersen RC. Spectrum of cognition short of dementia: Framingham Heart Study and Mayo Clinic Study of Aging. *Neurology* 2015; **85**: 1712–21.

11. Petersen RC, Caracciolo B, Brayne C, Gauthier S, Jelic V, Fratiglioni L. Mild cognitive

impairment: A concept in evolution. *J Intern Med* 2014; **275**: 214–28.

12. Busse A, Hensel A, Guhne U, Angermeyer MC, Riedel-Heller SG. Mild cognitive impairment: Long-term course of four clinical subtypes. *Neurology* 2006; **67**: 2176–85.

13. Ganguli M, Snitz BE, Saxton JA, Chang CC, Lee CW, Vander Bilt J, . . . Petersen RC. Outcomes of mild cognitive impairment by definition: A population study. *Arch Neurol* 2011; **68**: 761–7.

14. Fischer P, Jungwirth S, Zehetmayer S, Weissgram S, Hoenigschnabl S, Gelpi E, . . . Tragl KH. Conversion from subtypes of mild cognitive impairment to Alzheimer dementia. *Neurology* 2007; **68**: 288–91.

15. Chen P, Ratcliff G, Belle SH, Cauley JA, DeKosky ST, Ganguli M. Patterns of cognitive decline in presymptomatic Alzheimer disease: A prospective community study. *Arch Gen Psychiatry* 2001; **58**: 853–8.

16. Blazer D. Neurocognitive disorders in DSM-5. *Am J Psychiatry* 2013; **170**: 585–7.

17. Rabins PV, Lyketsos CG. A commentary on the proposed DSM revision regarding the classification of cognitive disorders. *Am J Geriatr Psychiatry* 2011; **19**: 201–4.

18. George DR, Whitehouse PJ, Ballenger J. The evolving classification of dementia: Placing the DSM-V in a meaningful historical and cultural context and pondering the future of 'Alzheimer's'. *Cult Med Psychiatry* 2011; **35**: 417–35.

19. Jones T, Hungerford C, Cleary M. Pharmacological versus non-pharmacological approaches to managing challenging behaviours for people with dementia. *Br J Community Nurs* 2014; **19**: 72–7.

20. Taft LB, Fazio S, Seman D, Stansell J. A psychosocial model of dementia care: Theoretical and empirical support. *Arch Psychiatr Nurs* 1997; **11**: 13–20.

21. Finnema E, Droes RM, Ribbe M, van Tilburg W. A review of psychosocial models in psychogeriatrics: Implications for care and research. *Alzheimer Dis Assoc Disord* 2000; **14**: 68–80.

22. Engel GL. The need for a new medical model: A challenge for biomedicine. *Sci* 1977; **196**: 129–36.

23. Rabins PV, Lyketsos CG, Steele CD. *Practical dementia care*. UK, Oxford University Press, 2006.

24. Samus QM, Johnston D, Black BS, Hess E, Lyman C, Vavilikolanu A, . . . Lyketsos CG. A multidimensional home-based care coordination intervention for elders with memory disorders: The Maximizing Independence at Home (MIND) pilot randomized trial. *Am J Geriatr Psychiatry* 2014; **22**: 398–414.

25. Spector A, Orrell M. Using a biopsychosocial model of dementia as a tool to guide clinical practice. *Int Psychogeriatr* 2010; **22**: 957–65.

26. Revolta C, Orrell M, Spector A. The biopsychosocial (BPS) model of dementia as a tool for clinical practice. A pilot study. *Int Psychogeriatr* 2016; **28**: 1079–89.

27. Kitwood T. The dialectics of dementia: With particular reference to Alzheimer's disease. *Ageing Soc* 1990; **10**: 177–96.

28. Hadas R. *Strange Relation: A Memoir of Marriage, Dementia and Poetry*. Philadelphia, Paul Dry Books, 2011.

29. Kitwood T. The experience of dementia. *Aging Ment Health* 1997; **1**: 13–22.

30. Kitwood T, Bredin K. Towards a theory of dementia care: Personhood and well-being. *Ageing Soc* 1992; **12**: 269–87.

31. Mitchell G, Agnelli J. Person-centred care for people with dementia: Kitwood reconsidered. *Nurs Stand* 2015; **30**: 46–50.

32. Sabat SR, Harré R. The construction and deconstruction of self in Alzheimer's disease. *Ageing Soc* 1992; **12**: 443–61.

33. Snyder L. *Speaking Our Minds: Personal Reflections from Individuals with Alzheimer's*. New York, Freeman, 1999.

34. Epp TD. Person-centred dementia care: A vision to be refined. *Can Alz Dis Rev* 2003; April: 14–18.

35. Macrae H. Managing identity while living with Alzheimer's disease. *Qual Health Res* 2010; **20**: 293–305.

36. Harrison C. Personhood, dementia and the integrity of a life. *Can J Aging* 1993; **12**: 428–40.

37. Johnston B, Narayanasamy M. Exploring psychosocial interventions for people with dementia that enhance personhood and relate to legacy: An integrative review. *BMC Geriatr* 2016; **16**: 77–102.

38. Kontos PC. Embodied selfhood in Alzheimer's disease: Rethinking person-centred care. *Dement* 2005; **4**: 553–70.

39. Fazio S, Mitchell DB. Persistence of self in individuals with Alzheimer's disease: Evidence from language and visual recognition. *Dement* 2009; **8**: 39–59.

40. Brooker D. What is person centred care in dementia? *Rev Clin Gerontol* 2004; **13**: 215–22.

41. Rosvik J, Kirkevold M, Engedal K, Brooker D, Kirkevold O. A model for using the VIPS

framework for person-centred care for persons with dementia in nursing homes: A qualitative evaluative study. *Int J Older People Nurs* 2011; **6**: 227–36.

42. Kogan AC, Wilber K, Mosqueda L. Person-centered care for older adults with chronic conditions and functional impairment: A systematic literature review. *J Am Geriatr Soc* 2016; **64**: e1–e7.

43. Fazio S, Pace D, Flinner J, Kallmyer B. The fundamentals of person-centered care for individuals with dementia. *Gerontologist* 2018; **58**; S10–S19.

44. Hagberg B. The dementias in a psychodynamic perspective. In Miesen B, Jones G, eds. *Care-Giving in Dementia: Research and Applications (Vol. 2)*. London/New York, Routledge. 1997; 14.

45. Brooker D, Droës RM, Evans S. Framing outcomes of post-diagnostic psychosocial interventions in dementia: The adaptation-coping model and adjusting to change. *WWOP* 2017; **21**: 13–21.

46. Bowlby J. *Attachment and Loss (Vol. 1)*. London, Hogarth Press, 1969.

47. Miesen BML. Alzheimer's disease, the phenomenon of parent fixation and Bowlby's attachment theory. *Int J Geriatr Psychiatry* 1993; **8**: 147–53.

48. Dröes R.-M, van der Roest HG, van Mierlo L, Meiland FJM. Memory problems in dementia: Adaptation and coping strategies and psychosocial treatments. *Expert Rev Neurother* 2011; **11**: 1769–82.

49. Hall GR, Buckwalter K C. Progressively lowered stress threshold: A conceptual model for care of adults with Alzheimer's disease. *Arch Psychiatr Nurs* 1987; **1**: 399–406.

50. Souren L, Franssen E. *Verbroken verbindingen: de ziekte van Alzheimer deel II. Praktische richtlijnen voor het omgaan met de Alzheimerpatiënt*. Amsterdam/Lisse, Swets & Zeitlinger, 1993.

51. Reisberg B, Ferris SH, de Leon MJ, Franssen ESE, Kluger A, Mir P, . . . Cohen J. Stage-specific behavioral, cognitive, and in vivo changes in community residing subjects with age-associated memory impairment and primary degenerative dementia of the Alzheimer type. *Drug Dev Res* 1988; **15**: 101–14.

52. Nolan MR, Brown J, Davies S, Nolan J, Keady J. *The Senses Framework: Improving Care for Older People through a Relationship-Centred Approach. Getting Research into Practice (GRiP) Report No 2*. Sheffield, University of Sheffield, 2006.

53. Warren JD, Hu MTM, Galloway M, Greenwood RJ, Rossor MN. Observations on the human rejection behaviour syndrome: Denny-Brown revisited. *Mov Disord* 2004; **19**: 860–2.

54. Wampold BE. How important are the common factors in psychotherapy? An update. *World Psychiatry* 2015; **14**: 270–7.

55. Randall WL. The anthropology of dementia: A narrative perspective. *Int J Geriatr Psychiatry* 2009; **24**: 322–4.

56. Pollitt PA. Dementia in old age: An anthropological perspective. *Psychol Med* 1996; **26**: 1061–74.

57. Young A. An anthropological perspective on medical knowledge. *J Med Philos* 1980; **5**: 102–16.

58. Oxlund B. The life course in a migrating world: Hybrid scripts of ageing and imaginaries of care. *Adv in Life Course Res* 2018; **38**: 72–9.

59. Kehoua G, Dubreuil C-M, Ndamba-Bandzouzi B, Guerchet M, Mbelesso P, Dartigues J-F, Preux P-M. People with dementia in sub-Saharan Africa. From support to abuse by caregivers: Results of EPIDEMCA-FU program in Congo. *Dement Geriatr Cogn Disord Extra* 2019; **9**: 163–75.

60. Mushi D, Rongai A, Paddick SM, Dotchin C, Mtuya C, Walker R. Social representation and practices related to dementia in Hai District of Tanzania. *BMC Public Health* 2014; **14**: 260.

61. Hashmi M. Dementia: An anthropological perspective. *Int J Geriatr Psy* 2009; **24**: 207–12.

62. Braun KL, Browne CV. Perceptions of dementia, caregiving, and help seeking among Asian and Pacific Islander Americans. *Health Soc Work* 1998; **23**: 262–74.

63. Henderson JN, Henderson LC. Cultural construction of disease: A supernormal construct of dementia in an American Indian tribe. *J Cross-Cult Gerontol* 2002; **17**: 197–212.

64. Henderson JN, Traphagan JW. Cultural factors in dementia: Perspectives from the anthropology of aging. *Alzheimer Dis Assoc Disord* 2005; **19**: 272–4.

65. Traphagan JW. Interpreting senility: Cross-cultural perspectives. *Care Manag J* 2005; **6**: 145–50.

66. Calia C, Johnson H, Cristea M. Cross-cultural representations of dementia: An exploratory study. *J Glob Health* 2019; **9**: 011001.

67. Chiu H, Tsoh J. Commentary on 'Dementia: An anthropological perspective' by Mahnaz Hashmi. *Int J Geriatr Psychiatry* 2009; **24**, 325–7.

68. Shimizu H. Beyond individualism and sociocentrism: An ontological analysis of the opposing elements in personal experiences of Japanese adolescents. *Human Devel* 2000; **43**:195–211.

69. Cohen L. *No Aging in India: Alzheimer's, the Bad Family, and Other Modern Things.* Berkeley, University of California Press, 1998.

70. Ikels C. Constructing and deconstructing the self: Dementia in China. *J Cross-Cult Gerontol* 2002; **17**: 233–51.

71. World Health Organization. Global Action Plan on the Public Health Response to Dementia, 2017–25. https://apps.who.int/iris/bitstream/handle/10665/259615/9789241513487-eng.pdf.3. [Accessed 11 November 2020].

72. Pitt B. *Psychogeriatrics: An Introduction to the Psychiatry of Old Age* (2nd edition). Edinburgh, Churchill Livingstone, 1982.

73. Andrews ES. Institutionalising senile dementia in 19th-century Britain. *Sociol Health Illn* 2017; **39**: 244–57.

74. Health Advisory Service. *The Rising Tide: Developing Services for Mental Illness in Old Age.* Sutton, Surrey: National Health Service, Health Advisory Service, 1982.

75. King's Fund Centre. *Living Well into Old Age: Applying Principles of Good Practice to Services for People with Dementia. Report Number 63.* London, King's Fund Publishing Office, 1984.

76. Poulshock SM, Deimling GT. Families caring for elders in residence: Issues in the measurement of burden. *J Gerontol* 1984; **39**: 230–9.

77. Pratt CC, Sclunall VL, Wright S, Cleland M. Burden and coping strategies of caregivers to Alzheimer's patients. *Fam Relat* 1985; **34**: 27–33.

78. Hirschfield MJ. Families living and coping with the cognitively impaired. In Copp LA, ed. *Care of the Ageing: Recent Advances in Nursing.* Edinburgh, Churchill Livingstone, 1981;159–67.

79. Hirschfield, MJ. Home care versus institutionalization: Family caregiving and senile brain disease. *Int J Nurs Stud* 1983; **20**: 23–32.

80. Sweeting HN. Caring for a relative with dementia: Anticipatory grief and social death. *Generations (Bulletin of the British Society of Gerontology)* 1991; **16**: 6–11.

81. Sweeting HN, Gilhooly MLM. Anticipatory grief: A review. *Soc Sci Med* 1990; **30**: 1073–80.

82. Woods RT. *Alzheimer's Disease: Coping with a Living Death.* London, Souvenir Press, 1989.

83. Nolan MR, Keady J. Training together: A challenge for the future. *J Dement Care* 1996; **4**: 10–13.

84. Kitwood T. *Dementia Reconsidered: The Person Comes First.* Bucks, Open University Press, 1997.

85. Davis R. *My Journey into Alzheimer's Disease.* Amersharn-on-the-Hill, Buckinghamshire, Scripture Press, 1989.

86. McGowin DF. *Living in the Labyrinth: A Personal Journey through the Maze of Alzheimer's Disease.* Cambridge, Mainsail Press, 1993.

87. Bartlett R, O'Connor D. From personhood to citizenship: Broadening the lens for dementia practice and research. *J Aging Stud* 2007, **21**: 107–18.

88. Swarbrick S, Khetani B, Riley C, Keady J. Reflections on the ethics of co-research alongside people living with dementia. *SAGE Research Methods Cases: Medicine and Health* 2020. Available online at https://dx.doi.org/10.4135/9781529709209

89. Shannon K, Bail K., Neville S. Dementia-friendly community initiatives: An integrative review. *J Clin Nurs* 2019; **28**: 2035–45.

90. Kaplan DB, Andersen TC, Lehning AJ, Perry TE. Aging in place vs. relocation for older adults with neurocognitive disorder: Applications of Wiseman's behavioral model. *J Gerontol Soc Work* 2015; **58**: 521–38.

91. Clark A, Campbell S, Keady J, Kuhlberg A, Manji K, Rummery K, Ward R. Neighbourhoods as relational places for people living with dementia. *So Sci Med* 2020. Available online at https://doi.org/10.1016/j.socscimed.2020.112927

92. Wimo A, Guerchet M, Ali G-C, Wu Y-T, Prina AM, Winblad B, . . . Prince M. The worldwide costs of dementia 2015 and comparisons with 2010. *Alzheimers Dement* 2017; **13**: 1–7.

93. Hampson C, Morris K. Dementia: Normal ageing, political cause or social construction. *Gerontol Geriatr Med* 2017; **1**: 555568.

94. Broda A, Bieber A, Meyer G, Hopper L, Joyce R, Irving K, . . . ActifCare Consortium. Perspectives of policy and political decision makers on access to formal dementia care: Expert interviews in eight European countries. *BMC Health Serv Res* 2017; **17**: 518.

95. Cloos P. Is there a pathological way of ageing? *Med Anthropol Theory* 2017; **4**: 60–9.

Starry Night Poem

Appreciative.
Very calm – and yet there's turmoil.
A little suspect, a little sinister,
something evil about it, that plant.
Confusing.

A star tastes delicious.
A star tastes like a milky way.

If I had a thought, I would but you're okay
so you can get away.

A star smells like peanut butter.
You've got to do it.

The stars sound like full heritage.
Everyone looks at a star and dreams.

A star sounds like a symphony.

The painting is soothing you could sleep happily.
I see bi-polar, I feel pity for the person
describing his feelings in the painting.

You can read a lot into Van Gogh's painting.

I like the sun the way it moves.
Oh my goodness!
Let me think about that now.

Not to count everything that you can use.

It looks like a storm.
Blue's my favorite color, as we can see.

'Starry Night Poem', *anonymous, from the Alzheimer's Poetry Project.* Dementia Arts: Celebrating Creativity in Elder Care, *Gary Glazner, Health Professions Press, 2014. Reprinted by permission of Gary Glazner.*

From History to Intervention
A Sociocultural Analysis of Dementia Stigma

Perla Werner, Pieter Vermeulen, Baldwin Van Gorp and Peter Simonsen

1 Introduction

Driven by the increasing number of persons with the disorder, dementia has been declared a major public health concern worldwide. In an effort to deal with this challenge, many countries have developed and adopted national dementia strategy programmes aimed at raising awareness and decreasing stigma. Accordingly, an increasing amount of research has been devoted to understanding the concept of stigma in the area of dementia and to examining its antecedents and revealing its consequences [1–2]. Despite these important advances, the literature on dementia stigma is still in its developing stages and is lagging behind the knowledge accumulated on the topic of stigma in the area of mental illnesses. An increased understanding of the concept will help answer the worldwide call to reduce dementia stigma and help turn the disease into a more liveable condition for people with dementia and their caregivers.

This chapter aims to make a modest contribution to the existing literature while trying to provide an explanation for *dementia stigma*, with special attention to *dementia public stigma*. We start with a brief summary of the knowledge accumulated in this area until today (Section 2). We follow by summarizing and critically discussing the historical roots of dementia stigma (Section 3), and then turn to a discussion of the mechanisms perpetuating it (Section 4). In the second half of the chapter, we turn to a number of different strategies to manage dementia stigma. We look at how literary engagements with dementia have expanded our imaginings and experiences of dementia (Section 5), which might open the way to a less stigmatizing approach to dementia. In a final section, we focus on existing efforts to address dementia stigma through education and contact and on how media might frame dementia in a more positive way (Section 6). We conclude by suggesting future steps to expand knowledge in this incipient area of study.

2 Dementia (Public) Stigma: Typology, Prevalence, Characteristics

Four main types of stigma are conceptually distinguished: self-stigma, courtesy stigma, structural stigma and public stigma. Self-stigma names the *internalization* of the stereotypes held by the general public towards people with devalued characteristics, such as people with mental illnesses. Courtesy stigma refers to the emotions and beliefs of those *surrounding* the stigmatized person, such as family members and professionals. Structural stigma, for its part, refers to the inequalities inherent in *social structures* that restrict the means and resources of stigmatized groups. Public stigma, finally, is defined as the cognitive, emotional and discriminatory attributions endorsed by the *general public* towards a group or a person with a disease or a disability [3].

It is this fourth kind of stigma that is central to this chapter, for three reasons (apart, of course, from the fact that the relation between dementia and society is the explicit focus of this book): it is the most common type of dementia stigma; it is the one that has attracted the most interest in stigma studies; and, finally, public stigma is at the core of the formation of the three other types of stigma, which means that reducing this type of stigma will help reduce the other types as well [4]. The strategies we survey in the second half of the chapter, which directly target public stigma, can then also be expected to have a more general beneficial impact on the complex interactions between different forms of stigma.

The (mostly quantitative) empirical literature shows that the prevalence of public stigma in the area of dementia is, surprisingly perhaps, moderate [5]. Regarding its characteristics, evidence shows that the most common *cognitive* beliefs or stereotypes attributed by the general public to a person with dementia are dangerousness and a lack of aesthetic propriety [6–7], while the most common *emotional* reactions are mostly positive and include principally sympathy, concern and a willingness to help. The main negative emotions are fear and uneasiness. Feelings of pity are also common, although its classification as a positive or negative emotion requires further examination. The main stigmatic behavioural reactions attributed by laypersons to persons with dementia are work-related and health-related discrimination, treatment coercion and institutionalization. Finally, studies indicate that laypersons belonging to cultural minorities and people having lower levels of education, lower levels of knowledge about the disease and limited contact with persons with dementia tend to report higher levels of dementia stigma [4].

3 The Historical Roots of Dementia Stigma

These empirical findings might differ from anecdotal accounts about dementia stigma. Especially the relatively moderate nature of public stigma and the prevalence of positive emotional reactions show that strategies to remedy stigma in this area are far from hopeless and can rely on positive emotional resources to achieve change. Elucidating the origins of the stigma concept as well as of the understanding of dementia across time throws further light on the phenomenon of dementia public stigma and allows us to gain a better grasp of the challenges facing efforts at destigmatization or stigma reduction. As this section shows, the concept of dementia stigma is strongly rooted in historical developments of the concept of stigma in general, as well as of historical changes in the understanding of dementia.

3.1 The Historical Development of the Concept of Stigma

The concept of stigma can be traced back to Greek and Roman societies, when the word was used to represent the physical marks put on specific groups to indicate their lower social status and deviance. During the second half of the twentieth century, the study of stigma in the area of mental illnesses evolved from descriptive investigations of laypersons' attitudes towards mental illnesses to the seminal conceptualizations developed by Erving Goffman, who provided a clear characterization of the concept. Defining stigma as a physical or figurative *mark* that deeply discredits its bearer and leads to discrimination, Goffman paved the way for the development of cognitive and sociological theories of stigma, such as attribution theory and modified labelling theory, which have guided researchers in the identification of the antecedents and consequences of stigma.

Attribution theory holds that stigmatic behaviour is determined by a complex cognitive-emotional-behavioural process, in which individuals' cognitive attributions or stereotypes about the person with a disease lead to negative emotional reactions (such as anger or fear), as well as to positive emotional reactions (such as sympathy and concern). Negative emotions are conceptualized in this theory as motivating hostility and rejection, leading to behavioural reactions such as increased discrimination; positive emotions, for their part, motivate positive behaviour such as a willingness to help. Expansions of the attribution model hold that increased familiarity with the mental disorder are associated with a decrease in discriminatory behaviour [8]. As we will see, this explains why a number of destigmatization strategies rely on familiarizing audiences with realities they may fear because of a lack of previous exposure. The *modified labelling theory* adds to this the insight that individuals *internalize* social labels in order to assess their disease diagnosis [9]. This leads to stigmatized people's withdrawal from social life and a weakening of their social network, making them even more vulnerable than a mere assessment of public stigma would suggest. Here again, it is clear that public stigma is deeply entangled with other forms of stigma – such as, most notably here, self-stigma.

Despite robust theoretical and empirical developments in the study and conceptualization of stigma, especially in the area of mental illnesses, its understanding in the area of dementia is emerging slowly, with the majority of the studies still being descriptive and a-theoretical. Scrutinizing the historical roots of dementia is crucial for advancing this line of research.

3.2 The Historical Roots of the Understanding of Dementia

Several explanatory models have been advanced in an effort to understand dementia. Across time, the meaning attributed to the disease has changed from an irreversible, incurable and hopeless condition to a more positive risk-reduction approach (see Chapter 8). As the general development of the concept of dementia is covered by the first chapter of this book, in this chapter we restrict our discussion to the interactions between those conceptual changes and the prevalence of stigma.

While the Greek philosophers generally view dementia as having an organic origin and as being an inevitable part of old age, it is not until the beginning of the nineteenth century that dementia begins to be framed as instigated by a disease. Following this change, the *biomedical* model became the dominant framework for understanding dementia: it stresses the pathological aspects of the condition and sees the pursuit of a cure as the first priority of professionals, decision makers and society. While moving away from the perception of dementia as an extreme but ultimately *normal* part of ageing to a conceptualization of dementia as a *pathological* process of the brain, this altered perspective provoked feelings of hopelessness and fear about the condition, emotions that, as we have seen, are closely associated with stigmatic views. Other aspects of the biomedical understanding of dementia, such as it being a hereditary or genetically determined condition, might equally have contributed to the devaluation and social distancing from persons who carry the gene or who are supposed to be more vulnerable to the development of the disease. As we explain later in this chapter, this means that efforts to destigmatize dementia – be it in the media or literature or through education or contact – have to move beyond this still dominant biomedical model.

The *biopsychosocial* model this book puts forward provides a different explanation of dementia. Centring on internal-level indicators (such as biomedical, personality-based and emotional factors), as well as on external-level ones (such as environmental elements) as the basis for understanding dementia, this model provides a more holistic and person-centred approach [10]. However, it is not immediately clear to what extent or even whether this perspective contributes to decreasing laypersons' stigmatic beliefs. As we explore in more detail in the next section, several authors have mentioned that concentrating on the person with dementia as an individual rather than as a group does not decrease perceptions that might encourage stigma, such as a dualistic view between body and mind [11], or does not change the perception of the person with dementia as 'different' or 'strange' [12].

A third and final modern perspective on dementia is the *sociocultural* one, which considers the meaning of dementia to be embodied and shaped by social and cultural contexts [13]. This framework has been used mainly to explain dementia in non-Western cultures. As mentioned in Chapter 1, research focusses on religious beliefs such as the disease being a 'divine punishment', a supernatural curse or the result of the 'evil eye', as well as on cultural values such as filial piety or individualistic (as opposed to collectivistic) tendencies. Here, it is important to remark that factoring in cultural frameworks might put a further 'mark' on the person with the disease and thus encourage laypersons' stigmatic beliefs. Even though this framework is not generally applied to Western societies, there is no reason to assume that sociocultural dynamics do not determine the stigma of people with dementia in these societies also, and that sociocultural changes might not become a main driver of destigmatization, as the second half of this chapter explores.

In addition to these three conceptualizations, a fourth perspective for the understanding of dementia is currently emerging. Driven by an enablement and equality-based approach, a *relational* model of disability is increasingly being applied to dementia [14]. Stressing the principles of self-determination, human rights and involvement in decision-making, this view of dementia is at the basis of two important policy and public health initiatives. The first advocates the development of social, environmental, organizational or virtual communities – so-called *dementia-friendly communities* – as a strategy for empowering, supporting, respecting the rights of and recognizing the full potential of persons with dementia and their caregivers. The notion of dementia-friendly communities is supported by the World Health Organization and by Alzheimer's Disease

International as a path to the normalization of dementia. It has been incorporated in the national dementia plans of many countries, even if, as we discuss in what follows, its ability to decrease stigma is uncertain. A second approach is based on the emerging knowledge about modifiable dementia risk factors such as adequate diet, physical activity, smoking and hypertension. It underscores the benefits of adopting healthy behavioural patterns as a way to reduce the risk of developing dementia. This is a proactive approach to the maintenance of cognitive functioning that places responsibility directly with the individual person. This might lead to an increase in stigmatic perceptions of blame and responsibility towards persons with dementia, who can be condemned for failing to change their lifestyles, and therefore to increased discrimination, as occurs in sociocentric societies (see Chapter 1). As with the other three conceptions of dementia, there is no clear-cut relation to destigmatization.

Regardless of the views and conceptualizations of stigma and dementia across time, dementia stigma continues to be at the core of public health discourse. If we want to confront that challenge, it is vital to gain insight into the mechanisms that perpetuate it.

4 Socio-structural Mechanisms Perpetuating Dementia Stigma

Social structures are a crucial factor in reducing or perpetuating stigma in a variety of conditions. In the case of dementia, language, media and socio-cultural structures play a central role in the permanency of negative stereotypes about persons with dementia. This section discusses these three elements in turn.

4.1 Language

Language is, among other things, a system of symbols bridging the social world with the inner world; it is a medium through which interior states of mind, emotions and thoughts can be externalized, but it is also a medium that allows public stigma to be internalized and that can lead to self-stigma. *Linguistic relativity philosophy* holds that language may shape and frame the way the public perceive and feel the world in general and persons with a disability in particular. This means that it is important to use appropriate

terminology. This need has been recognized for a long time in the area of mental illnesses, with the *person-first movement*, for instance, calling for replacing the phrase 'a mentally ill person' with 'a person with mental illness' [15]. This position recognizes that language can do real harm in perpetuating stigma, but it also stresses the hope that linguistic change may be an effective strategic move in a destigmatizing direction. Here, as we will see, literature and media have a role to play.

Indeed, in recent years we have witnessed several steps in this direction. As mentioned in Chapter 1, first, in 2013, the term 'dementia' was replaced in the *Diagnostic and Statistical Manual of Mental Disorders* (DSM-5) with the term 'major neurocognitive disorder'. This is a welcome change, as the term 'dementia', literally meaning 'being out of one's mind', brings connotations of madness and insanity, which undoubtedly increases stigmatic beliefs. Still, because the term 'dementia' is already widely established and much easier than 'major cognitive disorder', it is likely that it will continue to be used by laypersons, the media and presumably professionals also.

Second, following the interventions of the person-first movement in the context of other mental diseases, guidelines suggesting the use of adequate language to refer to persons with dementia have been published in Canada, the UK and Australia. These relate to the use of derogative or pejorative language (such as 'demented', 'madman' or 'dull brain'), as well as to the use of militaristic metaphors (such as 'the battle against dementia', 'dementia as an enemy' or even 'combating stigma'), and metaphors associated with natural disasters (such as dementia as a 'rising tide' or 'an emergent silent tsunami'). Again, in spite of these welcome developments, it should be noted that these metaphors are still common in professional publications as well as in the media.

4.2 The Media

Traditional media as well as online and social media are important sources of potentially stigma-enhancing information and images. Since media play a central role in shaping and perpetuating stigma, they can also do the opposite – that is, reduce stigmatic beliefs. In all media, including films, TV documentaries, news reports, theatre plays, memoirs, novels and policy documents, dementia is often presented as a burden and as particularly threatening both to the individual and to society. This prevalent so-called tragedy discourse is reflected, for example, in the imaging and use of metaphorical language, which contributes to the perception that dementia is a real horror [16]; it is, according to this way of speaking, a fate worse than death [17]. Dementia is like a monster that lurks in wait, strikes unexpectedly and kills its victims. Additionally, there are references to the plague or other infectious diseases, leading to associations of dementia with contagiousness and pandemics. Even stakeholders who fight the disease by investing in scientific research or making donations to charities and non-governmental organizations (NGOs) exacerbate this 'tragic' representation of dementia in the competition for scarce research resources and in fundraising: they also tend to use threatening language, and to invoke the vast proportions and the overwhelming and unstoppable force of a 'tsunami'.

The use of war imagery is also common in media coverage of dementia. Although not unique to dementia, it is uniquely stigmatizing in the case of this disorder. For instance, while equally common with other diseases such as cancer and HIV, the difference is that the use of this stigmatic imagery in dementia is reinforced by the framing of at least three related themes: mental illnesses, old age and care institutions. Because all of these themes are already given shape in the media in a strongly stereotypical and stigmatizing way, they reinforce each other when they are addressed simultaneously, as is the case of people with dementia (and this is not to deny the prevalence of early-onset dementia).

First, dementia has in common with other *mental disorders* that diagnostics are not self-evident. To the average media consumer, it is not directly visible what is going on, as they may lack the knowledge or ability to assess what is happening to a person with dementia. The seemingly capricious and incalculable nature of the disorder might therefore create anxiety and uncertainty.

Second, the stigma surrounding *old age* in many cultures reinforces dementia stigma. Although recent studies show that the stigma attributed to older persons with dementia is lower than the stigma attributed to a younger person with the disease [18], the media tend to keep cases of young-onset dementia out of sight.

Moreover, some authors argue that media portray older people of the fourth age frequently as weak and repulsive and as outsiders. This perception of 'real' old age is aggravated by contrasting it with competing narratives about the 'third age', which is described as a period of low risk of disease or disease-related disabilities, of high cognitive and physical functional capacities and of engagement in interpersonal relations and activities that create social value [19–20]. In a society where many issues are looked at from a cost-benefit perspective, the perception that the economic usefulness of the elderly is minimal and replaced with huge costs constitutes a problem for older persons with dementia, resulting in a further strengthening of the stigma.

Third, stereotypical ideas about *residential care centres* are both a source and a consequence of the stigma of old age. Nursing homes are the last living place before death. This makes it easier to share, in the news and on social media, stories about poor care, misuse and abuse. In literature and films, nursing home narratives typically depict nursing homes as places of fear and terror, and it is much rarer to see them depict nursing homes as places where new opportunities and relations arise.

Paying attention to studies assessing the portrayal of dementia in different media sources reveals a complex picture. For instance, a longitudinal study (1984–2008) of news and talk shows in the United States shows that facts regarding symptoms, causes and the diagnosis of Alzheimer's disease remain underexposed compared to personal stories about the disease [21]. Overall attention, in general, did increase over time, as was also shown by a study of German photographs accompanying news articles magazines in the period 2000–9 [22]. This research shows that the characters in the photos are mostly shown in an individualized context: people are portrayed in their home environment and with their personal belongings. Moreover, although the majority of the photographs depict older people, they mainly portray them with positive emotions.

Inconsistent findings emerge regarding the portrayal of persons with dementia in films. For example, studies that contrast the image of dementia in feature films with the lived reality of the condition have concluded that the cinematic representation is misleading in certain respects: it suggests, for instance, that moments of complete lucidity occur and moments of agitation do not [23], which does not fit the medically attested manifestations of dementia. Despite this finding, Cohen-Shalev and Marcus analyse three films released between 2008 and 2010 and conclude that instead of portraying only negative sides, these films in fact do pay attention to personhood [24].

4.3 Sociocultural Structures

The forces perpetuating dementia stigma do not operate in a sociocultural vacuum – they influence and are influenced by social structures and systems. *Structural stigma*, defined as the intentional or unintentional discrimination of persons with a disease by cultural norms, societal systems, social institutions' rules, guidelines and norms, has not been widely examined in the area of dementia. This lack of attention to intangible, supra-individual forces is not surprising since several characteristics of dementia seem to contradict values and norms that are central to many cultures, not least in the West. Firstly, there is increased *individualism*: people are socialized by stressing that they need to learn to stand on their own two feet and ultimately strive for self-fulfilment. The prospect in dementia of being dependent on others, losing autonomy and slowly deteriorating contradicts this norm and strengthens the stigma. Secondly, there is the importance and high value attached to *ratio and cognitive abilities* in contemporary society. Because dementia impairs the very ability to reason, the stigma is reinforced again. Humans are distinguished from animals and other living organisms by their cognitive abilities; as soon as these disappear, the human dimension fades away too, according to this reasoning. Thirdly, and relatedly, there is a long-standing *Cartesian dualism*, in which body and mind are seen as separate identities, and in which the body is perceived as subordinate to the mind. This dualistic perspective is propagated and cultivated in different religions, in which the individual is represented by the spirit or the soul, which is valued at a higher level than the body. Dementia is often portrayed negatively as taking away the mind or soul, as if what makes a person unique and valuable disappears behind the diagnosis, leaving a deformed body, an empty shell, a plant. This state of affairs explains why different images and discourses about dementia, in literature and the media, that unsettle dualistic, individualistic and ratio-centric stereotypes can play an important role in destigmatizing dementia, as we will see in Sections 5 and 6.

Economic norms and expectations may similarly increase stigmatic beliefs towards persons with dementia, especially in societies where some form of return on investment seems a requirement in all circumstances (quid pro quo), stigmatic beliefs towards elderly people may increase. This is especially true in economic systems, such as the one currently reigning in the West, where manual labour is estimated to be of less value than cognitive labour. In a knowledge society, a condition marked by cognitive diminishment is prone to stigma.

Despite the undeniable importance of sociocultural structures to the understanding of dementia stigma, there is a dearth of studies examining this topic. Recent studies in Israel found considerable stigma towards persons with dementia engrained in the welfare system as well as in the legal system [25–26]. Moreover, Stites and colleagues in a study examining lay-persons' discriminatory beliefs towards persons with dementia found that half of the participants consider that health insurance should be limited for persons with dementia, and that 25% of participants believe that research resources should not be devoted to this population [27]. Here again, it seems likely that a lack of direct experience (as a person with dementia or a caregiver) had stigmatizing consequences. As welfare states operate in a context of scarcity, and difficult decisions about allocation of resources and policy priorities are unavoidable, stigma makes it hard for dementia research and care to acquire a prominent place on research and welfare agendas (see Chapter 14).

When evaluating sociocultural contexts, dementia stigma poses an important concern. Foregrounding destigmatizing interventions can have a real impact on the way stigma is addressed at the social and individual levels. The rest of this chapter zooms in on such interventions, and points to different strategies used to bring about stigma reduction: first in literature, which can be considered a 'free zone' where social stereotypes can be negotiated and changed, and then in the context of intervention programmes that invest in education and contact and in the development of alternative images and discourses.

5 Literature and the Destigmatization of Dementia

Much art and literature has dealt in recent years with the topic of dementia from a variety of perspectives and in many different forms and genres. A general tendency in this body of work over the past half century is to increasingly emphasize that a dementia diagnosis is not necessarily an end-of-life-diagnosis, but that it is possible to imagine living with dementia and even under certain circumstances deriving new meanings and positive values. Interestingly, in some ways, some of the features that make dementia prone to stigma are also what make it attractive to artistic practitioners: its relative invisibility and inscrutability; its challenge to received ideas of selfhood, rationality and identity; and its irremediable, terminal nature. In a sense, the way art and literature attend to dementia in itself may contribute to destigmatization. By imagining what it might be like to live with the disease, whether as the person with the disease or as a caregiver, art and literature make audiences perceive individuals living with dementia as fellow humans. The following subsections present and evaluate three potentially destigmatizing literary strategies: empathy, complexity/ambiguity and forms that generate direct and sudden insight.

5.1 Literary Fiction: Empathy and Dementia

Remarkably often, works of fiction invite their readers to imagine a highly educated and highly rational character to have a diagnosis of dementia. In Matthew Thomas' novel *We Are Not Ourselves*, a neuroscientist receives a dementia diagnosis; in Alice LaPlante's *Turn of Mind*, a retired orthopaedic surgeon suffers from dementia and is accused of killing her best friend. The most famous example is Lisa Genova's bestselling novel *Still Alice* and its award-winning Hollywood movie adaptation featuring Julianne Moore. The novel offers the reader an empathetic identification with the brilliant and beautiful Alice Howland, who lives an enviably successful life both as a private person (wife and mother in privileged affluence) and as a professor of cognitive linguistics at Harvard University. As this character at age 50 experiences early-onset dementia, audiences come to a new

and perhaps richer awareness of dementia as something that could potentially affect them as well, but that may not necessarily be only catastrophic. Based on the author's (who holds a PhD in neuroscience from Harvard) expert knowledge, the novel does more than circulate scientific ideas: it offers the intimate perspective of a character who lets the reader share her gradual loss of cognitive functioning, control of memory and language especially, but also vicariously experience the approximation and renewed intimacy between Alice and her family.

The question whether works of literature and art can effectively contribute to the destigmatization of dementia is a speculative one: empirical studies of the effects on readers' opinions are rare and remain contested within the scholarly community. Tracking the engagement with a book like *Still Alice* on Goodreads.com – the leading social media site for sharing reading experiences – shows that ordinary readers report a destigmatizing effect. Of the 287,256 readers who have rated the novel, 47% gave it five stars out of five possible and 39% gave it four stars. More than 27,000 readers have left reviews of it. The most liked five-star review, by 'Annalisa' (469 likes as of 8 April 2020), opens: 'After you read this, you will never look at Alzheimer's the same again. Nor will you ever forget it. Oh the irony.' 'I lived Alice's story right along with her, crying when she cried and smiling at her accomplishments.' 'Genova has done a fabulous job bringing attention to this debilitating disease.' It is evident that the novel functions to create an affective community for readers (all of whom use female names) who have or fear to have personal contact with the disease, and for whom the novel is seen as providing unique insight into this condition. In comparison to other kinds of media representations of the disease, art and literature offer a more internal – and potentially more transformative – encounter with the reality of dementia.

A more direct way that literature and the arts can potentially aid the destigmatization of dementia is by impacting key players in the social systems that, as the previous section showed, all too often perpetuate stigma. Fictional texts can play a role in the training of doctors and nurses. The interdisciplinary field of the medical humanities (or the health humanities) has ample experience exposing doctors and health professionals to fictional texts that enrich and challenge their engrained ideas about particular diseases, which will carry over into their relation to patients and the care profession as a whole [28]. In the case of medical doctors, an appreciation of diverse positions and the complexity of the lived reality of disease has been shown to counter mis- and over-diagnosis, and to allow doctors to adopt different postures than that of the infallible expert [29]. We can mention a novel like *Elizabeth Is Missing* by Emma Healey, which is being used in nurses' training in the UK. The novel is partly narrated from the perspective of Maud, an ageing woman with dementia, and these parts of the novel invite the reader to adopt the same uncertain, limited and destabilizing perspective as the narrator. Other parts of the novel focus more on the perspective of the caregivers, most notably Maud's daughter, and evokes the plight of family members living with people with dementia. The novel has been credited with increasing nurses' empathy for and understanding of people with dementia. Because of the complex and multiple narrative perspectives, it also helps nurses reflect on and update their own engrained ideas about the experience of living with dementia [30].

However, the destigmatizing efforts of *Still Alice* and *Elizabeth Is Missing* risk missing their goals and reinforcing the stigma they want to undo. Goodreads reactions show that a considerable subset of readers object to the privileged social position of *Still Alice*'s protagonist, while *Elizabeth Is Missing*, in having Maud contribute to the solution of a decades-old crime, risks having its destigmatizing efforts spill over into an uncalled-for idealization of dementia [31]. As we argue in Section 6.3., a combination of a(n often negative) frame and a (more hopeful) counter-frame may lead to more convincing results. An alternative strategy that has been embraced by literary work is to destigmatize the contiguous elements, such as the care facility, that, as the previous section showed, exacerbate the stigma of dementia. Nursing homes are traditionally depicted as sites one wants to run away from (as in Jonas Jonasson's wildly popular novel *The Hundred-Year-Old Man Who Climbed Out of the Window and Disappeared*) because they enforce a dependency that is incompatible with values such as control and self-determination. Still, some novels and short fictions provide more nuanced and sometimes even hopeful representations of the care work carried out in and by these institutions which enable new forms of living for both the elderly and their adult children [32].

In Nobel Prize–winner Alice Munro's story 'The Bear Came over the Mountain', for instance, a woman with dementia's move to late-life housing allows her to escape a stifling marriage and to engage in new, meaningful relationships [33]. Not only is the caring home imagined as something other than a place of terror; in another destigmatizing move, dementia is credited with the ability to neutralize a surfeit of troubling memories. Similarly, research on Canadian and Scandinavian literature has established that contemporary fiction is increasingly intent on a more hopeful imagining of institutionalized late life [34].

5.2 Fiction and the Complexity of Dementia

The destigmatizing effects of efforts to portray the experience of dementia in an intimate way are never guaranteed, and the empathetic experience of dementia that fiction offers always threatens to reinforce rather than challenge stigma. For this reason, some approaches to literature and the arts have situated their destigmatizing potential elsewhere: not in a straightforward empathetic experience, but in an appreciation of complexity. A difficult, disorienting and morally complex work like Samuel Beckett's *Waiting for Godot*, for instance, has been seen as providing its audience with the disorientation and complexity of dementia – even if it remains contentious whether the author intended the work to be *about* dementia [35]. An increasing amount of scholarship investigates literary texts to use them as 'catalysts for deepening our understanding of the human condition and for challenging negative stereotypes and for critiquing the neglect and "othering" of those who are consigned to be a "burden"' [36–37]. Literary representations of dementia also have the capacity to highlight aspects of the dementia syndrome that are difficult to capture in accessible media frames.

The insight that people with dementia, until a fairly advanced stage of the condition, retain an experiencing self that continues to struggle to reflect on its situation is arguably best reflected in a novel like Dutch author J. Bernlef's *Out of Mind*, which is a first-person narrator's account of his own declining cognitive abilities, including his loss of language. Or, as stated previously, a novel like *Elizabeth Is Missing*, which alternates between the perspective of a narrator with dementia and the perspective of a caregiver, offers repetitions, frustration, misdirection and disorientation that end up telling us more of what it means to care for a person with dementia than scientific or mass media discourses could. By making the complexity of dementia palpable, literature can contribute to overcoming reductive stigmatizing and stereotypical images of it.

In general, dementia narratives have developed from negative and stigmatizing depictions that focus on loss of functionality to accounts that imagine dementia as a challenging but non-exceptional part of life. An example of the earlier 'stigmatizing approach' is B. S. Johnson's *House Mother Normal* (1973), which provides a thoroughly negative and stigmatizing image of people living with dementia as sufferers at the mercy of a ruthless and un-empathetic welfare system. This view of people with dementia as deeply scary and hardly human informs early dementia novels such as Margaret Forster's *Have the Men Had Enough?* (1989), Michael Ignatieff's *Scar Tissue* (1993), Mordecai Richler's *Barney's Version* (1998) and Jonathan Franzens' *The Corrections* (2001). Increasingly, however, fiction has come to diversify the representation of dementia. As medical doctor Gayatri Devi argues in *The Spectrum of Hope: An Optimistic and New Approach to Alzheimer's Disease and Other Dementias*, there is a 'spectrum' of dementia enabling many people to live perfectly ordinary and satisfying lives with their disease, but their stories rarely get told and instead public discourse (and that of arts and literature) tends to equalize late-stage dementia with dementia itself. Examples of novels attentive to different stages of dementia include, apart from *Elizabeth Is Missing* and *Still Alice*, Ian McEwan's *Saturday* (2005) and Matthew Thomas' *We Are Not Alone* (2014) [38].

5.3 Flashes of Insight: Graphic Novels, Memoirs, Poetry

Different genres have different affordances for contributing to the destigmatization of dementia. Especially *graphic novels* and *memoirs* have become an important artistic medium: the interaction of word and images offers opportunities to operate on the border of the speakable, imaginable and the knowable in experimental ways, which is especially relevant for a liminal condition

like dementia. Examples include Roz Chast's *Can't We Talk about Something More Pleasant?* (2014), which is an autobiographical narrative about Chast's father's dementia and the difficulties facing an adult child who must increasingly begin to take on parenting responsibilities for her own parents. Spaniard Paco Roca's *Wrinkles* (2007/15) explores a character's developing dementia, but complicates the customary emphasis on loss: increasingly, the reader gains access to the lives and imaginations of other characters in the dementia ward of the nursing home, whose dementia is different and not only associated with loss and anxiety, and who find themselves changing for the better in the meeting with the main character's dementia. Medical anthropologist and artist/writer Dana Walrath's graphic memoir of her mother, *Aliceheimer's: Alzheimer's through the Looking Glass* (2016), puts the powers of graphic literature to enrich and destigmatize dementia on full display. The inevitable decline narrative is countered by the daughter's story of regaining a meaningful relationship to a mother she had never felt close to. Walrath sees her book as offering a counter-frame to the dominant biomedical narrative of Alzheimer's disease. Instead of 'a horror story: people with the disease are perceived as zombies, bodies without minds, waiting for valiant researchers to find a cure', *Aliceheimer* presents the cohabitation of daughter and mother as 'a time of healing and magic' (p. 4). The work is explicitly imagined as capable of countering stigma: 'Stigma, silence, and social death surround rejected ways of being and echo through the hallways of hospitals, medical school lecture rooms, and textbooks. This is where stories and comics come in. They can rewrite the dominant narrative' (p. 5). The book presents enriching, surprising and often humorous experiences in short prose pieces, typically one page long, accompanied by visual artwork combining collage and drawings using *Alice in Wonderland* cut-outs. (see Figures 2.1 and 2.2). The brevity and humorousness of these elements is, for Walrath, what makes them especially effective: 'showing the faces, the lived experience, and the daily reality of those with Alzheimer's and other altered, different states removes the stigma and restores their humanity' (p. 6). Such short flashes of insight and connection offer a destigmatizing strategy that complements the empathy and the appreciation of complexity explored in the previous two subsections.

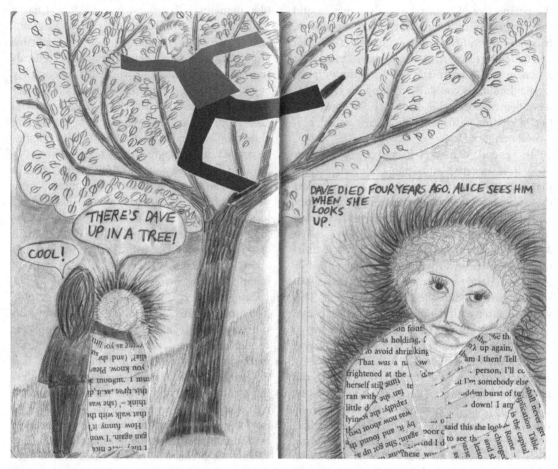

Figures 2.1 and 2.2 Illustrations from Dana Walrath's *Aliceheimer's: Alzheimer's through the Looking Glass* (used with permission)

The emphasis on short forms, fragmentariness and sub-semantic effects also characterizes *poetical* attempts to engage with dementia. Here, the development of the work of Tony Harrison is paradigmatic of a destigmatizing shift. Harrison's first poem about dementia, 'The Mother of the Muses' (1989), still unequivocally focusses on loss, fear and confusion, and on the final phase of the condition rather than the full spectrum. Harrison's much-quoted lines 'If we are what we remember, what are they / Who don't have memories as we have ours' come close to suggesting that 'they' are non-beings insofar as they have no memories. Harrison's *Black Daisies for the Bride* (1993) offers a more enabling picture of dementia, and like *Aliceheimer*, it not coincidentally does so by mixing different media: it is a film/poem mixing song, lyric, acting and documentary

film-making. The work combines actors with people with dementia, staging with documentary, and it makes visible the proximity between seemingly insignificant nursing rhyme poetry with radical avant-garde language experiments: both disrupt conventional ways of meaning-making and invite attention to non-traditional sites of significance (sounds, rhythms, movements). Harrison insists that there is a human being behind the (seemingly nonsensical) language, which does not have to be intended as poetry to count and matter as poetry, and which does not have to mean anything to be understood as possibly an indication of some form of joy and pleasure. The work features a key scene in which the actors who play the nurses dress up as young brides, as younger versions of the people with dementia, to underline the tension between

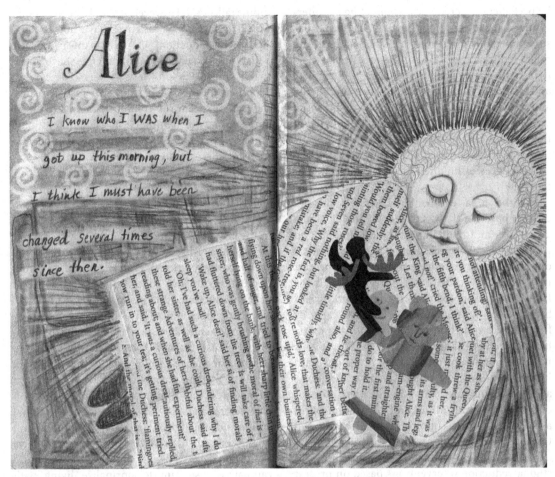

Figures 2.1 and 2.2 (cont.)

continuities and discontinuities of identity. *Black Daisies for the Bride* bestows a destigmatizing humanity on these individuals, even if this means bestowing, imagining and hypothesizing signs that are not readily discernible; this combination of imagination and recognition, it suggests, is key for dealing with literature, and also when it comes to interacting with and caring for people with dementia. Harrison's work displays a transition from a seemingly unthinking stigmatizing representation to a new attempt to use literature to explicitly destigmatize individuals living with dementia by showing them as individuals with resources, including creative and poetic resources. In that way, as this section has shown, it is exemplary of broader literary and artistic developments. Even if the real-world impact of these destigmatizing efforts remains

hard to assess, they complement the endeavours we foreground in the next section.

6 Addressing Stigma: Education, Contact, Alternative Discourses

In the area of mental illnesses, we find advocacy, government and community service groups leading the development of strategies to reduce public stigma. These efforts are based on the willingness to improve the quality of life of persons with mental illnesses and include three main types of interventions: education, contact and protest. *Educational* interventions are based on the assumption that increasing awareness and overcoming misinformation and ignorance through the provision of factual and evidence-based knowledge about the stigmatized condition will help challenge stereotypes. *Contact-based* interventions are founded on the rationale that exposure to persons pertaining to a stigmatized group might reduce laypersons' stigmatic beliefs by clarifying and erasing stereotypes, decreasing anxiety and increasing positive emotions such as empathy and understanding. Finally, *protest or social activism* strategies are rooted in the conviction that stigma can be discouraged by stressing its immoral grounds and by clearly criticizing the consequences of holding on to stigmatic stereotypes [39].

In the area of dementia, education and contact-based initiatives to reduce public stigma are scarce, and their impact is still limited and inconclusive, as we discuss next. To the best of our knowledge, there have not been any protest interventions yet. This might be related to the fact that, as we noted earlier, the importance of highlighting the human rights and the capacity for self-determination of people with dementia has only emerged in the past few years. This new understanding of dementia, together with increased knowledge about its early diagnosis and prediction, might soon increase the number of dementia organizations and advocacy groups, as today, in many countries, these are limited to caregivers' groups. As these developments occur, we might witness the flourishing of stigma-reduction interventions based on protest activities such as letter writing and public demonstrations.

6.1 Educational Dementia Stigma-Reduction Interventions

While several small-scale educational interventions have been developed, the most important and thorough initiative based on the principles of education to overcome dementia stigma is undoubtedly the Dementia Friends programme. Based on the principles of increasing awareness and knowledge about the disease, the Dementia Friends programme recruits volunteers and provides them with information about the disease with the aim of motivating them to spread it to other groups and thus reduce stigmatic beliefs [40]. Currently adopted by many countries with national strategic programmes, Dementia Friends initiatives have been implemented mainly with college students as the target population, and by providing information either through offline or

online talks [41]. However, it should be noted that up till today, these initiatives have not attained significant reductions in participants' stigmatic beliefs about dementia, although they have undeniably improved knowledge levels. These fairly sobering findings stem from two main reasons: the lack of structured valid instruments to assess empirically the concept of dementia stigma among laypersons, as well as the low to moderate levels of stigmatic beliefs about dementia, as stated earlier in this chapter.

6.2 Contact-Based Interventions

In the area of dementia stigma, the use of contact-based interventions was implemented mainly with intergenerational groups including young populations such as college students. The use of video or other media to bring audiences into contact with a person with dementia was adopted by several dementia anti-stigma campaigns in Japan, the UK, Australia and Israel [42]. Although there is little knowledge of how exactly they function, media campaigns are a viable method of putting a stigma-reducing approach into practice [43]. An Australian study shows that both national and local campaigns emphasize personhood and underscore that persons with dementia have rights and deserve dignity and respect [44]. Local campaigns also aim to normalize living with dementia more than national campaigns do, as they try to strengthen the social commitment of those directly affected.

While the hope informing these campaigns is that a greater exposure to and a deeper and more personal identification with persons with the disease will at least approach them in a more open and unprejudiced way, evidence accumulating from these interventions shows modest improvements in laypersons' stigmatic beliefs at best. This is not surprising, especially as the most successful component in contact-based interventions to reduce mental illness stigma is the direct live contact with a person with mental illness sharing personal life experiences. In the case of dementia, this is possible only with persons who retain their language and communication abilities and who probably find themselves at a relatively early stage of the disease. In a disease that, as we explain in the next subsection, is mainly framed by discourses stressing the loss rather than the preservation of cognitive abilities, exposure to a person with the disease might reinforce stigmatic stereotypes instead of reducing them. And moreover, as we stated earlier in the chapter, dementia public stigma is typically characterized by high levels of positive feelings towards the person with the disease. Exposure to such a person might erase such positive feelings and increase rather than decrease negative emotions, especially fear.

Thus, reducing laypersons' stigma in the area of dementia is a complex and challenging task. Knowledge accumulated until today shows that two of the most recommended strategies for other diseases – education and contact – might have a merely moderate or even a negative effect, as they might increase feelings of pity, helplessness and victimization towards persons with dementia. Called 'benevolence stigma', this phenomenon reinforces stigmatized persons' inability to make decisions by themselves and perpetuates their need to rely on authoritative figures [45]. Investing in the development of an alternative discourse for the understanding of dementia might provide an alternative strategy for reducing dementia public stigma.

6.3 Interventions Providing Alternative Discourses and Images

As stated earlier, the prevalent 'tragedy discourse' emphasizing the 'worst case' aspects of the disease, such as the progressive loss of cognitive abilities and the gradual but irrevocable process of deterioration in which people no longer recognize their loved ones, is very likely strengthening the stigma surrounding dementia [46]. The question then arises whether there are alternative discourses available that may reduce stigma. A possible alternative to the 'tragedy' discourse is the 'living well with dementia' discourse. In this discourse, personhood is emphasized, and encouraging the support from others makes it possible to deal with the condition. This is in line with policies that focus on early care planning, the promotion of 'ageing well', and the concept of dementia-friendly communities.

There are many examples of initiatives that want to promote and express these values. For instance, the 'living well with dementia' project in Stillorgan, Blackrock, in Dublin (Ireland), aims to build 'a community that respects, supports and empowers people with dementia; a community in which people with dementia are

socially and culturally valued'. In the domain of art and literature, such values are pursued through forms of interactive creativity. The TimeSlips project, for instance, develops a technique for collaborative storytelling, in which a visual cue (such as a painting or a photo) leads to responses that allow the group leader to construct a story with the participants. As the TimeSlips website puts it (under the slogan 'connect through creativity'): 'TimeSlips opens storytelling to everyone by replacing the pressure to remember with the freedom to imagine.' Other examples include Gary Glazner's Alzheimer's Poetry Project (APP), in which a call-and-response model is used to unlock hidden forms of creativity that may result in strengthening the dignity of the people with dementia involved, and John Killick's *Poetry and Dementia: A Practical Guide* (2018), which demonstrates that through poetry people with the condition can help others to look at different aspects of life from an unexpected angle [47]. From this perspective, identity and selfhood are situated more in playfulness, social interactions, embodied activities and forms of community than in rationality or self-consciousness. McParland, Kelly and Innes point out some pitfalls in this type of alternative approach. Sometimes, it seems to be a matter of just doing your best to maintain third-age (rather than fourth-age) status and continue to participate in a normal, active life [48]. This risks obscuring the undeniable negative aspects of the disorder.

The major risk of the 'living well' perspective is that the most vulnerable will be seen as the 'failed ones', and as a result, stigmatization is strengthened rather than reduced for this group. As McParland, Kelly and Innes note, 'dementia means different things to different people depending on their social context' (p. 259). To achieve a more nuanced image, they state, it is necessary to accept the paradoxical nature of this very complex condition. It is therefore important to break open the dichotomy between 'tragedy' and 'living well' and to *combine* several frames in the representation of dementia.

Van Gorp and Vercruysse distinguish a number of counter-frames that can counterbalance the dominant stigmatizing views on dementia [49]. A nuanced image of dementia, first of all, does not focus exclusively on the last stage of the disease. It covers aspects of life from the moment the

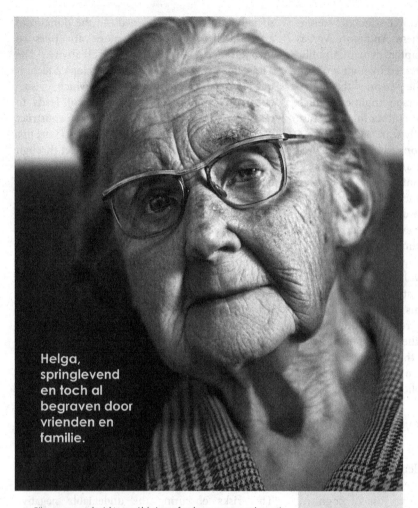

Figure 2.3 Advertisement designed by Tramway21 (tramway21.be) combining different frames and tested in an experimental study design (photo taken by Laura Baudoux, used with permission)

Helga,
springlevend
en toch al
begraven door
vrienden en
familie.

Bij mensen met de ziekte van Alzheimer of andere vormen van dementie gaat het geheugen er geleidelijk op achteruit. Toch zijn ze nog gevoelig voor emoties en voor de kwaliteit van menselijke relaties. Help hen geluk te vinden in de kleine dingen van het leven.

Antwoorden op uw vragen, zie www.**alzheimer**.org

Achter elke
Alzheimer-
patient schuilt een
mens die leeft.

diagnosis is made. Depending on the age at the time of diagnosis, life expectancy is on average seven to ten years (three years or less if the patient is 90 years or older), so time is still available to gain in quality of life. A useful counter-frame might then be 'seize the day'. Although there is an undeniable gradual decline in the number and nature of activities that are still possible, one could learn to enjoy the little things that make life still worth living, even with a diagnosis of dementia. Alternative forms of communication can be sought with people with dementia, which is, as in the poetry examples presented earlier, mainly non-verbal yet

meaningful. In this way, caregivers can get to know their loved ones during the process of illness in different and unexpected ways.

The deployment of a number of framing and counter-framing strategies, as discussed earlier, have been tried out in experimental research that explores to what extent these strategies can be used in awareness-raising campaigns. A combination of a frame that focusses on the problem with a counter-frame that offers a more positive and hopeful alternative perspective turns out to be the best choice to get the audience thinking and evaluating the campaign positively. Figure 2.3, for example, uses a combination of the heading

'Helga, already buried by her friends and family, and yet she's still alive' and the baseline 'Behind every person with Alzheimer's is a living person' [50].

Furthermore, the 'Unity' frame (which does not distinguish between body and mind) has proven useful and has led to positive attitudes towards people affected by dementia [51]. A frame that distinguishes between body and mind, in contrast, brings about emotions such as sadness and anger. Visual stimuli, especially the depiction of people with dementia, draw attention to the campaign image, as demonstrated by the use of eye-tracking technology. The image of an elderly person ensures that more attention is paid to the accompanying text on a campaign image. A younger adult holds the attention for a longer time, but directs the attention away from the text. The results of this type of research make clear that each building block of a message matters, as it can generate different effects with different target groups. Communication should therefore be tailored as closely as possible to the living world of the different target groups.

One example is the story of a woman who got to know her father through dementia as someone who liked to cuddle, whereas before he was always very distant from her. The ability to discover previously occluded aspects of a parent's character is also underlined in the literary genre of the filial dementia memoir, in which (often female) authors report on new physical and emotional intimacy with fathers who, because of reigning ideals of masculinity, were previously often aloof or simply absent (although one of the famous cases, Arno Geiger's *Der alter König in seinem Eksil*, in which a son gets to know his father through dementia, is written by a male author). As such, a ray of light appears in a life with dementia that is very often presented as pitch-black. Therefore, the German nationwide awareness-raising campaign Konfetti im Kopf (Confetti in the Head) tries to bring colour to the lives of people with dementia by making use of the motivating power of art, culture and direct encounters.

Another strategy to identify alternative perspectives consists in greater awareness that the perception of dementia is not determined solely by the actual symptoms of the condition; it is not simply a biological, but also a psychological, social and cultural condition. For example, in the context of informal care, reference is regularly made to the role reversal between parents and children ('reverse parenting'): parents should care for their children, but not the other way around. However, this is not a natural fact but a socially constructed norm. It is equally possible to look at informal care from the perspective of reciprocity. Parents take care of their young children, and later in life it is the children's turn to take care of their parents. Similarly, people with dementia who play with a doll or use the tablecloth to wipe their mouth in the restaurant are a source of shame only to the extent that they are viewed from a normative perspective. It is also possible to see a person with dementia playing with a doll as the liberating falling away of social inhibition. The adults, then, can return to the carefree and playfulness of their childhood. Wanting to prevent this type of situations in public at all cost can increase the social isolation of people with dementia. In other words, how dementia is perceived and conceived has real impacts on the lived experiences of citizens with dementia. This also means that changing perceptions matters.

7 Conclusion: Future of Dementia Stigma

The aim of this chapter was to familiarize the reader with the historical and sociocultural origins of dementia public stigma, its conceptualization, perpetuation mechanisms and interventions to reduce it. Undoubtedly, we are at a unique turning point. Promoted by initiatives of leading worldwide bodies in the area of dementia, such as Alzheimer's Disease International, Alzheimer's Europe and the World Health Organization, public health attention on the topic is at its peak. Still, conceptual, methodological and strategic limitations continue to obstruct the successful translation of this interest into productive research and intervention initiatives. Some of the questions remaining are: First, do we have a clear understanding of dementia public stigma, or are we sticking to conceptualizations developed in relation to other conditions? Are we, in other words, missing the uniqueness of dementia stigma? Second, to what extent will recent, socially oriented and positively inclined views of dementia affect dementia stigma?

Third, do we even have reliable and valid instruments to assess dementia stigma? And fourth, why is the impact of interventions to reduce dementia stigma so modest?

Our approach to dementia stigma needs to walk a fine line between assuring the problem is urgent without representing it as hopeless, and valorizing it as a distinct way of life and underlining the very real challenges it involves. Because the stigma surrounding dementia might partly be due to the dramatization of the disorder, it might be tempting to opt for a more extensive form of deproblematization of the disorder. This is, however, not a panacea either. In the contested book *The Myth of Alzheimer's*, the authors state unequivocally that dementia is a normal far-reaching form of natural ageing of the brain [52]. Searching for a cure for Alzheimer's would therefore be a futile quest for a 'cure' for ageing in general. Because the search for this holy grail is pointless, the authors argue for a radical shift in attention: away from the stubborn desire to find a cure for the disease to prevention and especially caregiving. For all the good intentions powering this destigmatizing effort, it again risks exacerbating the stigma and trivializing the condition. In any case, there is a paradox that needs to be taken into account – namely, that dramatizing the condition contributes to the stigma, whereas deproblematizing can result in the disorder being disguised in such a way that it seems no longer necessary to pay attention to it. As a result, the limited resources available for scientific research might go to, for instance, research into cancer, a disease that is less easily perceived as being primarily age related.

This is only one of the challenges future engagements with dementia stigma will need to reckon with. Another key challenge is to involve people with dementia more in ethically responsible ways in research into dementia perceptions. A further challenge is to develop more sophisticated and dementia-specific methods to understand both the causes and the mechanisms behind stigma. Further, and as we underlined in the sections on literature and media, the cognitive processing of text and image remains to a large extent a black box. All of these challenges remain, and if efforts at destigmatization insist that dementia is not a hopeless and meaningless condition, they should never fool us into believing that living with dementia is easy.

References

1. Herrmann LK, Welter, E, Leverenz, J, et al. A systematic review of dementia-related stigma research: Can we move the stigma dial? *The American Journal of Geriatric Psychiatry* 2018; **26**: 316–31.

2. Nguyen T, Li X. Understanding public-stigma and self-stigma in the context of dementia: A systematic review of the global literature. *Dementia* 2018; **19**: 148–81.

3. Corrigan PW, Kosyluk KA. Mental illness stigma: Types, constructs, and vehicles for change. In Corrigan, PW, ed. *The Stigma of Disease and Disability: Understanding Causes and Overcoming Injustices*. Washington, DC, American Psychological Association, 2014; 35–56.

4. Werner P. Stigma and Alzheimer's disease: A systematic review of evidence, theory, and methods. In Corrigan, PW, ed. *The Stigma of Disease and Disability: Understanding Causes and Overcoming Injustices*. Washington, DC, American Psychological Association, 2014; 223–44.

5. Werner, P, Kalaitzaki AE, Spitzer N, et al. Stigmatic beliefs towards persons with dementia: Comparing Israeli and Greek college students. *International Psychogeriatrics* 2019; **31**: 1393–1401.

6. Stites, SD, Rubrighr JD, Karlawish J. What features of stigma do the public most commonly attribute to Alzheimer's disease dementia? Results of a survey of the U.S. general public. *Alzheimer's & Dementia: The Journal of the Alzheimer's Association* 2018; **14**: 925–32.

7. Corrigan PW, Green A, Lundin R, et al. Familiarity with and social distance from people who have serious mental illness. *Psychiatric Services*. 2001; **52**: 953–8.

8. Link B, Cullen F, Struening E, et al. A modified labeling theory approach to mental disorders: An empirical assessment. *American Sociological Review* 1989; **54**: 400–23.

9. Kitwood T. *Dementia Reconsidered: The Person Comes First*. Buckingham, Open University Press, 1995.

10. Van Gorp B, Vercruysse T. Frames and counter-frames giving meaning to dementia: A framing analysis of media content. *Social Science & Medicine* 2012; **74**: 1274–81.

11. Gerritsen D, Oyebode J, Gove, D. Ethical implications of the perception and portrayal of dementia. *Dementia* 2016; **17**: 596–608.

12. Hillman A, Latimer J. Cultural representations of dementia. *PLoS Medicine* 2017; **14**: e1002274.

13. Young JA, Lind C, Orange JB, Savundranayagam MY. Expanding current understandings of

epistemic injustice and dementia: Learning from stigma theory. *Journal of Aging Studies* 2019; **48**: 76–84.

14. Granello DH, Gibbs TA. The power of language and labels: 'The mentally ill' versus 'people with mental illnesses'. *Journal of Counseling & Development* 2016; **94**: 31–40.

15. McParland P, Kelly F, Innes A. Dichotomising dementia: Is there another way? *Sociology of Health & Illness* 2017; **39**: 258–69.

16. Zeilig H. Dementia as a cultural metaphor. *The Gerontologist* 2013; **54**: 258–67.

17. Werner P, Raviv-Turgeman L, Corrigan PW. The influence of the age of dementia onset on college students' stigmatic attributions towards a person with dementia. *BMC Geriatr* 2020; **20**: 1–6.

18. Higgs P, Gilleard C. Frailty, abjection and the 'othering' of the fourth age. *Health Sociology Review* 2014; **23**: 10–19.

19. Rowe JW, Kahn RL. Successful aging. *The Gerontologist* 1997; **37**: 433–40.

20. Kang S, Gearhart S, Bae, HS. Coverage of Alzheimer's disease from 1984 to 2008 in television news and information talk shows in the United States: An analysis of news framing. *American Journal of Alzheimer's Disease & Other Dementias* 2010; **25**: 687–97.

21. Kessler EM, Schwender C. Giving dementia a face? The portrayal of older people with dementia in German weekly news magazines between the years 2000 and 2009. *The Journals of Gerontology: Series B* 2012; **67**: 261–70.

22. Gerritsen DL, Kuin Y, Nijboer J. Dementia in the movies: The clinical picture. *Aging & Mental Health* 2014; **18**: 276–80.

23. Cohen-Shalev A, Marcus E. An insider's view of Alzheimer's: Cinematic portrayals of the struggle for personhood. *International Journal of Ageing and Later Life* 2012; **7**: 73–96.

24. Strier R, Werner P. Tracing stigma in long-term care insurance in Israel: Stakeholders' views of policy implementation. *Journal of Aging & Social Policy* 2016; **28**: 29–48.

25. Werner P, Doron I. Alzheimer's disease and the law: Positive and negative consequences of structural stigma and labeling in the legal system. *Aging & Mental Health* 2016: **21**: 1206–13.

26. Stites SD, Rubrighr, JD, Karlawish J. What features of stigma do the public most commonly attribute to Alzheimer's disease dementia? Results of a survey of the U.S. general public. *Alzheimer's & Dementia: The Journal of the Alzheimer's Association* 2018; **14**: 925–32.

27. Whitehead A, Woods A. Introduction. In Whitehead A, Woods A, eds. *The Edinburgh Companion to the Medical Humanities*. Edinburgh, Edinburgh University Press, 2016; 1–31.

28. Bleakley A. *Medical Humanities and Medical Education: How the Medical Humanities Can Shape Better Doctors*. Abingdon, Routledge, 2015.

29. Bladon H. Using fiction to increase empathy and understanding in dementia care. *Nursing Times* 2019; **115**: 47–9.

30. Vermeulen P. *Homo sacer/homo demens*: The epistemology of dementia in contemporary literature and theory. In Krüger-Fürhoff I, Schmidt N, Vice, S, eds. *The Politics of Dementia: Forgetting and Remembering the Violent Past in Literature, Film, and Graphic Narratives*. Berlin, De Gruyter, 2020; 39–54.

31. Simonsen P. The terror of dementia in Ian McEwan's *Saturday*. In Chivers S, Kriebernegg U., eds. *Care Home Stories: Aging, Disability, and Long-term Residential Care*. Bielefeld, Transcript, 2017; 175–90.

32. Jamieson S. Reading the spaces of age in Alice Munro's 'The bear came over the mountain'. *Mosaic: An Interdisciplinary Critical Journal* 2014, **47**: 1–17.

33. Simonsen P. *Livslange liv: Plejehjemsromaner og pensionsfortællinger fra velfærdsstaten*. Odense, Syddansk Universitetsforlag, 2014.

34. Casey B. Dementia and symbiosis in *Waiting for Godot*. In Maginess T, ed. *Dementia and Literature: Interdisciplinary Perspectives*. Abingdon, Routledge, 2018; 37–52.

35. Maginess T. *Dementia and Literature: Interdisciplinary Perspectives*. Abingdon, Routledge, 2018.

36. Swinnen A, Schweda M, eds. *Popularizing Dementia: Public Expressions and Representations of Forgetfulness*. Bielefeld, Transcript, 2015.

37. Swaffer K. Foreword. In Maginess T., ed. *Dementia and Literature: Interdisciplinary Perspectives*. Abingdon, Routledge, 2018; xi–xiii.

38. Devi G. *The Spectrum of Hope: An Optimistic and New Approach to Alzheimer's Disease and Other Dementias*. New York, Workman, 2017.

39. Rüsch N, Xu Z. Strategies to reduce mental illness stigma. In Gaebel W, Rössler W, Sartorius N, eds. *The Stigma of Mental Illness: End of the Story?* Cham, Springer, 2017; 451–67.

40. Phillipson L, Hall D, Cridland E, et al. Involvement of people with dementia in raising awareness and changing attitudes in a dementia friendly community pilot project. *Dementia* 2019; **18**: 2679–94.

41. Buckner S, Darlington N, Woodward M, et al. Dementia friendly communities in England: A scoping study. *International Journal of Geriatric Psychiatry* 2019; **34**: 1235–43.

42. Werner P, Schifmann KI, David D, AboJabel H. Newspaper coverage of Alzheimer's disease: Comparing online newspapers in Hebrew and Arabic across time. *Dementia* 2019; **18**: 1554–67.

43. Werner P, Schiffman, KI. Exposure to a national multimedia Alzheimer's disease awareness campaign: Assessing stigmatic beliefs towards persons with the disease. *Int J Geriatr Psychiatry* 2918; **33**: 336–42.

44. Haapala I, Carr A, Biggs S. What you say and what I want: Priorities for public health campaigning and initiatives in relation to dementia. *Australas J Ageing* 2019; **38**: 59–67.

45. Fominaya AW, Corrigan PW, Rusch N. The effects of pity on self- and other-perceptions of mental illness. *Psychiatry Research* 2016; **241**: 159–64.

46. Herrmann LK, Welter E, Leverenz J, et al. A Systematic review of dementia-related stigma research: Can we move the stigma dial? *The American Journal of Geriatric Psychiatry* 2016: **26**: 316–31.

47. Killick J. *Poetry and Dementia: A Practical Guide.* London, Jessica Kingsley, 2018.

48. McParland P, Kelly F, Innes A. Dichotomising dementia: Is there another way? *Sociology of Health & Illness* 2917; **39**: 258–69.

49. Van Gorp B, Vercruysse T. Frames and counter-frames giving meaning to dementia: A framing analysis of media content. *Social Science & Medicine* 2012; **74**: 1274–81.

50. Van Gorp B, Vercruysse T, Van den Bulck, J. Toward a more nuance perception of Alzheimer's disease: Designing and testing a campaign advertisement. *American Journal of Alzheimer's Disease and Other Dementias* 2012; **27**: 388–96.

51. Cuadrado F, Antolí A, Rosal-Nadales M, Moriana JA. Giving meaning to Alzheimer's disease: An experimental study using a framing approach. *Health Communication* 2020; **35**: 447–55.

52. Whitehouse PJ, George D. *The Myth of Alzheimer's.* New York, St. Martin's Press, 2008.

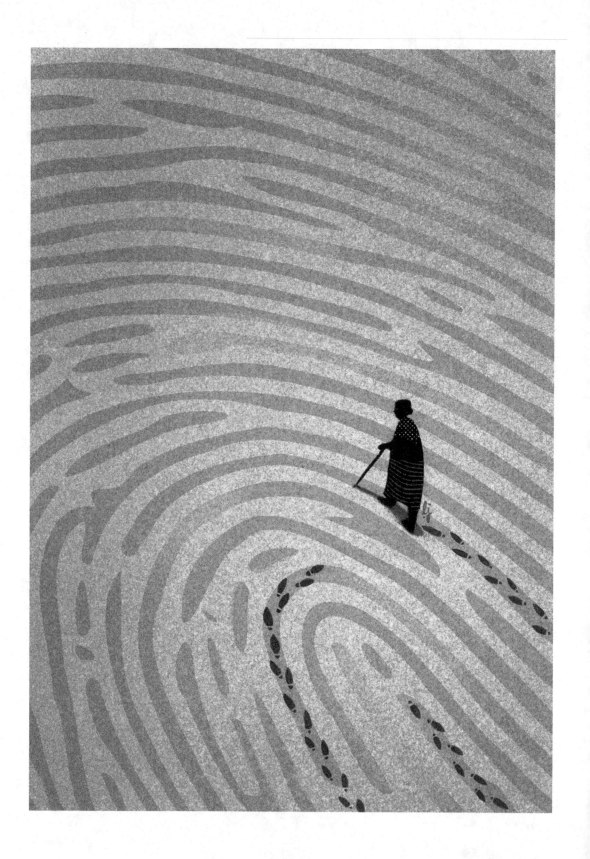

Chapter 3

Personhood, Identity and Autonomy

Bart Pattyn and Peter Hacker, with commentary from Ursula Basset, Mathieu Vandenbulcke and Rose-Marie Dröes

Bart Pattyn, Peter Hacker

The confrontation with the dementia process is harsh. With Alzheimer's disease (AD), the first symptoms seem harmless: the person is often scatterbrained, does not come up with the right word, forgets what he or she had just planned – things that can happen to anyone – but over time those episodes follow more quickly, and relatives and friends find that something unusual is going on. The common ground from which conversations and joint activities are coordinated crumbles and the shared principles, thoughts and memories that formed the anchor points of everyday interactions become increasingly inaccessible to the person with dementia. Due to the limited access to a common understanding of what is at stake, it becomes more and more difficult for persons with dementia to participate perspicuously in an interaction.

In these circumstances, people often ask 'philosophical' questions. How come someone standing right in front of us isn't really there? Has the dementia process only made it more challenging to get through to that person, or is his or her personality fraying apart? It is when we are lost that we start to ponder.

In this chapter, we discuss some assumptions that shape our attitudes towards people with dementia. There are many such assumptions. Take for instance the concern of a healthcare provider to make sure that persons with dementia can always make their own decisions. For them, showing respect for a person is equivalent to showing respect for their autonomy. For other caregivers, the first thing to consider may be the fact that the person with dementia feels safe and happy and is not in distress. For them, it is self-evident that in all circumstances, someone's well-being needs to take precedence. Other caregivers believe that persons with dementia should be able to function in their familiar environment for as long as possible because they intuitively assume that our identity is determined by what we personify in our habitual

social environment. Others assume that we always should prioritize what the person with dementia desires, even if what is desired does not meet what is socially accepted. For them, it is wrong to impose our moral expectations on others. All of these care options are based on implicit assumptions concerning what is essential for human beings in general.

In psychological and social science theories, assumptions about what a human being naturally needs are more prominent because part of these theories is built on these kinds of assumptions. The person-centred care approach, for example, starts from a particular assumption about what being a person means and what it takes to be a person [1]. Something similar applies to psychoanalytic theories. They rely on a specific view of human desire. It is from such a perspective that the behaviour of people with dementia has been linked to failing defence mechanisms [2]. Theories based on the importance of basic trust will associate the anxiety of people with dementia with the fear of losing the confidence that they acquired as a child through affective attachment to loving parents [3]. In theories in which well-being is linked to pleasure based on affective and sensory contact, one also starts from a specific conception of what human well-being implies.

Assumptions about what it means to be a full human being are also prominent in legislation. The first principle of the United Nations (UN) Convention on the Rights of Persons with Disabilities, for instance, offers a clear example of this when it confirms as its first principle 'respect for inherent dignity, individual autonomy including the freedom to make one's own choices, and independence of persons' [4].[1] The assumption is that in

---

[1] According to this Convention, persons with disabilities 'include those who have long-term physical, mental, intellectual or sensory impairments which in interaction with various barriers may hinder their full and effective participation in society on an equal basis with others' (Article 1).

order to be considered a full person, human beings must be able to make decisions for themselves.

Discussions about the public perception of dementia are based on assumptions about what a fulfilling human life amounts to. It is, for instance, believed that the framework from which the general public perceives dementia is too negative because in our Western culture, the importance of cognitive functions is overestimated while the affective and sensitive aspects of a person's personality are supposed to be underestimated [5]. That would imply that it remains possible to have a fulfilling life based on emotional and sensitive contact only. Due to the overvaluation of cognitive skills, the notion of dementia has a stigmatizing character, which is why it is argued that the public perception of dementia should be adjusted. The implicit assumption is here that emotional aspects of someone's personality can flourish even if the cognitive functions are low.

Surveying these informal philosophical assumptions, it seems relevant to subject them to a more formal philosophical analysis. We plan to do so by clarifying the concepts on which some of these assumptions are built.

Concept clarification consists in explaining how a particular concept can licitly be used. That use is constrained. Words do not mean whatever you want them to mean. That is why concept clarification will enable us to identify cases in which concepts are being applied beyond their licit limits. We are all easily tempted to use concepts beyond the bounds of their proper application, thereby misleading ourselves and our interlocutors often without being aware of it. This is also the case when we use concepts such as 'self', 'mind', 'person' and 'autonomy' [6]. Making those inaccuracies visible should make it possible to adjust a series of common but misleading philosophical assumptions on which some of our attitudes towards people with dementia rely.

In the context of discussions about dementia, some conceptual misunderstandings appear to be based on a language-induced deception. The reason for such delusion is often our tendency to spontaneously regard things that we can denote with a noun or with a personal pronoun as an independent entity, even if this 'objectification' is conceptually nonsensical. Grammatically, we can make what we designate with a noun or a personal pronoun function as the subject or the object of a sentence and in this way ascribe all kinds of properties and activities to it. We can do this without appearing unusual, strange or unnatural, even if the particular reality we refer to with that noun cannot in practice be regarded as an independent entity. For example, the contradiction we make between body and mind appears to be based mainly on a deception induced by language. Let us explain the nature of that deception with the concept of 'self'.

'Self' – The word 'self' was initially used in situations where one wanted to emphasize that it was indeed about that very person or object that one was talking, as in 'He did not leave it to someone else: he preferred to do it himself.' 'Self' was and is also used as a possessive and as a reflexive pronoun (oneself). In all of these cases, the concept of 'self' represents the person or object to which reference is made with emphasis, possessive or reflexive. Language, however, allows the use of 'self' independently of any attached pronoun in a select range of contexts. It is perfectly all right to talk about 'someone's true self' or 'someone's better self'. When people started to do that, the impression was created that someone's 'self' does not coincide with the subject. Instead, it seems to refer to a being or entity to which one can attribute characteristics that differ from those of the person. Philosophers further enhanced that supposed independence when they assumed in Locke's footsteps that what guarantees the continuity of one's 'self' is something that does not coincide with the living human being. A person's 'self' would be the product of what someone imagines to be the inner subject or 'owner' of experience. Instead of continuing to think of the word 'self' as a part of a pronoun immediately referring to the person, 'self' became the designation of a separate being or entity. It appears to be about something that does not necessarily undergo the same changes as the living human being. The fact that 'self' can be used in an objectifying way does not, of course, mean that we always use the concept in a misleading way. With this personal pronoun we usually refer to a concrete private person and not to an objectifiable item belonging to that person.

Regarding the philosophical assumptions that underlie conceptions of dementia, the distorting use of the term 'self' has given rise to the appearance that, despite the neurological damage caused by the dementia process, a person's 'self' appears as something that can remain itself unchanged. If there were an independent entity or a particular item in our mind that we may call 'our self', that would make sense, but there is not. The licit use of 'self' is simply to refer to aspects of our nature, not to any kind of being or entity.

'Body' and 'mind' – Such an 'objectification' has also occurred with respect to the concepts of 'body' and 'mind'. 'A's body' and 'A's mind' can function as the subject of a sentence which makes it appear as if such phrases refer to something substantial. Furthermore it is grammatically all right to say that we *have* a body and equally in order to say that we *are* a body. This is the source of much confusion, as it raises the question of the relation between the body I am (this particular animate spatio-temporal continuant) and the body I have? For how can what I am also be something I have? Clarity dawns when one realizes that all of our talk of the body I have is in fact no more than talk of my somatic characteristics. If NN has a lithe, athletic, beautiful body, then she is lithe, athletic and beautiful. If NN has a frail, ageing and weak body, then he is frail, ageing and weak. Something similar holds of our talk about our mind or someone's mind. It appears superficially to be talk about something associated with a person's body (as Cartesian dualists argue). But if the use of 'mind' is carefully examined, it becomes evident that this is no more than a way of speaking of a range of a human being's intellectual, cognitive, cogitative and volitional acts and activities. For a thought to cross one's mind is for a thought to occur to one; to have something in mind is to think of something; to make up one's mind is to decide; to use one's mind is to think; to be in two minds about something is to be undecided; to be in half a mind to do something is to feel inclined to do it; to call something to mind is to remember, and for something to slip out of one's mind is to forget. To do something mindlessly is to do it without thought, to lose one's mind is to lose one's rational faculties and so on. All of our talk of the mind is a manner of speaking of our rational faculties and their exercise. In short, all of our talk of the mind and body a person *has* is talk of intellectual and somatic features of a living human being, not talk of two separate entities that stand in some baffling relationship to each other.

Nevertheless, people rely on all kinds of dualist assumptions, and if one looks back in the past, one will find that dualist principles were more the rule than the exception. After all, in Western history, there have hardly been periods when the opposition between soul and body has not been assumed. In Christian doctrine, this opposition was taken for granted because almost all theologians proceeded from the Neoplatonic and Augustinian distinction between the visible, material and perishable reality on one hand, and the invisible, immaterial and imperishable reality on the other. The body was supposed to be part of material reality while the soul belonged to the spiritual world.[2] The fact that in the early modern period intellectuals distanced themselves from scholastic philosophy did not lead to the elimination of dualism. On the contrary, the classical dualist view of man was radicalized under the influence of Descartes. According to Descartes, the material world consists of material substance (*res extensa*) and is the subject of physical laws. The human body belongs to this sphere of reality. The human mind, on the other hand, is a substance that does not occupy physical space and is therefore not subject to physical laws (*res cogitans*). In that sense, according to Descartes, body and mind belong to two completely separate spheres of reality.[3]

Naive Cartesian dualism may make us smile, but it should not be overlooked that the assumptions many modern scientists use to explain human behaviour are no less dualist. For example, when neurologists suggest that they can explain how people think, feel or desire based on physiological processes, they implicitly assume that the physiological and psychological realms of reality form two mutually independent spheres. This distinction is similar to that of Descartes. However, unlike Descartes, they do not assume that the spiritual sphere directs the material one, but the other way around: what people think, feel and

---

[2] Neoplatonic dualism initially proved difficult to reconcile with Christian beliefs about incarnation, trinity and physical resurrection that gave rise to all kinds of dogmatic disagreements. In the Middle Ages, some theologians were inspired by Aristotle's hylomorphism. However, the distinction between the earthly and the heavenly was interpreted almost unanimously from the Neoplatonic conceptual framework.

[3] Because apparently body and soul are nevertheless related to each other, Descartes was forced to indicate how the two spheres are connected. He assumed he could identify the point of interaction with an organ in the brain, specifically the pineal gland. This is the standard view of Cartesianism. But it is arguable that he was a trialist, rather than a dualist (see [7]).

desire is determined by physical, chemical or physiological processes. Indeed, thinking, feeling and longing are based on a series of physical, chemical and physiological processes, and those processes are the necessary conditions for thinking, feeling or longing. However, it is a bridge too far to consider these processes as sufficient conditions for how we think, feel or desire. The fact that the amygdala in my brain causes a freeze or a flight response will not make me understand what it means to be scared. Likewise, the fact that there is a certain amount of dopamine in my nervous system can not explain what counts as happiness. The fact that we can indicate more precisely which physiological processes accompany feeling anxious or happy does not make our ordinary dealing with anxiety or happiness redundant. Physiological and psychological explanations are not mutually exclusive. They are complementary. They highlight aspects of the same act, event, activity or process.

Dualist views are still prevalent today, not only because from a scientific point of view it is easily assumed that what people think, feel or desire can be explained on the basis of physiological processes. At least as misleading is the premise that our mind can function on its own. The notion that what we experience psychologically does not depend on the nature of our body has been fuelled by numerous philosophical considerations, not least by Locke's conception of personal identity. As indicated, Locke believed that the continuity of a person's identity is independent of his or her body because it is guaranteed by his or her memory, implying that even if a person's consciousness were to be transferred to another body, the continuity of his or her personal identity would be ensured. Locke's' account is misleading, as we have already discussed. The fact that I have forgotten that I was the one punching someone in the face yesterday does not undo the fact that it was me. Nevertheless, Locke's ideas have often been taken into consideration because people are tempted to assume that our psychological properties alone constitute who and what we are. That we can experience anything independently of our being living spatio-temporal continuants with powers of intellect, will and feeling is incoherent. What we experience and feel is based on what we perceive physically. Therefore the world will appear differently if a child or an adult experiences it, a man or a woman, a tall or a small

human being.[4] For all kinds of cognitive and emotional functions, we need to be in good shape. We cannot reason sensibly when we are in shock, drunk or exhausted, and our particular physical aversions, fears, lust and passions are no less physical than they are psychological. From that perspective, the idea that we could retain our personality if we were able to transfer our mind or consciousness to any other body seems absurd. That is why we use all kinds of expressions in terms of which we describe what happens to us physically to make clear what we are going through psychologically. We say, for example, that our heart is beating faster with excitement, or that we are breathless with effort or blushing with embarrassment. These descriptions cannot be understood as purely physical or as purely psychological. They are descriptions of what we experience psychosomatically. That is ultimately what we are: psychosomatic creatures, with physical and psychological powers, physical and psychological attributes.

The conceptual clarification regarding the contrast between body and mind has consequences for how we perceive what happens to someone with dementia. The damage to a person's neurological system cannot be understood as the damage to an entity distinct from the individual. It is damage to the person himself or herself. The self or the mind of a person is not something on its own that operates within its own sphere vis-à-vis other aspects of our personality. In the same way, when I am suffering from a disease, it is not just my body that is suffering: it is me.

Cognition and emotion – Just as body and mind do not belong to separate realities, neither does our cognitive and affective nature. Thought operations and emotions do not function independently of each other. They intervene and determine each other's content and quality. The motivation for answering, objecting or checking something is usually attitudinal or emotional, and

---

[4] Aristotle was aware of the absurdity of this misunderstanding. He wrote, 'saying that the psyche is angry is of the same order as saying that the psyche weaves or builds'. According to him, it is misleading to say that the psyche regrets, learns or thinks. Ultimately, it is the human being who does that with his psyche in the sense in which a human being does things with his talents. Aristotle did not have the concept of a person, which emerged only in Rome. He spoke simply of human beings or men.

the shades of what we feel are determined by the nuanced differences between what we can cognitively distinguish. We do not think without feeling the relevance of what we are thinking, and our attitudes and emotions would be poorly differentiated without our conceptions. That means that if a person's cognitive abilities change, his or her feelings inevitably change as well. In that sense, it is misleading to assume that cognition and affection belong to separated spheres. If something goes wrong cognitively, it will often immediately have an effect on what occurs emotionally and vice versa.

Identity – The concept of identity has at least two distinct uses. On one hand, the term 'identity' is used in the context of questions about someone's numerical identity, such as: 'Is the person I met yesterday really the person who stands before me today?' As indicated, contrary to what Locke suggested, a person's numerical identity seems to be guaranteed by the continuity of his or her existence as a living human being and not by what the person concerned remembers. In our everyday interactions, we seldom experience the determination of a person's numerical identity as problematic. It is only in situations when we do not recognize someone, for example, that we doubt whether that person is the one we had in mind.

However, 'identity' can also refer to what someone is because of his or her position, function or standing in a personal relation or in an institutional setting. Lydia is, for instance, someone's friend, colleague or mother while she is also a neighbour and a citizen. The identity of a person in this context is determined by the formal and informal norms and expectations that fix a person's status within a web of social interactions. It is in this sense that we speak of a person's sense of identity – that is, of their conception of who they are and what they stand for.

To make sure of someone's numerical identity, we know what to focus on. Our passports contain passport photos to check whether we are indeed the person we purport to be. If that is not sufficient, biometric identification techniques can be used based on, for example, fingerprints or iris recognition. It is less obvious to assure ourselves of someone's status in a relation. Since all relations in which people stand to each other are particular, there doesn't seem to exist an objective conception of someone's social identity. What

a person means to me will never fully correspond to what he or she means to you. However, that doesn't mean that we are condemned to constant misunderstandings about each other's roles or functions. In most of our interactions, we are well aware of what we can expect from each other from a common perspective. That awareness seems to be a precondition for the success of our interaction. Indeed, if we could not share the same idea of each other's function, we would not be able to coordinate our common interactions, evaluate each other's initiatives and monitor our own behaviour. In all of our interactions we trust that each of us is aware of what we want to obtain in that shared interaction and how each of us can contribute to realizing it. Since most of what we do is part of an interaction, there are hardly situations where we are not implicitly aware of how our social identity is perceived from a particular common perspective. We know what is expected from us as a member of a family, as a customer in a store, as a colleague among peers, as a passerby on the sidewalk etc. Even in many informal, short-lived interactions, we know how we are expected to meet the situation and to respect the rules and norms that guide our behaviour. In our daily life, our conception of a person's social identity is therefore not based on the heterogeneous collection of subjective impressions that each of us has separately, but on assumptions, beliefs and judgements we share in the course of our interactions.

This observation has some consequences. It implies, for instance, that if we cannot address a situation from a shared perspective, we will not be able to realize how each of us is supposed to be perceived within the context of our interaction. The ability to estimate from a common point of view how someone comes across seems to be crucial, not only to realize *someone else's* but also *our own* social identity in a particular interaction. People cannot realize their own status vis-à-vis the status of others if they cannot participate in the common understanding of the interaction.

Another consequence of the observation that our identity is illuminated by a shared perspective is that nobody can fully control his or her own status. The recognition of our social identity will be determined by what our social environment agrees it to be. To be taken seriously we depend on our companions or our fellow citizens. They need to give us a chance to be acknowledged as a full interlocutor. It is from this perspective that Erving Goffman, the sociologist who developed the core concepts we use today in research on stigma, framing and identity, stressed the vulnerability of our identity. He illustrated with numerous observations how we can lose face – sometimes by accident, sometimes by our own failure, sometimes by a lack of collaboration or by bad intentions of our interlocutors [8]. In our intimate relations, we have the tendency to protect each other from this kind of trouble. Decent people will offer someone who ends up in an embarrassing situation a way out. They will protect their fellow citizens who fail to perform their role or present themselves properly. But people can be cruel. They can ridicule, stigmatize or destroy someone's reputation. All of this illustrates how dependent we are on the sympathy and solidarity of others to preserve the respectability of our identity.

A third consequence of our observation is that in order to be a reliable player, you need to know the game. If you want to participate in a conversation, you need to understand what someone is talking about. If you want to be trusted with a particular responsibility, your fellow human beings need to trust that you realize what that responsibility implies. You can only actively participate in an interaction if you can show that you know the rules that structure the common understanding from which the interaction partners assess the meaning of what is at stake in that interaction.

The principles on which the structure of a common understanding in an interaction is based cannot be derived from what is empirically observable. These principles seem to have the same conventional status as the imaginary lines that we project between the stars so that each of us can distinguish the same constellations. People can only realize what is happening from a common perspective if they know the concepts, conventions or rules that they are expected to use to structure what is at stake from a common viewpoint. The concepts we use to coordinate our perception and our interactions are derived from language. Language offers all kinds of ready-to-use formats that help us organize reality in a shared way. It presents scripts and expectation patterns that help us 'read' situations in a common way. Depending on the circumstances, the concepts we use to coordinate our interactions and communication will be spontaneously

enhanced and fine-tuned until we mutually trust that they fit the situation naturally. This is not something we do consciously. It is part of the way we ordinarily make sense of reality.[5]

Participating in a common understanding is not only intellectually but also emotionally important. As Donald Winnicott has aptly described, we will only invest emotionally in what is at stake insofar as we can merge into the game from which we can attribute meaning to that reality along with the companions with whom we can share what we realize. People are affectively involved with reality to the extent that they can attribute shared emotional meaning to specific aspects of reality [10]. Winnicott observed that those who cannot or insufficiently participate in a shared engagement lose part of their emotional interest in the world and become indifferent. If the capacity to be involved in a common enterprise is wholly lost, there can be only limited awareness of and, as a consequence, only limited interest in what happens.

When family, friends or acquaintances informally ask 'philosophical' questions about what is going on with the identity of the person with dementia, they do not worry about that person's numerical identity. No one doubts whether a person will remain the same numerically during the dementia process. Rather, it is the fading presence of the person they used to interact with that worries family members, friends and acquaintances; it is their inadequate capacity to play the role they used to play and to function as a full interlocutor; it is their inability to participate in their previous engagements; it is the withering away of emotional interest in what they cared about. For a long period between the first diagnosis and the last phase of the disease, the person with dementia's interactions with their social

---

[5] Goffman observed that when we ask what is happening, we are not so much interested in the empirical details of the event as we are curious to know how we are supposed to understand the situation. For example, if people are nervously crammed in a shopping street, we will be eager to know if the fuss is about a spectacular clearance sale, a sudden incident or a demonstration. The importance of getting the frame right is about finding out if we are on the same wavelength. The three different conceptualizations imply three different interaction patterns. Getting it right is vital because if we frame the situation in the wrong way, we will look foolish [9].

environment function as before and their participation hardly changes. There are of course moments when the interaction falters – for example, when the person becomes distracted or cannot follow a train of thought properly. In such circumstances, people are spontaneously inclined to jump in and stand up for each other. When someone seems to be going astray, we usually take it for granted in conversation to supplement broken lines of reasoning, to articulate the unfinished phrase, to explain the missed presuppositions and the like. That well-intentioned support can sometimes be perceived as inappropriate. People may be inclined to take the initiative of a person with dementia too quickly; out of impatience they give their interaction partners too little time to decide for themselves what to do. Patronizing interventions can be experienced as humiliating. Of course, this does not alter the fact that attentive support will allow a person with dementia to participate longer in his or her usual interactions with others. Another factor that perpetuates participation is the stability of the context in which that interaction takes place. When an interaction is part of a set of fixed and familiar rituals embedded in a person's daily routine, the initiative the person with dementia is expected to take will be supported by habit formation. Removing someone from their familiar sphere of interaction will therefore be accompanied by a decline in personal initiative. Towards the end of the dementia process, periods in which the person is no longer fully aware of his or her status within the framework of a specific relationship will alternate with clear periods in which the person is aware of this, and those moments are in a relationship often experienced as healing. At the end of the process, relatives, friends and caregivers observe that the person with dementia exhibits a growing incapacity to realize how what happens and what is discussed makes sense. That incapacity manifests itself in different ways: they fail to access a collective memory that could enhance the understanding of an anecdote; they fail to realize the relevance of a concept that is crucial for the interpretation of an event; they can no longer understand a certain rule or they don't realize the repercussion of a convention. In this situation, of course, the person with dementia continues to be a father or mother, husband or wife, neighbour or friend. But he or she is no longer aware of these social roles and can no longer fulfil them. Nevertheless, his or her children, partner, neighbour or friend still stand in the complementary relation to them, a relation that carries with it a manifold of obligations of care.

Person – The term 'person' is often used to refer to a human individual in general – for example, when we specify the number of persons for a hotel reservation or when we verify the maximum number of persons who can occupy a lift.

The term, however, has also a specific meaning. 'Person' is also used to refer to an individual who can be held liable for his or her own moral or legal decisions or behaviours. In that context, 'person' signifies an autonomous human being with powers of rationality, sensitive to reasons for thinking, feeling and acting, responsible for their actions. We don't grant very young children such a person status, since no one expects them to be answerable for their actions in the same way as adults. We will assume someone oversees them and takes responsibility for them. Obviously, this does not mean that we do not consider them intrinsically valuable human beings, nor that we are no longer prepared to take into account their personal views, decisions or wishes. It just means that we do not assign them the same responsibility status as most of our fellow citizens. When decisions have to be made that concern people who can stand up for themselves, we want them to be involved in that decision-making process. Even if we have a certain expertise from which we know what is good for them, it would be wrong to compel them to follow our lead. If we respect them as persons and they agree that we should advise them, we will invite them to share a perspective on their situation from which our advice will appear reasonable to them, and only when they themselves want what we think they should do will we feel confident to proceed. Such agreements can only be made if a person can participate on an equal standing, in a shared understanding as someone who can speak for themselves.

The particular meaning of 'person' corresponds with its etymological meaning. 'Person' was derived from the Greek word for stage mask (*prosōpon*) that was gradually used figuratively to refer to a person's role in a play [11]. Stoics generalized that reference when they drew attention to the fact that in life, every individual plays a specific role and needs to answer the expectations connected to it. According to the Stoics, it is essential to meet these expectations as best as possible, without wanting to determine the role that defines those expectations. The term 'person' was later used in the legal context for the role someone takes in a trial – for example, the role of the complainant or the role of the accused. It was gradually assumed that all citizens have a legal personality except slaves, called *aprosōpos*.

In the modern age, the concept of the person was set against the background of Descartes' and Locke's views. These views gave rise to a web of misconceptions from which one could not easily free oneself. Kant was one of the few intellectuals who could put Locke's view into perspective. 'A person', Kant wrote, 'is a subject whose actions can be imputed to him. Moral personality is, therefore, nothing other than the freedom of a rational being under moral laws.' To which he added: 'Psychological personality is merely the ability to be conscious of one's identity in different conditions of one's existence' (6.224) [12]. According to Kant, people have intrinsic value because they are persons. In the words of Kant himself:

> A human being is a being of slight importance and shares with the rest of animals, as offspring of the earth, an ordinary value. Although a human being has, in his understanding, something more than they and can set himself ends, even this gives him only an *extrinsic* value for his usefulness … But a human being regarded as a *person*, that is as a subject of a morally practical reason, is exalted above any price; for as a person he is not to be valued merely as a means to the ends of others, but as an end in himself, that is he possesses a *dignity* (an absolute inner worth) by which he exacts *respect* for himself from all other rational beings in the world. *(6. 434f.)*

This definition of a person will raise questions about the consequences of the process of dementia. If at the end of the process it becomes difficult for an individual with dementia to participate as an autonomous actor, can that individual still be considered a person? Since we are used to call all human beings persons in the broad sense of the word, this question will be perceived as disturbing only for those who associate the human dignity of human beings with their status as autonomous and responsible individuals, as Kant would have it. But is the connection between human dignity and autonomy justified? We will answer this question in the course of clarifying the concepts of autonomy and respect.

Autonomy – People are autonomous when they are free to make their own decisions and take responsibility for them. Autonomy, freedom and responsibility are concepts that presuppose each other. It is because a person can decide autonomously and freely what to do that he or she can be held liable for it.

Some philosophers wonder whether autonomy, freedom and responsibility are meaningful concepts because they suppose that everything, including human behaviour, is determined. Recent neurological research has increased public interest in that statement, but the question of whether there is such a thing as 'free will' is anything but new. In the sixteenth and seventeenth centuries, this issue was a central point of contention in the context of a theological discussion about predestination, and at the end of the eighteenth century, the denial of free will was the pivot of radical materialistic Enlightenment thinking. It is, of course, impossible within the scope of this chapter to go into that philosophical discussion in detail. However, there is a particularly much-referenced contribution which provides a relevant starting point in this matter. In 'Freedom and Resentment', Peter Strawson demonstrated that nothing could provide good reasons for abandoning our ordinary notions of freedom and responsibility [13]. In ordinary life, we praise people for their meritorious deeds and blame them for what we consider reprehensible, and we find these reactive attitudes justified. We do make a distinction between what is coerced and what one could freely decide and we consider not everyone fit to take full responsibility. That is how freedom and responsibility make sense in our ordinary interactions. This observation as such does not refute the idea of someone who takes an objectifying attitude (an attitude in which we abstract from how we are involved with each other in ordinary life) and beliefs that all what happens is determined, but the fact that it may seem inconsistent from an objectifying attitude to consider people autonomous, free and responsible is not a sufficient reason to give up the way we interact and organize our lives naturally.

Strawson seems to be right. Even the philosopher who explains in front of a full auditorium that the concepts of autonomy, freedom and responsibility are illusory because everything people do is determined will not get away with this statement when his partner accuses him of having cheated. In our ordinary lives, we know what responsibility means. We know whom we can consider a reliable autonomous actor. We realize that someone who cannot participate in the shared understanding of the meaningfulness of our interactions will not be able to take full responsibility of his or her acts because they will not be able to fully realize the relevance of what they are saying or doing. Without this participation, an individual is still able to act. However, he or she will not be trusted to attune that behaviour to the expectations that apply within mutual involvement. It is only when people trust that you know how the game is played, or that you know what will be considered appropriate and inappropriate within a given context, that you will be accepted as someone who can act in a responsible way as an equal respondent.

The fact that the way we can function as autonomous actors presupposes a relational context implies that we depend on our fellow humans for the success of much of what we do, communicate or represent. If someone threatens to fall out, bystanders can help that individual to play his or her role or to take up his or her function without losing face. Within a family or among friends and trusted acquaintances, the permanent structure of the usual interactions can continue to guarantee the interpretation of the role that the person with dementia has within these different common understandings, even if that person is no longer capable of performing this interpretation himself or herself. Among people who are deeply involved in a family or as friends and acquaintances, the interaction patterns can uphold the place and status of the person with dementia even if the personal initiative of the person with dementia has deteriorated significantly. To keep up these patterns, however, requires a lot of energy and engagement of the family, friends and acquaintances. As for so many other aspects of care, the starting point for supporting someone's 'autonomy' is uneven. Some people have a loving partner, live in a close-knit family or are related as friends or neighbours. Others live alone, are part of a broken family, have few loyal friends and no contact with residents. The capacity to support what an individual wants to personalize is limited. Sooner or later, there will come a time when there is no other alternative for the person than to be treated without much mutual understanding. In this sense, the dementia process confronts people with finitude: limits of the interactions, limits to the kind of role one can play and limits to one's freedom, responsibility and autonomy.

Respect – Showing respect to people can mean different things depending on the context. We use the concept of respect when we value someone in a particular sense – for example, because of his or her talents, achievements or responsibilities. However, respect also applies in a universal sense: we know that we should respect human beings as human beings. Indeed, it seems to us quite natural that we should deal with a human individual differently than with an object or an animal. Although this realization is fragile, we know that when we deal with a human being, whether newly born or old, whether alert or confused, rich or poor, criminal or righteous, we should respect it as a human being. That realization manifests itself before we reflect on its meaningfulness. We do not ask ourselves if that being meets the criteria to be considered human. People can indeed think about what qualities are characteristic of a human being, but when they do that, they do so in a world where it is already clear what a human being is. Indeed, some philosophers doubt whether we should continue to respect that pre-reflective conception. For them, it is questionable whether people who have lost their rational capacities and are no longer aware of themselves have more value than, for example, intelligent animals. They believe that we should give up our 'speciesist' assumptions when determining that value [14]. As long as these thoughts only concern purely theoretical reflections, these statements may be tolerated. However, prioritizing the life of an injured dog over the life of a human being who has lost his or her rational capacities in practice would be considered a transgression.

We also know that wherever we can we should respect human beings as persons. This fact has undoubtedly strengthened our reverence for human dignity, but it is important to recognize the difference between the concept of a person and the concept of a human being. 'Person' is a status concept while 'human being' is a substance concept. Human beings qualify as persons because their powers of rationality and reasonableness and their sensitivity to reasons for acting, feeling and thinking enable them to be an individual who can decide and can speak for themselves in a answerable and responsible way. We do not respect someone as a person only because of his or her cognitive or emotional qualities, but also because those cognitive and emotional powers enable them to realize what matters in the context of their interactions. When someone doesn't realize what's going on, there is no point in trusting him or her as someone who knows what he or she is responsible for. That is why we do not consider very young children or those with severe mental problems accountable for their behaviour and why we expect someone else to take responsibility for what they do. If someone is not or is no longer able to participate in an involvement from which one can decide what is needed, we suppose that it will be the partner, the supervisor or the caregiver who will have to decide what needs to be done for him or her. However, ceasing to trust that someone can participate in our common understanding doesn't necessarily imply that we deny his or her human dignity.

Losing the ability to realize autonomously what kind of decisions and behaviour make our mutual interaction work is never abrupt, except in cases with traumatic brain injury or other forms of acute brain damage. Acquiring or losing the ability to be an independent and accountable person is often determined by a gradual process. In some dementias, even at an advanced stage, confused and more lucid moments alternate. It is not always obvious when someone can't speak up for himself or herself. Because of this, the denial of someone's status of being an accountable person in the strict sense can often be contested. In legal discussions, however, the status of being accountable is of importance, as is discussed in another contribution.

1 The Juridical Take on Personhood, Identity and Autonomy

Ursula Basset

What, if anything, is translated into the legal approach to personhood, identity and autonomy? International law seizes the underlying philosophical debates and takes a stand on them by choosing a specific phrasing – hence the phrase 'lay down the law'.

Personhood is probably one of the most remarkable contentions of law.[6] Law does not understand personhood as relying on a human being able to be autonomous and make its own decisions. The UN Universal Declaration of Human Rights, Article 1, is not derived from personhood, but from being human: 'All human beings are born free and equal in dignity and rights' [18]. Further on, Article 6 reads: 'Everyone has the right to recognition everywhere as a person before the law.' The background of this landmark wording relies on the horrors of two world wars, which were still fresh in the memories of the drafters [19]. Being human has ever since been the only requisite to be entitled to claim recognition to legal personhood as a universal human right [20]. The Convention on the Rights of Persons with Disabilities, in Article 12, comes back to this radical approach: 'States Parties reaffirm that persons with disabilities have the right to recognition everywhere as persons before the law.'

We should be deeply impacted by the radicalness of a legal disposition that feels the urge to specify that every human being has, by the mere fact of being and belonging to the human species, an entitlement to qualify as a person. And this is phrased as an obligation imposed 'universally'. There is a certain 'moral passion' behind the Declaration, which is meant to be a stark and powerful statement [21].

The 'recognition' of personhood means the pre-existence of personhood beyond the law: recognition is a sort of agreement with an acceptance and an acknowledgement. It also may indicate admiration and respect. It means that it is not in the hands of each local legal system to decide who is a person and who is not based upon any other basis than the fact of being human, whatever the stage of human development is, whatever the state of mind is, whatever the age is, whatever the race is, whatever the sex is. It is probably the broadest possible meaning of personhood.

Then again, philosophers might say that everything comes back to the meaning of 'human being'. Law has to be interpreted by its most ordinary

---

[6] Let us recall the UNESCO report consisting of a questionnaire sent to a philosophers' committee, composed by Mahatma Gandhi, Pierre Teilhard de Chardin, Benedetto Croce, Chung Su Lo, Aldous Huxley, S. V. Puntambekar, Ralph Gerard, Salvador de Madariaga, F. S. C. Northrop and J. M. Burgers, among others.

meaning. In that sense, a human being is just a living creature belonging to the species *Homo sapiens.*

Even more strikingly, Article 12 specifically implies that persons with disabilities are full human persons and therefore entitled to the status of personhood before the law [22]. In a way, this statement disrupts the association between legal capacity and legal personhood. Even if the use of the word *reaffirm* implies that there is no new recognition of a right [23], but a confirmation of previous legal provisions, in this context, Article 12 refutes any possible intrinsic association between full mental fitness or autonomy to decide and the right to be fully recognized as a person.

Identity has had another interesting turn when it comes to international law. It made its official appearance in international law in the International Convention on the Rights of the Child, Article 8.:

> 1. States Parties undertake to respect the right of the child to preserve his or her identity, including nationality, name and family relations as recognized by law without unlawful interference. 2. Where a child is illegally deprived of some or all of the elements of his or her identity, States Parties shall provide appropriate assistance and protection, with a view to re-establishing speedily his or her identity.

Much has been written about this article, which sometimes called the Argentinian clause because it was proposed by the Argentinian member to the drafting commission, and because it is closely related to Argentinian history of forced disappearances and illegal adoptions [24].

The right to personal identity deepens the meaning of the legal recognition of personhood. It means that who or what a person is or chooses to be has legal implications [25]. While the recognition of legal personhood means acknowledging the common basis of humanity, the recognition of identity deals with the specifying traits of each human being: his or her cultural background, relations, beliefs, race, religion, political ideas, membership of a certain family, sex and nationality. It also means the projection of this identity in his or her biography: what he or she chooses to be, the knowledge and understanding of his or her parentage, commitments to family, intellectual capacity and talents.

The wording of the Convention on the Rights of the Child is particularly interesting because it spells out a number of *elements* of human identity that one might be selectively deprived of and a correlative obligation of the State to provide *appropriate assistance and protection* in view of *re-establishing speedily* the deprived element. This interesting approach of identity might be well understood as a development of the recognition of legal personality. By Article 6 of the Universal Declaration of Human Rights, international law demands recognition of all human beings, no matter who they specifically are or choose to be. By Article 8 of the Convention on the Rights of the Child, it demands the recognition of each singular person, of his or her choices and traits.

The placement of the right to identity within the Convention on the Rights of the Child by no means restricts this recognition to children. International law has understood that the right to identity (as the quest for one's own origins) does not decrease with age.[7] The social dimension of the right to identity becomes apparent by its recording (nationality, identity records and the documentation derived from registration). Recording is enormously important because it is the gate to access every other human right. All of this sends us back to the numerical sense of identity (identification).

However, it is apparent that this meaning of identity is not consistent with the idea of identity as discussed earlier. The blurring of identity, the increasing absence of self-consciousness and the

---

[7] ECHR, Case of *Jäggi* v. *Switzerland*, Application 58757/00, 13 July 2006, paras. 38 and 40: 'The Court considers that persons seeking to establish the identity of their ascendants have a vital interest, protected by the Convention, in receiving the information necessary to uncover the truth about an important aspect of their personal identity. At the same time, it must be borne in mind that the protection of third persons may preclude their being compelled to make themselves available for medical testing of any kind, including DNA testing … The Court must examine whether a fair balance was struck between the competing interests in this case … Although it is true that, as the Federal Court observed in its judgment, the applicant, now aged 67, has been able to develop his personality even in the absence of certainty as to the identity of his biological father, it must be admitted that an individual's interest in discovering his parentage does not disappear with age, quite the reverse.'

memories of the person subject to earlier dementia stages is a phenomenon law has not yet addressed. It is an unfathomable depth of human drama towards which law remains speechless.

As for *autonomy*, there is an extraordinarily rich legal debate on how it should be understood. First, we do not find the word in the main international law treaties. It is construed as a positive obligation springing out of the protection of privacy [26]. Hence, the definition of autonomy from a legal point of view is a hard task. The European Court of Human Rights (ECHR) made the connection between privacy and autonomy in the case of *Friedl* v. *Austria* (ECHR, 1996), in which it held: 'Although no previous case has established as such any right to self-determination as being contained in Article 8 of the Convention, the Court considers that the notion of personal autonomy is an important principle underlying the interpretation of its guarantees.' This interpretation should be framed within the European Convention. Within the frame of the Inter-American human rights system, the Inter-American Court has interpreted it in a similar manner, making personal autonomy derive from Article 7 of the American Convention of Human Rights (which deals with privacy and dignity) [27].

Autonomy has since been related to the concept of legal capacity, often hinting at children's rights. However, autonomy is also linked to the right of personal development and self-determination. As such, autonomy makes its entrance in UN international law in the Convention on Persons with Disabilities. In its preamble, the Convention recognizes 'the importance for persons with disabilities of their individual autonomy and independence, including the freedom to make their own choices'. It is also a general principle of the Convention. Article 3 enshrines the principle of 'respect for inherent dignity, individual autonomy, including the freedom to make one's own choices, and independence of persons. The States shall take actions to promote self-respect, dignity and autonomy of the person' (Article 16). State parties will also require health professionals to provide care 'raising awareness of the human rights, dignity and autonomy' of persons with disabilities.

Surprisingly, the Convention adopts an individualistic approach to autonomy, precisely when a relational framework is most needed in order to achieve resilience. That is probably why it has been said that 'autonomy does not equate to detachment or complete independence from others; it includes relying on other individuals for support' [28]. Hence the proliferation of new approaches that choose the wording 'relational autonomy' over 'personal autonomy' [29–33]. Concerning decision-making, persons with progressive cognitive disabilities have been presented with several alternatives to make an autonomous decision – advanced directives, shared decision-making and decisions by proxy – as a way to bypass the fading of cognitive abilities.

In a word, law is a witness to the tragedy of a human person whose inner self is slowly fading. It derives from the philosophical debates that underlie the intersection between personhood, identity and autonomy. International law spoke up on behalf of every human being, going beyond any philosophical debate. It is reasonable to assume that law protects to a higher standard, to make sure no human being is left out: this is nowadays also called a right to citizenship. Everyone has a right to have rights.

However, law seems speechless when it comes to a fading identity. This could be a magnificent sign of respect or just a sign that law is taken aback by dementia. The turn is taken when it comes to agency. Since much of law revolves around agency, ascertaining the competence to decide and legal capacity become key issues to the recognition of human dignity. It all comes down to ascertaining, because if a person is not fully competent to make choices, dignity also means adequate protection, support and care.

The legal take of international law describes a careful attempt to address the manifold dilemmas brought by dementia. There is an equalizing and non-discriminatory approach to grant personhood: every human being, without regard to their cognitive abilities, has equal right and dignity. It is a beautiful point of departure. From then on, dignity relies on recognizing to the fullest extent possible the right to self-determination and personal autonomy, providing with means to bypass the finitude, whether by anticipating directives or by a shared decision-making process.

2 Clinical Reflections on Personhood, Identity and Autonomy

Mathieu Vandenbulcke and Rose-Marie Dröes
The approaches of philosophers and clinicians are complementary. Philosophers develop theoretical concepts and apply them to the real world, whereas clinicians think empirically and seek concepts that make sense of clinical phenomena. In doing so, clinicians probably prioritize interpretations that they consider beneficial for their patients. Together, these approaches may reveal the polysemic nature of concepts such as self, identity and personhood.

As Bart Pattyn and Peter Hacker point out, the concept 'self' is often used to refer to the nature of a person. In the dementia field, the comparison is often made between the 'now' self and the 'then' self of yesteryear. This is reflected in statements such as 'he is no longer himself' or 'he is still himself despite the loss of memory'. The philosophical approach clarifies that someone's self by definition coincides with the subject. In that sense, a statement such as 'he is no longer himself' represents a *contradictio in terminis*, as a person cannot 'not be' what that person coincides with. A positive reading of this inconsistency is that someone with dementia 'is' always himself. However, being himself at any stage of dementia does not mean that the nature of that person, or his personality, remains unchanged, as might be erroneously suggested by an objectified use of 'the self' as an entity that belongs to a person and could remain undamaged by the dementia process. On the other hand, the radical differentiation between the formerly intact 'then' self and the current 'now' self with dementia is a misrepresentation as well and continuities are often manifest. This is nicely articulated by a carer who reflected on his father's Alzheimer's disease. 'In the two years that followed the loss of his supposed "self", I can't stop finding it' [33]. To respect and to enhance the residual self-consciousness as much as possible may even be one of the most important points of attention in the intercourse with people with dementia. Of course, as noted, this is not to deny that crucial changes occur during the dementia process. But even then, one could question whether this should be seen as a complete loss of personal identity. Lesser argues that identity is not

momentary and that personal identity should include 'boundedness' or connections to both the past and the future [34]. According to this reasoning, a person's identity can and should be preserved by others. The psychodynamic interactive adaptation-coping model [35, 36] describes how in people with dementia a revision of their identity and self image (i.e. taking into account their disabilities therein) is necessary to find a new equilibrium, as is the case with chronic diseases in general [37], to experience continuity between past, present and future, and to prevent an identity crisis and withdrawal in the past focussing only on the former self (see also [38,39]). Supporting people in the process of adjustment and preserving identity and positive self image is one of the goals of psychosocial care based on this theoretical model.

Similarly to consequences of objectification of the self, Pattyn and Hacker point out that the objectification of the concepts body and mind may suggest that they are separate entities rather than descriptions of the same reality. They remind us that dualistic assumptions are still visible today and continue to influence our thinking. Indeed, a striking example is a heated discussion on whether dementia should be classified as a mental disorder or a disease of the central nervous system in the international classification of diseases (ICD) [40]. Another way of thinking is that the brain equates the mind, called physicalism. An example given by Pattyn and Hacker is that neurologists sometimes suggest that they can explain human behaviour based on brain activity. Although this might be an over-interpretation – most neurologists describe associations between cerebral processes and mental experiences without claiming that they are mutually exclusive or claiming causality in one direction or another – it is indeed important to pay attention to the complementarity of physiological and psychological explanations of phenomena in the counselling of people with dementia. The fact that someone repeats himself is related to atrophy of the brain structures that are important for memory, but does not exclude other additional reasons. Brain atrophy does not explain why someone keeps asking about her mother's engagement ring. The fact that someone with Alzheimer's lives in the past is explained by Ribot's law, which states that the loss of autobiographical information decreases as one returns in time, but that does not explain why person x feels secure while believing to be with his mother and person y is frightened by being convinced that his father is present. As pointed out by Pattyn and Hacker, understanding the pathological brain process does not lead to an understanding of the person's world of experience.

Along the same line of reasoning, Pattyn and Hacker highlight that cognition and emotion have an intrinsic relationship, rather than being separate entities. They argue that 'we do not think without feeling the relevance of what we are thinking, and our emotions would be poorly differentiated without our conceptions'. Although one can doubt if we always feel the relevance of what we are thinking, also, for example, when we are daydreaming or let our thoughts run wild, this interconnectedness and the consequences of disconnection become apparent in certain forms of dementia. For instance, persons with frontotemporal dementia lack the kind of feelings, such as shame or guilt, normally associated with thinking in certain contexts, leading to unexpected and inappropriate behaviour. Also, despite often normal physiological responses, persons with frontotemporal dementia are not able anymore to label or conceptualize their emotions. Conversely, in early to moderate AD, there is no significant change in the ability to report emotions or to discriminate between emotions despite the cognitive impairment, although the loss of memories can of course lead to people also forgetting the emotional experiences they had. But it is certainly true that remaining memories and thoughts do elicit associated emotions and that situations in which one had strong emotions are better memorized and recalled. On the other hand, although cognition and emotions are intrinsically linked in many ways, some core aspects of emotions are spared compared to cognitive processes in the majority of dementias. This has to do with the neurodegeneration affecting disproportionately the cerebral cortex involved mainly in cognitive processes with relative sparing of subcortical areas where most aspects of emotions are processed. Denying this difference in impairment of cognition and emotion implies denying the architecture of our mental apparatus, leading to unjustified sobering messages to persons with dementia who find comfort in retaining emotional life.

Identity is determined by several factors and can be described in many ways. Pattyn and Hacker focus on the status someone acquires in relation to others, referred to as social identity, which is relevant in the context of dementia, not because relationship is all that is left to persons with dementia, but because this is an essential characteristic of all our lives. They argue that a person's social identity is based on assumptions, beliefs and judgements that we share in the course of interactions. As a common understanding of the interaction is compromised by dementia, the social identity is increasingly at risk when the dementia progresses. To mitigate the impact on status, the social environment has the tendency to support and protect the person with dementia during interactions, as noted by the authors. However, as Pattyn and Hacker point out, our status is dependent on the (support, communication and empathic skills of the) social environment we belong to and is difficult to control. An important consequence in our experience is that many persons with dementia withdraw from social life and interactions in order to preserve their social status. Also, people delay or conceal a diagnosis of dementia because of fear being stigmatized. 'It's a strange life when you "come out" – people get embarrassed, lower their voices and get lost for words', wrote the novelist Terry Pratchett after he was diagnosed [41]. Langdon et al. interviewed persons with early-stage dementia and cited one of them: 'I didn't tell anybody, because they will treat me differently' [42]. So the paradox is that sharing would make the person a lesser person. This has little to do with the person with dementia himself or herself, but with the malignancy of the social environment as Thomas Kitwood puts it, devaluating the person with his varied social roles to a person with only one role – that is, being a patient. Research by Lion et al. [43] suggests that there are differences in experienced stigma between countries and cultures and that it is associated with social support and quality of life. Dependent on the stage of dementia and personality, the initiative to withdraw is taken by the person with dementia himself ('I withdraw because I don't feel involved in what they are talking about' [44]) or their families. In either way, the impact of such isolation on quality of life is usually high. From an empirical point of view, the idea that identity is dependent on a common understanding of interaction and on shared concepts, conventions and rules is interesting but doubtful at the same time. The lack of insight in how one is perceived by others in certain dementias would then be a consequence of lacking a common understanding rather than of functional disability.

Another interesting point the authors raise is the loss of emotional interest when people with dementia cannot participate any longer in shared engagement. Apathy, which is the behavioural correlate of loss of interest, is often regarded as a neuropsychiatric symptom resulting from dysfunction in brain circuits involved in cognition, motivation and reward, and less so from an interpersonal point of view which can be a starting point for therapy. It is indeed known that an overly demanding environment can lead to the person with dementia to withdraw into himself or herself, which is often typified as apathetic behaviour. Sometimes this behaviour also seems like a coping strategy to limit or prevent feelings of insufficiency and shame which one would experience when failing in activities [35]. On the other hand, apathy can also be a depressive reaction when coping fails.

Pattyn and Hacker draw our attention to a distinction between the use of the word 'person' in a general sense and a strict etymological interpretation of the concept 'person' in the context of dementia. According to the latter approach, to be a person, one needs to play a certain role in society and be accountable for one's actions. The sobering conclusion by Pattyn and Hacker for persons with advanced dementia is, then, that they cannot be considered persons anymore. This is of course socially inacceptable and the opposite of the intention of the person-centred approach of Kitwood, which is about treating any human being with dementia as a full person with the same value as any other person, despite cognitive impairment. It is also in contradiction with the Convention on the Rights of Persons with Disabilities, which states that persons with disabilities are full human persons and therefore entitled to the status of personhood before the law (see also Basset in this chapter). You may also wonder if it is true that a person with advanced dementia no longer plays a role in the lives of others, his spouse who cares for him daily, his children who love him and professionals who treat him with respect. Relatedly, the authors question the connection between autonomy and dignity, and point to the philosophical idea that respect for human beings is something

pre-reflective. They make a distinction between respect for human dignity and respect for a person in the narrow sense, which they make conditional on a mutual awareness of the interaction. Yet involvement of the person with dementia is often created by partners or caregivers based on advance care planning and/or by holding an imaginary consultation that takes into account the pre-dementia view of this person in an effort to continue to show respect to the person. This is also the idea behind continuing efforts to make shared decisions instead of substituted decisions in more advanced stages of dementia.

More generally, it is clear that the clarification of concepts and arguments has heuristic value for clinicians and can be useful for clinical practice. However, a narrow approach to concept clarification, such as an approach that is purely based on the etymological origin of concepts, can also lead to unfortunate adjustment of attitudes towards persons with dementia.

References

1. Kitwood T. *Dementia Reconsidered: The Person Comes First*. Buckingham, Open University Press, 1997.

2. Hagberg B. The dementias in a psychodynamic perspective. In Miesen B, Jones G, eds. *Care-Giving in Dementia: Research and Applications*. London/New York: Routledge, 1997; 2.14: 14–35.

3. Miesen B. Alzheimer's disease, the phenomenon of parent fixation and Bowlby's attachment theory. *International Journal of Geriatric Psychiatry* 1993; 8(2): 147–53.

4. Convention on the Rights of Persons with Disabilities and Optional Protocol, Article 3, a.

5. Post SG. *The Moral Challenge of Alzheimer's Disease*. Baltimore, Johns Hopkins University Press, 1995.

6. Hacker PMS. *Human Nature: The Categorical Framework*. Oxford, Blackwell, 2007.

7. Cottingham J. Cartesian trialism (repr.). In his *Cartesian Reflections*. Oxford, Oxford University Press, 2008.

8. Goffman E. *The Presentation of Self in Everyday Life*. New York, Doubleday, 1959; *Stigma: Notes on the Management of Spoiled Identity*. Saddle River, NJ, Upper Prentice-Hall, 1963.

9. Goffman E. *Frame Analysis: An Essay on the Organization of Experience*. New York, Harper & Row, 1974.

10. Winnicott DW. *Playing and Reality*. London, Tavistock, 1971.

11. Trendelenburg A. A contribution to the history of the word person. *The Monist* 1910; **20**: 336–63.

12. Kant I. *The Metaphysics of Morals*, ed. M. Gregor. Cambridge, Cambridge University Press, 2017.

13. Strawson P. Freedom and resentment. *Proceedings of the British Academy* 1962; **48**: 1–25.

14. Singer P. *Animal Rights*. New York, HarperCollins, 1975.

15. Brooker D. What is person centred-care in dementia? *Reviews in Clinical Gerontology* 2004; **13**: 215–22.

16. Mitchell G, Agnelli J. Person-centred care for people with dementia: Kitwood reconsidered. *Nursing Standard* 2015; **30**(7): 46–50.

17. Universal Declaration of Human Rights, UN, Paris 10 December 1948, General Assembly, Resolution 217 A.

18. Glendon MA. *A World Made New: Eleanor Roosevelt and the Universal Declaration of Human Rights*. New York, Random House, 2001; Preface.

19. Universal Declaration of Human Rights, UN, Article 16, International Covenant on Civil and Political Rights, adopted 16 December 1966, General Assembly Resolution 2200 A.

20. Langlois AJ. Human rights universalism. In Hayden P, ed. *The Ashgate Research Companion to Ethics and International Relations*. London and New York, Routledge, 2019, Chapter 12, p. 201.

21. Quinn G, Arstein-Kerslake A. Restoring the 'human' in 'human rights': Personhood and doctrinal innovation in the UN disability convention. In Gearty C, Douzinas C, eds. *The Cambridge Companion to Human Rights Law*. Cambridge Companions to Law. Cambridge, Cambridge University Press, 2012; 36–55.

22. Arstein-Kerslake A. *Restoring Voice to People with Cognitive Disabilities*. Cambridge, Cambridge University Press, 2017; 23.

23. Van Bueren G. *The International Law on the Rights of the Child*. Leiden, Martinus Nijhoff, 1998; 118.

24. Marshall J. *Human Rights Law and Personal Identity*. Abingdon and New York, Routledge, 2014.

25. Ziegler K., *Human Rights and Private Law: Privacy As Autonomy*. London, Bloomsbury, 2007; 38.

26. IACtHR. *Cuadernillo de Jurisprudencia de la Corte Interamericana de Derechos Humanos*, p. 31.

27. IACtHR. Case 'Instituto de Reeducación del Menor' Vs. Paraguay. Excepciones Preliminares, Fondo, Reparaciones y Costas. 2 September 2004. Serie C No. 112, par. 147.

28. Herring J. *Law and the Relational Self*. Cambridge, Cambridge University Press, 2019.

29. Lornellino P. *Community Autonomy and Informed Consent*. Cambridge, Cambridge Scholars, 2015.

30. Herring J. *Relation Autonomy and Family Law*. Heidelberg, New York, Dordrecht and London, Springer, 2014.

31. Nedelsky J. *Law's Relations: A Relational Theory of Self, Autonomy and the Law*. Oxford, Oxford University Press, 2011.

32. Mackenzie C, Stoljar N. *Relational Autonomy: Feminist Perspectives on Autonomy, Agency and the Social Self*. Oxford, Oxford University Press, 2000.

33. Aquilina C, Hughes JC. The return of the living dead: Agency lost and found? In Hughes JC, Louw SJ, Sabat SR, eds. *Dementia: Mind, Meaning and the Person*. New York, Oxford University Press, 2006; 143–61.

34. Lesser AH. Dementia and personal identity. In Hughes JC, Louw SJ, Sabat SR, eds. *Dementia: Mind, Meaning and the Person*. New York, Oxford University Press, 2006; 55–61.

35. Dröes RM. In Beweging; over psychosociale hulpverlening aan demente ouderen. Academic thesis. Vrije Universiteit Amsterdam, Intro, Nijkerk, 1991.

36. Dröes RM, Van Mierlo LD, Meiland FJM, Van der Roest HG. Memory problems in dementia: Adaptation and coping strategies, and psychosocial treatments. *Expert Reviews Neurotherapeutics* 2011; **11**(12): 1769–82.

37. Samson A, Siam H. Adapting to major chronic illness: A proposal for a comprehensive task-model approach. *Patient Educ Couns.* 2008 Mar; **70**(3): 426–9. doi: 10.1016/j.pec.2007.10.018. Epub. 2007 Dec. 21. PMID: 18096353

38. Van der Wulp JC. Verstoring en verwerking in verpleeghuizen; belevingswereld en conflicten van hen die hun verdere leven in een verpleeghuis doorbrengen. Academic thesis. Universiteit Utrecht, Intro, Nijkerk, 1986.

39. Moos RH, Tsu VD. The crisis of physical illness: An overview. In Moos RH, ed. *Coping with Physical Illness: Current Topics in Mental Health*. Boston, Springer, 1977. https://doi.org/10.1007/978-1-4684-2256-6_1

40. Gaebel W, Jessen F, Kanba S. Neurocognitive disorders in ICD-11: The debate and its outcome. *World Psychiatry* 2018 Jun; **17**(2): 229–30.

41. Werner P. Stigma and Alzheimer's disease: A systematic review of evidence, theory, and methods. In Corrigan PW, ed. *The Stigma of Disease and Disability: Understanding Causes and Overcoming Injustices*. Washington, DC, American Psychological Association, 2014; 223–44.

42. Langdon SA, Eagle A, Warner J. Making sense of dementia in the social world: A qualitative study. *Social Science & Medicine* 2007; **64**(4): 989–1000.

43. Lion KM, Szcześniak D, Bulińska K, Evans SB, Evans SC, Saibene FL, . . . Rymaszewska J. Do people with dementia and mild cognitive impairments experience stigma? A cross-cultural investigation between Italy, Poland and the UK. *Aging & Mental Health* 2020; **24**: 6947–55. doi: 10.1080/13607863.2019.1577799

44. Holst G, Hallberg IR. Exploring the meaning of everyday life for those suffering from dementia. *American Journal of Alzheimer's Disease and Other Dementias* 2003; 18(6): 359–65.

The Tongues
George Oppen

of appearance
speak in the unchosen
journey immense
journey there is loss in denying
that force the moments the years
even of death lost
in denying
that force   the words
out of that whirlwind his
and not his strange
words surround him

Living Meaningfully with Dementia

Laura Dewitte, Gørill Haugan, Mathieu Vandenbulcke
and Jessie Dezutter

1 Meaning in Life and Its Benefits

1.1 What Is the Psychological Experience of Meaning in Life?

Since the early days of ancient Greek philosophy, through twentieth-century existentialism and phenomenology, up to the modern take of Monty Python, philosophical thinkers have been agonizing over the question of whether human life on earth has an ultimate meaning, and what that meaning could possibly be. More recently, the issue of meaning has become a topic of keen interest in mainstream psychology. Since the second half of the twentieth century, psychologists have started to acknowledge the importance of experiencing one's own life as meaningful, regardless of the answer to the philosophical question of the meaning of life in general. In contrast to the latter, the subjective experience of meaning – called meaning in life – can be studied empirically from a psychological perspective.

Current psychological research on meaning in life mostly relates to the fields of existential and positive psychology. This contemporary work finds important foundations in the work of existential-humanistic psychotherapists and psychologists such as Frankl [1, 2], Maddi [3], Maslow [4] and Yalom [5]. They proposed that searching for meaning in life is a fundamental quest for humans and that the failure to find meaning is a major source of mental ill being. Building on these foundational works, contemporary existential psychologists still approach meaning in life largely from the perspective that finding meaning in a chaotic world, and in difficult times and adversity, is one of the major challenges or 'existential givens' that humans face during their life [6, 7]. Since the new millennium, these psychologists have been joined in their interest for the concept of meaning by

researchers from the field of positive psychology. In contrast to the existential perspective, this field focusses on the brighter side of life, on human potential, happiness, strengths and flourishing [8]. Accordingly, positive psychologists have investigated meaning in life mostly as a trait-like tendency to experience meaning in everyday life – a tendency believed to be relatively stable, albeit more variable than a personality characteristic, and related to positive psychological functioning.

While dissecting the psychological experience of meaning has proved not so straightforward, meaning researchers have made important advancements in the past decennia. Two broad focusses can be discerned: a first line of research has focussed on what meaning is derived from, what the most common *sources* of meaning are [9, 10]. Sources of meaning are personally relevant life domains, activities or internal states that make life meaningful and therefore guide people's action [11–14]. While there is of course considerable individual variation in the sources that contribute to life's meaningfulness, the most central sources for most people can be captured under a number of broad overarching categories such as work, health, creativity, personal growth, leisure, religion and spirituality. However, as demonstrated in various populations, interpersonal relationships with family and friends represent the most important source of meaning in life for most people [9, 11, 15–19].

A second line of research has focussed on what meaning in life is; that is which *components* are included or involved in perceived meaning. Earlier works have treated meaning and purpose largely as synonymous whereas researchers have now come a long way in more precisely disentangling the different components of meaning. An important foundation for the current understanding of meaning in life was provided by Reker and

Wong [20], who suggested that meaning could be divided into a cognitive, motivational and emotional component. Since then, several variations and extensions have been presented [e.g. 21–24]. Recently, a tripartite conceptualization of meaning in life is gaining momentum. In this view, experiencing meaning in life means having (a) a sense of being directed by valued life aims (i.e. purpose in life), (b) a sense that life matters and is worth living (i.e. significance) and (c) a sense that life is coherent and comprehensible (i.e. coherence) [25–27]. Purpose in life then reflects the motivational component and coherence the cognitive component of meaning. Significance, on the other hand, is regarded as an evaluative and not emotional component, so therein lies the biggest difference with the view proposed by Reker and Wong [20]. Importantly, these three components are not entirely separate but closely interconnected and blending into one another.

In addition to the work on sources and components, other approaches have framed the experience of meaning more broadly. A now widely acknowledged distinction, for example, is between the *presence* of meaning in life and the *search* for meaning in life [28]. The term 'presence of meaning' encompasses whether individuals perceive their lives as significant, purposeful and coherent, and is often regarded as a highly desired psychological *quality* ('my life is meaningful') [29]. The term 'search for meaning', on the other hand, refers to people's efforts to establish or increase their understanding of the meaning and purpose of their lives: it refers to the *process* of how individuals develop their sense of meaning in life ('how can I make my life more meaningful?') [29, 30].

Another stream of literature has focussed on *meaning-making processes* in the face of threats to meaning such as stressful or traumatic situations [31, 32]. An important meaning-making model distinguishes global meaning from situational meaning [31]. The former represents the complex system of global beliefs and goals that an individual holds, and the latter represents the meaning that this individual encounters in specific situations. When these situational experiences and evaluations are not in line with the global meaning system, meaning-making processes are engaged in an attempt to solve the discrepancy and alleviate distress [31, 33].

1.2 The Many Benefits of Experiencing Life As Meaningful

Over the past decades, evidence for the benevolent role of experiencing meaning in life for optimal human functioning is accumulating. Across different study designs, research shows clear and consistent associations between experiencing one's life as meaningful and a wide range of outcomes of physical health, psychological distress and psychological well-being. With regard to physical health, meaning has been associated with better outcomes in both objective measures of health (e.g. recovery from surgery, survival in chronic diseases, reduced risk of stroke, mortality) and subjective measures of health (e.g. self-reported health, disability, pain, physical symptoms) [34–37]. Up to now, research on explaining mechanisms has been more limited, though. Preliminary findings suggest that meaning in life may work its benefits on health through the promotion of better health behaviour (e.g. more exercise, sleep, healthier diet, less smoking and drinking), better stress-response system functioning and stress-buffering and better immune system functioning [35, 38, 39]. Concerning psychological functioning (both psychological distress and well-being, which are regarded as related but separate dimensions rather than the opposite poles of the same dimension), the presence of meaning in life relates consistently and positively with outcomes of well-being and negatively with outcomes of psychological distress. For example, higher levels of meaning are associated with positive affect and emotions, global happiness, psychological adjustment, life satisfaction, quality of life and self-esteem [40]. One of the most recurring and persistent findings is that meaning in life is negatively related to depressive symptoms and depression [40].

Although most research linking meaning in life and psychological functioning has been cross-sectional, there is a modest increase in studies examining meaning in life over time. Psychological views advance meaning in life as a predictor rather than a consequence of well-being [e.g. 20, 39]. In line, longitudinal studies suggest that higher meaning predicts less depressive symptoms over time, but depressive symptoms do not predict lower meaning [41–43]. These findings were replicated in a sample of chronic pain patients where meaning also positively predicted life satisfaction over time [44], as well in a sample of African-Americans, where it also predicted higher positive affect over time [42].

Furthermore, within the literature focussing on meaning-making processes, maintaining a sense of meaning in life has been shown to be of particular importance in adapting to changing circumstances and dealing with challenges and stressors in life, such as bereavement, chronic illness or psychological trauma [33, 45–47]. In this regard, meaning might be an especially valuable resource in old age and has indeed been forwarded as an important aspect of ageing well [48].

1.3 Meaning in Life As a Strength and Resource for Older Adults without Dementia

Older adults often have to deal with losses associated with ageing, such as functional disability, health problems, loss of friends and family members, retirement and changing roles in society, making late life a challenging life stage for many. At the same time, many older adults seem to cope surprisingly well and show high levels of life satisfaction [49]. Similarly, research has shown that older adults even report *higher* levels of meaning in life than younger adults [50]. However, some findings suggest this might depend on the specific component of meaning that is being assessed and the specific measure that is used. For example, the component of purpose in life has been found to decrease slightly in older adults, although still less than might be expected when considering the challenges of old age [51, 52]. This is in line with some theoretical ideas framing late life as a stage where older adults can adapt to their circumstances, come to terms with their lives lived and cultivate a more contemplative, deepened and mature sense of meaning in life [53–57]. Empirical work shows that this sense of meaning remains highly important in this population, contributing to an impressive range of physical and psychological outcomes of late life well-being, both cross-sectionally [51, 58, 59] and over time [60–62]. Perhaps particularly relevant for older adults, increasing evidence suggests that greater meaning in life, specifically sense of purpose, may

be protective against cognitive decline in older adults without a cognitive disorder [63–66]. It is therefore reassuring that many older adults can retain a strong sense of meaning despite life challenges.

A population that is of particular interest is the large group of older adults living in nursing homes. On one hand, older adults in nursing homes are often confronted with a multitude of additional changes and losses in life [48]. Compared to their counterparts in the community, they have shown more vulnerability to depressive symptoms, depression and suicidal behaviour [67, 68], physical health problems, worse psychological well-being and lower levels of meaning in life [62, 69]. Importantly, this does not mean that moving to a nursing home *causes* these issues. Older adults with more severe physical and mental health problems are also more likely to move to a nursing home to receive professional care. However, it does indicate that this population and their caregivers could be in need of additional support in dealing with these issues. While in general levels of meaning in life may be lower in nursing homes, retaining higher levels of meaning might be especially protective in this context. Studies have shown that nursing home residents who experience higher meaning in life reported fewer physical and emotional symptoms such as insomnia, nausea and depressive symptoms [70, 71] and higher emotional and functional well-being [37, 72]. Another study even showed that the association between meaning in life and psychological well-being was stronger for nursing home residents than for community-dwelling older adults [69], which emphasizes the importance of meaning for the potentially vulnerable population of older adults in nursing homes.

Unfortunately, relatively few studies on meaning or related topics focus specifically on a nursing home setting. Even more problematic perhaps, residents with cognitive difficulties or dementia are often excluded at the outset, with many inclusion criteria mentioning the 'cognitively intact' [62]. This is not only problematic from a moral perspective, but it also leaves a very pertinent question unanswered: how is meaning in life experienced by older adults with dementia, and is it still important?

2 Meaning in Life in Dementia: Preserved, Challenged, or Lost?

2.1 The Role of Cognitive Functioning in Experiencing Meaning in Life

Examining the conceptualization of meaning in life more closely reveals a strong emphasis on cognitive aspects of meaning. Steger [40] refers to a cognitive component of meaning in life, which includes holding 'a strong set of related memories that coalesce into a continuous narrative, defensible theories about how the world works' (p. 2). Reker and Wong [20, 48] appoint the cognitive component as the cornerstone of their three-component model, directly influencing the other two components. Additionally, the Meaning Maintenance Model – a prominent meaning-making model – is described in very cognitive terms, proposing that making meaning requires detecting and repairing incongruences between stimuli in the environment and internal working models of how the world works [32]. Baumeister, Vohs et al. [73], in their turn, state that 'happiness is about the present whereas meaning is about linking events across time, thus integrating past, present, and future' (p. 509). Krause [74] states that 'developing a sense of meaning is hard work that entails a number of complex cognitive functions. For example, meaning making requires complex reasoning skills, keen insight, and the capacity to be persistent. In order to perform these cognitive functions, a person must exercise a reasonable amount of focus, concentration, and control over their thought processes' (pp. 67–8).

In sum, many leading scholars seem to agree that experiencing meaning in life involves complex cognitive skills, such as integrating past, present and future, reflecting on and making abstraction of the self and the world, and planning and coordinating complex sequences of behaviours and activities. Consequently, some scholars suggest that when confronted with cognitive decline, an individual's ability to generate and sustain a sense of meaning in life might be compromised [74–76]. Empirical investigations of this assumption are relatively scarce. Some neuroimaging evidence showed that higher functional connectivity in the medial temporal lobe of the brain was related to higher meaning in life scores [77]

and a series of experiments showed that inviting people to mentally simulate events in the past/ future enhanced meaning in life ratings; for simulations of high subjective quality, meaning was rated even stronger [77, 78]. In discussing their findings, Vess, Hoeldtke et al. [78] suggest that older adults who experience deficits in episodic memory and/or future thought may therefore be vulnerable to declines in meaning in life. Another study on sense of purpose showed that lower scores on working memory, perceptual speed and semantic memory predicted declines in purpose over time [75]. In contrast, Takkinen and Ruoppila [79] found no evidence for higher levels of meaning in a group of older adults with higher cognitive abilities as compared to a group with lower cognitive abilities. These mixed findings trigger a pertinent question: are people with dementia destined to lose meaning in life because of their decreasing cognitive capacities?

2.2 Meaning under Pressure in Dementia

A number of studies indirectly suggest that older adults with dementia may indeed experience challenges in finding or maintaining meaning. Reflecting on and understanding who you are, what the world is like and how you fit in it is believed to be a central part of the experience of meaning [13]. However, even in the early stages of Alzheimer's disease, older adults have shown reduced ability to reflect on the behaviours, thoughts and feelings of self and others, making it more difficult to understand both the social and internal worlds [80]. Similarly, a qualitative interview study on everyday life in dementia identified difficulties in staying in touch with others, staying in touch with oneself and staying engaged in significant activities and interests; three sub-themes demonstrating how dementia affected important foundations of the participants' lives [81]. A small questionnaire study showed that older adults with more severe dementia reported weaker personal identity and reduced membership in social groups [82].

Having such fundamental parts of your life and sense of self affected will likely put a strain on the meaningfulness experienced in your life. One of the earliest works on the subjective experience of people with dementia described how people with dementia 'can experience a profound, existential sense of emptiness and absence which is related to the actual or anticipated damage to their sense of self' [83]. A more recent qualitative study described the 'fragmented existence' of older adults living alone with dementia, evidenced by a loss of coherence and meaning: 'Things that were once important in life, such as hobbies, clubs and travel, appear to lose meaning. This is followed by feelings of loneliness and forgetfulness that seem to cloud the meaning of life' [84]. There may be particular challenges involved in receiving a dementia diagnosis at a younger age [85]. Although research focussing specifically on meaning in life in this population is sorely lacking, some studies on the general experiences of adults living with young- or early-onset dementia have described how the diagnosis can be experienced as particularly threatening in this population, as it is perceived as premature and 'out of time' [86]. In early old age, such an unexpected dementia diagnosis is likely to more strongly interfere with long-term goals and aspirations for the future. In this way, early-onset dementia may be associated with an amplified sense of meaninglessness through greater perceived loss of social roles, relationships and meaningful activities [86, 87]. Taken together, these studies paint a poignant picture of how dementia can have the power to erode meaning in the lives of people struggling to cope with their condition.

2.3 Meaning Retained in Dementia

Importantly, other works have demonstrated great resilience in the ability to experience meaning in dementia. Some qualitative studies focussing on understanding life with dementia or coping with the disease concluded that meaning was a central theme in the narratives of participants. These accounts describe how older adults with dementia retain a continued sense of self and engagement with life, revealing a balance between finding meaning by staying engaged in important and valued activities on one hand, and finding new meaning by adapting to challenges on the other [88–95]. A recent in-depth phenomenological study from our lab zoomed in specifically on the experience of meaning in life from the insider perspective of older adults living with Alzheimer's disease [96]. We found that 'continuing to participate in the dance of life as oneself' reflected the essence of meaning in life for older adults with

Alzheimer's disease. Four intertwined constituents illuminated this essence further: (1) feeling connected and involved, (2) continuing everyday life as oneself, (3) calmly surrendering and letting go and (4) desiring freedom, growth and invigoration. Participants' stories highlighted how their meaning in life was partly influenced by dementia, but far from completely determined by it. Participants described challenges and worries of losing the ability to participate in the dance of life, but the majority expressed at least as much resilience and optimism about the meaningfulness of their lives.

Recent studies have now started to shed light on the sources that contribute to the sense of meaningfulness for people with dementia. Overall, meaning in life for people with dementia seems fuelled by largely the same sources as for other populations. When responding to an open-ended question on meaning, the most frequently mentioned sources of meaning were family, interpersonal relationships, work and health [97]. Some additional themes also emerged that gained more significance, such as the value of home and of being cared for. Another interesting trend could be noticed in this study concerning the component of purpose in life: our participants spoke relatively little of future-oriented purpose (as purpose is mostly conceptualized within meaning literature), but more often mentioned a sense of fulfilled purpose, which nonetheless still gave important meaning to the present. This finding can explain why certain themes pertaining to the past, such as work, were still highly relevant for participants' meaning in life, and it highlights the need to understand meaning and its components within the developmental context of specific age groups [97].

In a closed-ended questionnaire study, health, family and society/community were identified as the three most meaningful sources, followed by interpersonal relationships, work and spirituality/religion [98]. Interestingly, a path analysis revealed that two sources significantly predicted overall meaning in life scores: society/community and personal growth. This finding suggests that it remains important to invest in the personal development of people with dementia and to combat the idea that growth becomes irrelevant for this population. This also resonates with the findings of our qualitative phenomenological study, in which the desire for free exploration and growth emerged as one of the core constituents of the experience of meaning [96]. The centrality of family and close relationships for meaning aligns well with previous qualitative works describing how these contribute to a sense of belonging, value, contribution and reciprocal support [90, 91, 99].

Additional support for the notion that a loss of cognitive abilities does not necessarily mean a loss of meaning comes from a recent longitudinal quantitative study from our lab. In three measurement waves spanning two years, we found no compelling evidence that the experience of meaning in life as reported by older adults with Alzheimer's disease was significantly related to their cognitive abilities or cognitive decline. Meaning in life was measured using the Presence of Meaning subscale (short form) of the Meaning in Life Questionnaire [100], a widely used validated scale which allows participants to give their own interpretation of how they understand the term 'meaning', through general items such as 'I have a clear sense of what makes my life meaningful.' Meaning-in-life scores were not related to relative between-person changes in cognitive functioning as investigated in cross-lagged analyses, and not related to individual change (i.e. slope) in cognitive functioning over time as investigated in latent growth curve analyses [101]. This was the case for a measure assessing general cognitive status, as well as for measures of specific cognitive functions (with the exception of one positive association between first-wave working memory scores and second-wave meaning in life). While lack of evidence for an effect does not equal evidence for the lack of an effect and thus further work is needed on this front, these findings suggest, in line with the qualitative descriptions, that the decreasing cognitive capacities of people with dementia do not doom them to a loss of meaning, and that retaining a sense of meaning with dementia remains possible.

2.4 The Importance of Meaning in Life for People with Dementia

Our recent findings not only demonstrate that meaning can be maintained despite cognitive decline in dementia; we also found preliminary evidence that the experience of meaning in life remains important for the psychological functioning of older adults living with dementia.

Cross-sectional analyses of the first measurement occasion of our longitudinal quantitative study showed that participants who more strongly endorsed that they experienced meaning in life also had significantly higher scores of life satisfaction and reported significantly fewer depressive symptoms [102]. Interestingly, exploratory analyses revealed an interaction between meaning in life and cognitive status in predicting depressive symptoms and life satisfaction. More specifically, the relationship between meaning and both life satisfaction and depressive symptoms was stronger for residents with lower cognitive abilities. While these exploratory findings should be interpreted with caution, they may indicate that experiencing life as meaningful becomes not less but *more* important for psychological health when living with dementia. This finding is in line with the theoretical view of meaning in life as a psychological resource for facing challenges and losses in life [33, 46, 103].

Even more convincing perhaps, longitudinal cross-lagged analyses of our three-wave data revealed that older adults with Alzheimer's disease who reported higher meaning in life at one point in time scored significantly lower on depressive symptoms one year later [101]. In the opposite direction, depressive symptoms did not predict meaning in life over time. In contrast, meaning in life did not directly predict later life satisfaction over and above the predictive effect of depressive symptoms on life satisfaction, but this model did show an indirect effect of meaning in life scores on life satisfaction through lower depressive symptoms. In sum, this study provided an important first indication for the idea that meaning in life can not only be retained for people with dementia, but is an important predictor of healthy psychological functioning in this population as well.

These findings lend first quantitative support to the idea that meaning in life is a relevant predictor of healthy psychological functioning of people with dementia. This idea was already advanced by Dröes and colleagues [104] 15 years ago when they established in an exploratory qualitative study that people with dementia identify being useful and having meaning in life as a central part of their quality of life. More recently, Van Vliet and colleagues performed focus groups with participants with young-onset dementia and found that retaining a sense of usefulness and engagement was highly important to participants and connected to a sense of accomplishment and enjoyment [105].

Taken together, empirical studies on meaning in life for people with dementia are still scarce, but the modest increase noticeable in recent years can be framed within a broader tendency: while a deficit-oriented framework focussing mainly on symptom control dominated the literature on dementia in the past, dementia researchers are now increasingly acknowledging the importance of attending to the well-being and psychological strengths and resources of people with dementia as a separate dimension of their functioning [106–109]. Positive psychological concepts such as flourishing, wisdom, humour, agency, resilience, growth, optimism, spirituality and meaning in the context of dementia are on a steady rise, as is research showing their importance for the well-being of people with dementia [110, 111].

3 Understanding Meaningfulness in Dementia: Beyond a Hypercognitive View

The foregoing discussion reveals an apparent contradiction between the cognitive declines that people with dementia experience and their retained sense of, or even drive for, meaning. Somehow, the common assumption that progressive cognitive decline equals a progressive loss of a meaningful life seems inadequate and in conflict with how people with dementia view their lives [92].

From a deficiency perspective, it could be argued that when people with dementia report experiencing their lives as very meaningful, this reflects denial and lack of awareness of losses and difficulties. However, such explanation denies the self-determination of people with dementia and the fact that they remain experts of their own experience. Thorgrimsen et al. [112] convincingly point out that 'whether a person has insight or not is typically based on what is defined as "reality" by another person with greater power or status than the person interviewed' and that 'the subjective world is not directly accessible in any individual, whether they have dementia or not' (p. 202). Furthermore, it has become a widely accepted tenet in psychological research that sustaining a certain level of positive illusions about oneself, the future and one's control over life is a normal aspect of human functioning in general, which

can be beneficial for well-being [113, 114]. Such positive illusions should not be seen as outright false beliefs, but rather as positive interpretations of a situation which could perhaps be more readily interpreted as negative [113]. Of particular interest, such illusions have been suggested to be adaptive in finding meaning in adversity such as a severe illness [115, 116]. In this sense, positive illusions may be compared to what Frankl [2] called a tragic optimism or 'saying yes to life in spite of everything ... the human capacity to creatively turn life's negative aspect into something positive or constructive' (pp. 161–2). Therefore, from an existential perspective, it might be true that people with dementia are challenged more strongly to make positive sense of the things that are happening. However, the ability to do so should not be disregarded as invalid. On the contrary, it exemplifies the extraordinary ability of humans to find meaning in any situation.

From a capacity perspective, the predominant conceptualizations of meaning may simply be too narrow to capture the meaning experience of people with dementia. Post [117, 118] has warned against the hypercognitive preoccupation of our society that leads to a persistent bias against people with dementia, a 'hypercognitive snobbery' with potentially dangerous consequences: 'If we pass by the person with dementia just once and reach superficial conclusions, we fail morally' [118]. He suggests that with advancing cognitive difficulties, the person with dementia should be increasingly understood in terms of affect and relations [119]. In what follows, we argue that the affective and relational aspects of meaning provide an important perspective on how to understand, and thus support, meaning in life for people with dementia. Importantly, these aspects may become more prominent in dementia, but they are not assumed to be specific to the meaning experience of older adults with dementia alone. In some psychological views, affective and relational aspects of meaning have been proposed to constitute an essential part of meaning in life for people in general. However, these aspects have received relatively little consideration in dominant models of meaning in comparison with more cognitive aspects.

3.1 Meaning As Felt Sense

Some views of meaning have received less attention in mainstream meaning research but have been influential within psychotherapy research. The idea that higher-order cognitive processing may not be a prerequisite for experiencing meaning resonates well with Gendlin's [120, 121] conception of meaning as an implicit, holistic, bodily felt sense. Greenberg and Pascual-Leone [122], who describe the construction of personal meaning through different levels of processing, elaborate this idea further. In their view, an implicit bodily felt sense of meaning results from automatic, tacit processes which are primarily triggered by emotional experience: 'At any moment, a variety of affectively based schemes, formed from a person's inwired emotion response system and prior emotional experience, and cued by the situation, are activated in the internal field. ... The felt sense itself results from an automatic dynamic synthesis of affective and cognitive processes that contributes to the individual's internal complexity' (pp. 171–2). A next level of more conscious processing and reflection on meaning can then take place, but is not necessary for the felt sense of meaning to arise.

Recently, some scholars have tried to revive this view and integrate it into existing meaning theory. Hill et al. [123, 124] recently forwarded a felt sense of meaning as a fourth component to the tripartite view, defined as an intuitive experience, an immediate and affective perception of meaning in life. A similar argument can be recognized in the work of Heintzelman and King [125, 126], who proposed that a sense of meaning can arise not only from effortful reflective processes, but also from intuitive processes. These authors argue that meaning as an intuitive phenomenon, rooted in intuitive processes, has been neglected in psychological research in favour of meaning as an active construction. However sometimes, they propose, a feeling of meaning is just there, without any need to understand why or how it became: 'Acknowledging the potentially nonrational, intuitive nature of the feeling of meaning would allow for a greater understanding of the experiences that seem innately and even inescapably meaningful' (p. 476). They argue for a broadened understanding of meaning, acknowledging the feeling of meaning as a phenomenological state, a felt sense that can arise as an intuitive impression. Relatedly, in his work on experiential-existential psychotherapy, Vanhooren [127] distinguishes between a macro-, meso- and micro-dimension of meaning. The macro-dimension of meaning refers to an ultimate, transcendental, existential meaning; the meso-dimension to meaning in one's self- and world view and one's life story; and the micro-dimension to an experiential, felt sense in the here and now. These dimensions interact with one another but are also differentiated, which provides another way of understanding how a felt sense of meaning can remain after elements of the larger narrative are disrupted in dementia.

Of course, we do not deny the role of cognitive processes in the development of a felt sense of meaning. This felt sense will arise from a synthesis of both affective and cognitive processes, but it does not require higher-order cognitive abilities to be intact. Furthermore, these cognitive abilities should not be understood too strictly. According to Salthouse [128], completing cognitive tests such as the ones used to measure the cognitive status of people with dementia requires a level of novel processing and cognitive flexibility that is rarely needed in the daily life of older adults, where they can rely on their extensive experience for many of the real-life problems they encounter. The narrow focus of classical cognitive tests does not capture elements of a broader view of cognitive skills that older adults acquire throughout life, such as practical or pragmatic intelligence and wisdom [e.g. 129, 130].

The term 'embodied cognition' is also relevant in this regard. Several scholars have proposed the relevance of embodiment for maintaining a sense of self, coherence, continuity and meaning in dementia [131–133]. Matthews [133] explores this notion using the phenomenological philosophy of Merleau-Ponty, according to whom people can be understood as body-subjects: we are at the same time biological creatures and subjects that think, reflect and communicate. The reflecting subject cannot be seen separate from the body or vice versa; they are a unified whole. Accordingly, thoughts and reflections should not be regarded as some kind of inner world because they do not exist separate from the physical body but are essentially embodied. In fact, the body precedes the subject in some sense. We first exist as creatures in the world, pre-reflectively, and only then can begin to reflect on this existence. In some existential views, this reflection is not necessary for meaning to arise, as meaning is inherently tied to existence, rather than to reflection on existence [e.g. 2]. Bellin [134] notes: 'meaning through being is the part of meaning in life that transcends internal cognitive processes to the experience of mattering, not because of something external that a person did but rather because the meaning is tied to the person's very existence' (p. 226). During the course of life, we develop conscious thoughts, reflections, response patterns, expectations and habits, which in time become 'sedimented' or embedded into what Kontos and Martin [131] call 'habits of the body' (p. 291). In these unconscious, embodied ways of being and doing in the world, meaning can be retained for a long time after cognitive decline has set in.

Even in the very severe stages of dementia, these embodied meanings can be recognized – that is, if we stop to carefully observe, listen and appreciate. An inspiring example was provided by Kontos [135], who performed an eight-month ethnographic investigation of the lives of 13 residents in long-term care, in more severe stages of dementia. The author describes how the residents demonstrated attention to their physical self-presentation and to social conventions (e.g. saying 'thank you' and covering the mouth when coughing) and how they showed affection and caring among each other, enjoyment in singing and dancing and effective gestural, non-verbal communication. These examples show how residents were aware of and engaged with their surroundings, and interacted with each other and their surroundings in a meaningful way. These interactions were of course impacted by their cognitive decline, but had not become random or meaningless: there was an observable coherence, significance and purpose to their actions and engagements. The author discusses how the residents retain selfhood by an embodied interaction with the world: 'selfhood emanates from the body's power of natural expression, and manifests in the body's inherent ability to apprehend and convey meaning', an ability that is manifested 'below the threshold of cognition' [135].

3.2 Meaning As Socially Constructed within Relationships

Meaning is not only an embodied felt sense, it is also an extended experience: one that is in constant interaction with the external environment beyond our bodies. A crucial aspect of this immediate environment are the people surrounding us. In the introduction of their excellent and thought-provoking book *Dementia: Mind, Meaning, and the Person*, editors Hughes, Louw and Sabat [136] argue that people with dementia 'have to be understood in terms of relationships, not because this is all that is left to them, but because it is characteristic of all of our lives' (p. 17). Meaning in life is not merely a private inner experience; it is constructed in the social encounters with others. Constructing narratives of our life to render it coherent and meaningful is not a solitary act; our life narratives are co-written with other people. Meaning emerges in the interaction between the inner and outer world, in a 'shared space of meaning' (p. 19). This is, for example, visible in a qualitative study with repeated interviews and observations of five older adults (without dementia) at a primary care unit [137]. The findings here point out that creating togetherness and belonging is a crucial way to construct meaning. The authors describe how engagement in everyday activities with others creates an 'enacted togetherness' which is closely related to narrative meaning-making. Doing things together with others elicits feelings of safety and value and gives opportunities to create meaningful experiences in daily activities.

When cognitive difficulties start challenging 'standard' ways of communication, we are invited to support people with dementia in constructing meaning on their own terms. Robertson [94], for example, points to the rich and creative meaning-making processes that remain possible and pleads for an engagement 'with the varieties of ways that a person makes sense of their experiences, to avoid discounting those narratives that challenge the conventions of a "good" story' (p. 529). Similarly, Hydén and Örulv [138] draw attention to non-verbal aspects of storytelling and to the message that people with dementia are trying to convey in their stories: even if the higher-order temporal organization of a story is missing, 'the moral point of the lived life' (p. 212) is often present. That is, the person with dementia is communicating something important about the kind of person he or she used to be and how he or she wishes to be seen today. In this regard, we as conversation partners of people with dementia are also invited to become a more active, engaged participant; one that takes a collaborative stance and helps to proactively provide 'scaffolds' that support the shared meaning-making process [139]. In this way, meaning in life in dementia not only remains possible on the felt-sense micro-dimension, but can in interaction with others also be actively supported on the meso-dimension of a meaningful life narrative – which can in turn be expected to positively reinforce the felt sense of meaning [127].

The vital role of other people in constructing meaning in life also relates to the centrality of *connectedness* for meaning in life [e.g. 140, 141]. In this regard, attending to the quality of day-to-day interactions of people with dementia and those surrounding them is a priority for supporting meaning in life [96, 142]. For older adults with dementia living in a nursing home, the quality of interaction and connectedness with daily care staff is of central importance. Empirical studies have already demonstrated that these nurse–resident interactions are strong predictors of a sense of meaning in life for residents without dementia [143, 144].

Relationships with romantic partners are crucial to consider as well. According to McGovern [145], meaning-making processes in couples where one of the partners is living with dementia 'are not restricted to verbal exchanges, but rather can include interactions and sense-based perceptions. Accordingly, meaning-making processes can be determined, not only by cognitive ability, but also by embodied communication' (pp. 679–80). Tasks of daily care between intimate partners who are dealing with dementia together can be understood as a type of meaning-making process that stimulates a shared sense of purpose and commitment that can be beneficial for the well-being of both partners [145]. An intimate caregiving bond does not only contribute to a sense of meaning for the partner with dementia; many caregiving partners can derive a sense of meaning and purpose from their caregiving experiences, especially when they feel competent and motivated in their tasks, experience love and personal growth, and can embrace the changes coming along with the caregiver role [146, 147]. Research shows that those who can find meaning in caring for their partner with dementia also experience less caregiver burden and more caregiver gains [148, 149].

In sum, a social constructionism view of meaning invites us to reflect on how we interact with people with dementia and consider its consequences. In how we talk and behave, we have the power to support, build or reinvent the shared space of meaning, or to erode it. In this sense, it is our moral responsibility to assist people with dementia in continuing to write their story and to remind them of the continued meaningfulness of their lives, a responsibility that needs to be socially and societally supported [118]. This of course triggers the question of how we should go about this task.

4 Supporting Meaning in Life in Dementia

While interventions focussing on meaning and purpose have been employed regularly in the psychological counselling of people with a life-threatening illness such as cancer [e.g. 150], meaning-centred interventions for people with dementia are few and far between. However, some pioneering initiatives show promising results. For example, a number of recent studies (including two randomized controlled trials) have demonstrated the potential of meaning-focussed reminiscence and life story work for enhancing meaning and well-being in people with dementia [151–153]. These types of interventions may be especially useful in helping people with dementia review meaningful memories, discuss goals for the future and (re)connect to their overall life story. Related to the relevance of meaningful memories for supporting meaning, a recent experimental study suggests that inducing a sense of nostalgia may also enhance a sense of meaning in life in people with dementia [154].

A great challenge for both formal and informal caregivers of people with dementia, however, is how to support people with dementia in maintaining a programme of meaningful activities and experiences *on a daily basis*. While a considerable number of studies have focussed on meaningful activities for people with dementia, a recurring problem in this literature is the lack of a precise definition or position of what meaningful activity entails, often generalizing the meaningfulness of certain activities across the entire population of people with dementia [155, 156]. However, what constitutes meaningful activity will differ between individuals. Moreover, perspectives of family and professional caregivers on what meaningful activities are can differ from the perspective of people with dementia [91]. As activities can only be meaningful when evaluated as such by the person with dementia, involving them in the decisions on their daily activity schedule is crucial.

A recent review of meaningful activity for people with dementia emphasizes the importance of activities that do more than provide pleasure in the moment but also address the fundamental psychological needs of older adults, such as the need for life review, intergenerational relationships, sense of control and achievement and creativity [157]. Another review study, focussing specifically on research from the perspective of people with dementia themselves, identified connectedness as a prime underlying element of meaningful activity, which included being connected to the self and to others, as well as to the environment [158]. A sub-theme of the latter was feeling connected to nature. The relevance of nature for meaning in life was recently also supported in an interview study that evaluated the benefits of nature-based activities in the Netherlands [159]. A broad range of positive consequences were identified by people with dementia and their caregivers, including a sense of meaning in life.

The majority of studies on meaningful activity emphasize some element of connectedness with others, social interaction, sense of belonging. As emphasized in the previous section, supporting meaning in life thus requires considering the daily social context and interactions of the person with dementia. For example, in the nursing home context, nurse–resident interaction in the form of warm communication (both verbal and nonverbal) and meaningful dialogue is a key resource for supporting meaning in life, and for identifying what is meaningful for each specific resident [160]. Careful training and education of both professional care staff and informal caregivers, enhancing awareness of these underlying relational mechanisms, is crucial in this regard.

To support meaningful experiences and activities on a day-to-day basis, these activities must be embedded within a broad, widely supported approach to dementia – that is, one that casts off the influence of traces left by the biomedical paradigm that dominated dementia care for a long time in the past, and instead acknowledges the physical, psychological, social *and* existential needs of people with dementia. A biopsychosocial-existential model of care [160–162] takes a holistic view of well-being and incorporates attention for all domains that may be relevant in supporting a good life with dementia. Such an approach aligns well with related views of care that emphasize attending

to the whole person with dementia, such as person-centred or whole-person care [142, 163, 164]. Explicitly adding the existential dimension emphasizes the importance of caring for the existential needs and questions that older adults deal with at the end of life, especially when living with a terminal disease.

In line with these views, the available research on meaning in life for people with dementia reviewed in this chapter invites reflection on the overvaluation of cognitive abilities in contemporary psychological theories of meaning and demonstrates the relevance and importance of the experience of meaning in life for older adults with dementia, warranting more attention for this psychological concept in future dementia research and care approaches.[1]

References

1. Frankl VE. *Man's Search for Meaning: An Introduction to Logotherapy.* London, Hodder and Stoughton, 1968.

2. Frankl VE. *Man's Search for Meaning: Revised and Updated.* New York, Washington Square Press, 1984.

3. Maddi SR. The existential neurosis. *Journal of Abnormal Psychology* 1967; 72(4): 311–25.

4. Maslow AH. *Toward a Psychology of Being.* 2nd ed. New York, D. Van Nostrand Company, 1968.

5. Yalom ID. *Existential Psychotherapy.* New York, Basic Books, 1980.

6. Greening T. Existential challenges and responses. *The Humanistic Psychologist* 1992; 20(1): 111.

7. Batthyany A, Russo-Netzer P. Psychologies of meaning. In Batthyany A, Russo-Netzer P, eds. *Meaning in Positive and Existential Psychology.* New York, Springer, 2014; 3–22.

8. Seligman ME. *Authentic Happiness: Using the New Positive Psychology to Realize Your Potential for Lasting Fulfillment.* New York, Free Press, 2002.

9. Debats DL. Sources of meaning: An investigation of significant commitments in life. *Journal of Humanistic Psychology* 1999; 39(4): 30–57.

10. Wong PTP. Implicit theories of meaningful life and the development of the personal meaning profile. In Wong PTP, Fry PS, eds. *The Human Quest for Meaning: A Handbook of Psychological*

---

[1] This chapter builds on the general introduction and discussion of the PhD dissertation of the first author: 'Losing memory, losing meaning? Towards a deeper understanding of meaning in life in older adults with Alzheimer's disease'.

Research and Clinical Applications. Mahwah, NJ, Lawrence Erlbaum, 1998; 111–40.

11. Delle Fave A, Brdar I, Wissing MP, Vella-Brodrick DA. Sources and motives for personal meaning in adulthood. *The Journal of Positive Psychology* 2013; 8(6): 517–29.

12. Bar-Tur L, Savaya R, Prager E. Sources of meaning in life for young and old Israeli Jews and Arabs. *Journal of Aging Studies* 2001; 15(3): 253–69.

13. Schnell T. The Sources of Meaning and Meaning in Life Questionnaire (SoMe): Relations to demographics and well-being. *The Journal of Positive Psychology* 2009; 4(6): 483–99.

14. McDonald MJ, Wong PT, Gingras DT. Meaning-in-life measures and development of a brief version of the Personal Meaning Profile. In Wong PTP, ed. *The Human Quest for Meaning: Theories, Research, and Applications.* New York, Routledge, 2012; 357–82.

15. Glaw X, Kable A, Hazelton M, Inder K. Meaning in life and meaning of life in mental health care: An integrative literature review. *Issues in Mental Health Nursing* 2017; 38(3): 243–52.

16. Lambert NM, Stillman TF, Baumeister RF, Fincham FD, Hicks JA, Graham SM. Family as a salient source of meaning in young adulthood. *The Journal of Positive Psychology* 2010; 5(5): 367–76.

17. Grouden ME, Jose PE. How do sources of meaning in life vary according to demographic factors? *New Zealand Journal of Psychology* 2014; 43(3): 29–38.

18. O'Connor K, Chamberlain K. Dimensions of life meaning: A qualitative investigation at mid-life. *British Journal of Psychology* 1996; 87(3): 461–77.

19. Pedersen HF, Birkeland MH, Jensen JS, Schnell T, Hvidt NC, Sørensen T, et al. What brings meaning to life in a highly secular society? A study on sources of meaning among Danes. *Scandinavian Journal of Psychology* 2018; 59(6): 678–90.

20. Reker GT, Wong PTP. Aging as an individual process: Toward a theory of personal meaning. In Birren J, Bengston V, eds. *Emergent Theories of Aging.* New York, Springer, 1988.

21. Baumeister RF. *Meanings of Life.* New York, Guilford Press; 1991.

22. Wong PTP. Toward a dual-systems model of what makes life worth living. In *The Human Quest for Meaning.* New York, Routledge, 2013; 49–68.

23. Derkx P. The future of humanism. In Copson A, Graylin A, eds. *The Wiley Blackwell Handbook of Humanism.* Hoboken, NJ, Wiley & Sons, 2015; 426–39.

24. Baumeister RF, Landau MJ. Finding the meaning of meaning: Emerging insights on four grand

questions. *Review of General Psychology* 2018; 22(1): 1–10.

25. Martela F, Steger MF. The three meanings of meaning in life: Distinguishing coherence, purpose, and significance. *The Journal of Positive Psychology* 2016; 11(5): 531–45.

26. George LS, Park CL. Meaning in life as comprehension, purpose, and mattering: Toward integration and new research questions. *Review of General Psychology* 2016; 20(3): 205–20.

27. Heintzelman SJ, King LA. (The feeling of) meaning-as-information. *Personality and Social Psychology Review* 2014; 18(2): 153–67.

28. Steger MF, Frazier P, Oishi S, Kaler M. The meaning in life questionnaire: Assessing the presence of and search for meaning in life. *Journal of Counseling Psychology* 2006; 53(1): 80.

29. Steger MF, Kawabata Y, Shimai S, Otake K. The meaningful life in Japan and the United States: Levels and correlates of meaning in life. *Journal of Research in Personality* 2008; 42(3): 660–78.

30. Steger MF, Kashdan TB, Sullivan BA, Lorentz D. Understanding the search for meaning in Life: Personality, cognitive style, and the dynamic between seeking and experiencing meaning. *Journal of Personality* 2008; 76(2): 199–228.

31. Park CL, Folkman S. Meaning in the context of stress and coping. *Review of General Psychology* 1997; 1(2): 115–44.

32. Heine SJ, Proulx T, Vohs K. The meaning maintenance model: On the coherence of social motivations. *Personality and Social Psychology Review* 2006; 10(2): 88–110.

33. Park CL. Making sense of the meaning literature: An integrative review of meaning making and its effects on adjustment to stressful life events. *Psychological Bulletin* 2010; 136(2): 257–301.

34. Czekierda K, Banik A, Park CL, Luszczynska A. Meaning in life and physical health: Systematic review and meta-analysis. *Health Psychology Review* 2017; 11(4): 387–418.

35. Roepke AM, Jayawickreme E, Riffle OM. Meaning and health: A systematic review. *Applied Research in Quality of Life* 2014; 9(4): 1055–79.

36. Ryff CD, Heller AS, Schaefer SM, Van Reekum C, Davidson RJ. Purposeful engagement, healthy aging, and the brain. *Current Behavioral Neuroscience Reports* 2016; 3 (4): 318–27.

37. Haugan G. Meaning-in-life in nursing-home patients: A valuable approach for enhancing psychological and physical well-being? *Journal of Clinical Nursing* 2014; 23(13–14): 1830–44.

38. Ong AD, Patterson A. Eudaimonia, aging, and health: A review of underlying mechanisms. In Vitters⊘ J, ed. *Handbook of Eudaimonic Well-Being*. International Handbooks of Quality-of-Life. Cham, Springer, 2016; 371–8.

39. Hooker SA, Masters KS, Park CL. A meaningful life is a healthy life: A conceptual model linking meaning and meaning salience to health. *Review of General Psychology* 2018; 22(1): 11–24.

40. Steger MF. Experiencing meaning in life: Optimal functioning at the nexus of well-being, psychopathology, and spirituality. In Wong PTP, ed. *The Human Quest for Meaning: Theories, Research, and Applications*. 2nd ed. New York, Routledge, 2012; 165–84.

41. Disabato DJ, Kashdan TB, Short JL, Jarden A. What predicts positive life events that influence the course of depression? A longitudinal examination of gratitude and meaning in life. *Cognitive Therapy and Research* 2017; 41(3): 444–58.

42. Park CL, Knott CL, Williams RM, Clark EM, Williams BR, Schulz E. Meaning in life predicts decreased depressive symptoms and increased positive affect over time but does not buffer stress effects in a national sample of African-Americans. *Journal of Happiness Studies* 2020: 1–13.

43. Mascaro N, Rosen DH. Assessment of existential meaning and its longitudinal relations with depressive symptoms. *Journal of Social and Clinical Psychology* 2008; 27(6): 576–99.

44. Dezutter J, Luyckx K, Wachholtz A. Meaning in life in chronic pain patients over time: Associations with pain experience and psychological well-being. *Journal of Behavioral Medicine* 2015; 38(2): 384–96.

45. Park J, Baumeister RF. Meaning in life and adjustment to daily stressors. *The Journal of Positive Psychology* 2017; 12(4): 333–41.

46. Janoff-Bulman R. Posttraumatic growth: Three explanatory models. *Psychological Inquiry* 2004; 15(1): 30–4.

47. Davis CG, Nolen-Hoeksema S, Larson J. Making sense of loss and benefiting from the experience: Two construals of meaning. *Journal of Personality and Social Psychology* 1998; 75(2): 561–74.

48. Reker GT, Wong PTP. Personal meaning in life and psychosocial adaptation in the later years. In Wong PTP, ed. *The Human Quest for Meaning: Theories, Research, and Applications*. 2nd ed. New York, Routledge, 2012; 433–56.

49. Gana K, Bailly N, Saada Y, Joulain M, Alaphilippe D. Does life satisfaction change in old age: Results from an 8-year longitudinal study. *Journals of Gerontology Series B: Psychological Sciences and Social Sciences* 2012; 68(4): 540–52.

50. Steger MF, Oishi S, Kashdan TB. Meaning in life across the life span: Levels and correlates of meaning in life from emerging adulthood to older adulthood. *The Journal of Positive Psychology* 2009; 4(1): 43–52.

51. Pinquart M. Creating and maintaining purpose in life in old age: A meta-analysis. *Ageing International* 2002; 27(2): 90–114.

52. Hill PL, Weston SJ. Evaluating eight-year trajectories for sense of purpose in the health and retirement study. *Aging & Mental Health* 2019; 23(2): 233–7.

53. Tornstam L. Gero-transcendence: A reformulation of the disengagement theory. *Aging Clinical and Experimental Research* 1989; 1(1): 55–63.

54. Tornstam L. Gerotranscendence: The contemplative dimension of aging. *Journal of Aging Studies* 1997; 11(2): 143–54.

55. Cohen GD. *The Mature Mind: The Positive Power of the Aging Brain*. New York, Basic Books, 2005.

56. Leder D. Aging into the spirit: From traditional wisdom to innovative programs and communities. *Generations* 1999; 23(4): 36.

57. Hupkens S, Machielse A, Goumans M, Derkx P. Meaning in life of older persons: An integrative literature review. *Nursing Ethics* 2018; 25(8): 973–91.

58. Volkert J, Härter M, Dehoust MC, Ausín B, Canuto A, Da Ronch C, et al. The role of meaning in life in community-dwelling older adults with depression and relationship to other risk factors. *Aging & Mental Health* 2019; 23(1): 100–6.

59. Steptoe A, Fancourt D. Leading a meaningful life at older ages and its relationship with social engagement, prosperity, health, biology, and time use. *Proceedings of the National Academy of Sciences* 2019; 116(4): 1207–12.

60. Reker GT. Prospective predictors of successful aging in community-residing and institutionalized Canadian elderly. *Ageing International* 2002; 27(1): 42–64.

61. Krause N. Evaluating the stress-buffering function of meaning in life among older people. *Journal of Aging and Health* 2007; 19(5): 792–812.

62. Irving J, Davis S, Collier A. Aging with purpose: Systematic search and review of literature pertaining to older adults and purpose. *The International Journal of Aging and Human Development* 2017; 85(4): 403–37.

63. Kim G, Shin SH, Scicolone MA, Parmelee P. Purpose in life protects against cognitive decline

among older adults. *The American Journal of Geriatric Psychiatry* 2019; 27(6): 593–601.

64. Wingo AP, Wingo TS, Fan W, Bergquist S, Alonso A, Marcus M, et al. Purpose in life is a robust protective factor of reported cognitive decline among late middle-aged adults: The Emory Healthy Aging Study. *Journal of Affective Disorders* 2020; 263: 310–17.

65. Boyle PA, Buchman AS, Barnes LL, Bennett DA. Effect of a purpose in life on risk of incident Alzheimer disease and mild cognitive impairment in community-dwelling older persons. *Archives of General Psychiatry* 2010; 67(3): 304.

66. Windsor TD, Curtis RG, Luszcz MA. Sense of purpose as a psychological resource for aging well. *Developmental Psychology* 2015; 51(7): 975.

67. Gleeson H, Hafford-Letchfield T, Quaife M, Collins DA, Flynn A. Preventing and responding to depression, self-harm, and suicide in older people living in long term care settings: a systematic review. *Aging & Mental Health* 2019; 23(11): 1467–77.

68. Anstey KJ, Von Sanden C, Sargent-Cox K, Luszcz MA. Prevalence and risk factors for depression in a longitudinal, population-based study including individuals in the community and residential care. *The American Journal of Geriatric Psychiatry* 2007; 15(6): 497–505.

69. Fry PS. Religious involvement, spirituality and personal meaning for life: Existential predictors of psychological wellbeing in community-residing and institutional care elders. *Aging & Mental Health* 2000; 4(4): 375–87.

70. Haugan G. Meaning-in-life in nursing-home patients: A correlate with physical and emotional symptoms. *Journal of Clinical Nursing* 2014; 23(7–8): 1030–43.

71. Van der Heyden K, Dezutter J, Beyers W. Meaning in life and depressive symptoms: A person-oriented approach in residential and community-dwelling older adults. *Aging & Mental Health* 2015; 19(12): 1063–70.

72. Haugan G. Life satisfaction in cognitively intact long-term nursing-home patients: Symptom distress, well-being and nurse-patient interaction. In Sarracino FM, ed. *Beyond Money: The Social Roots of Health and Well-Being*. New York, Nova Science, 2014.

73. Baumeister RF, Vohs KD, Aaker JL, Garbinsky EN. Some key differences between a happy life and a meaningful life. *The Journal of Positive Psychology* 2013; 8(6): 505–16.

74. Krause N. Thought suppression and meaning in life: A longitudinal investigation. *The International Journal of Aging and Human Development* 2007; 64(1): 67–82.

75. Wilson RS, Boyle PA, Segawa E, Yu L, Begeny CT, Anagnos SE, et al. The influence of cognitive decline on well-being in old age. *Psychology and Aging* 2013; 28(2): 304.

76. McKnight PE, Kashdan TB. Purpose in life as a system that creates and sustains health and well-being: An integrative, testable theory. *Review of General Psychology* 2009; 13(3): 242–51.

77. Waytz A, Hershfield HE, Tamir DI. Mental simulation and meaning in life. *Journal of Personality and Social Psychology* 2015; 108(2): 336.

78. Vess M, Hoeldtke R, Leal SA, Sanders CS, Hicks JA. The subjective quality of episodic future thought and the experience of meaning in life. *The Journal of Positive Psychology* 2017; 13(4): 419–28.

79. Takkinen S, Ruoppila I. Meaning in life in three samples of elderly persons with high cognitive functioning. *The International Journal of Aging and Human Development* 2001; 53(1): 51–73.

80. Simm LA, Jamieson RD, Ong B, Garner MW, Kinsella GJ. Making sense of self in Alzheimer's disease: Reflective function and memory. *Aging & Mental Health* 2015; 21(5): 501–8.

81. Holst G, Hallberg IR. Exploring the meaning of everyday life, for those suffering from dementia. *American Journal of Alzheimer's Disease & Other Dementias* 2003; 18(6): 359–65.

82. Jetten J, Haslam C, Pugliese C, Tonks J, Haslam SA. Declining autobiographical memory and the loss of identity: Effects on well-being. *Journal of Clinical and Experimental Neuropsychology* 2010; 32(4): 408–16.

83. Bender M, Cheston R. Inhabitants of a lost kingdom: A model of the subjective experiences of dementia. *Ageing and Society* 1997; 17(5): 513–32.

84. Svanström R, Sundler AJ. Gradually losing one's foothold: A fragmented existence when living alone with dementia. *Dementia* 2015; 14(2): 145–63.

85. Harris PB. The perspective of younger people with dementia: Still an overlooked population. *Social Work in Mental Health* 2004; 2(4): 17–36.

86. Greenwood N, Smith R. The experiences of people with young-onset dementia: A meta-ethnographic review of the qualitative literature. *Maturitas* 2016; 92: 102–9.

87. Rostad D, Hellzén O, Enmarker I. The meaning of being young with dementia and living at home. *Nursing Reports* 2013; 3(1): e3-e.

88. Menne HL, Kinney JM, Morhardt DJ. 'Trying to continue to do as much as they can do': Theoretical insights regarding continuity and meaning making in the face of dementia. *Dementia* 2002; 1(3): 367–82.

89. Westius A, Kallenberg K, Norberg A. Views of life and sense of identity in people with Alzheimer's disease. *Ageing & Society* 2010; 30(7): 1257–78.

90. Genoe MR, Dupuis SL. The role of leisure within the dementia context. *Dementia* 2014; 13(1): 33–58.

91. Harmer BJ, Orrell M. What is meaningful activity for people with dementia living in care homes? A comparison of the views of older people with dementia, staff and family carers. *Aging and Mental Health* 2008; 12(5): 548–58.

92. Phinney A. Horizons of meaning in dementia: Retained and shifting narratives. *Journal of Religion, Spirituality & Aging* 2011; 23(3): 254–68.

93. Beard RL, Knauss J, Moyer D. Managing disability and enjoying life: How we reframe dementia through personal narratives. *Journal of Aging Studies* 2009; 23(4): 227–35.

94. Robertson JM. Finding meaning in everyday life with dementia: A case study. *Dementia* 2014; 13 (4): 525–43.

95. Steeman E, Tournoy J, Grypdonck M, Godderis J, De Casterlé BD. Managing identity in early-stage dementia: Maintaining a sense of being valued. *Ageing & Society* 2013; 33(2): 216–42.

96. Dewitte L, Van Wijngaarden E, Schellekens T, Vandenbulcke M, Dezutter J. (2021). Continuing to participate in the dance of life as oneself: The lived experience of meaning in life for older adults with Alzheimer's disease. *The Gerontologist* 2021; 61(7): 1019–29.

97. Dewitte L, Schellekens T, Steger MF, Martela F, Vanhooren S, Vandenbulcke M, Dezutter J. What can we learn about the concept of meaning in life from older adults with Alzheimer's disease? A directed content analysis study. *Journal of Happiness Studies* 2021; 22: 2845–71. https://doi .org/10.1007/s10902-020-00351-4.

98. Dewitte L, Vandenbulcke M, Schellekens T, Dezutter J. Sources of well-being for older adults with and without dementia in residential care: Relations to presence of meaning and life satisfaction. *Aging & Mental Health* 2019: 1–9.

99. Trevitt C, MacKinlay E. 'I am just an ordinary person . . .': Spiritual reminiscence in older people with memory loss. *Journal of Religion, Spirituality & Aging* 2006; 18(2–3): 79–91.

100. Steger MF, Samman E. Assessing meaning in life on an international scale: Psychometric evidence for the Meaning in Life Questionnaire-Short Form among Chilean households. *International Journal of Wellbeing* 2012; 2(3): 182–95.

101. Dewitte L, Hill PL, Vandenbulcke M, Dezutter J. The longitudinal relationship between meaning in life, depressive symptoms, life satisfaction, and cognitive functioning for older adults with Alzheimer's disease. European Journal of Ageing (accepted).

102. Dewitte L, Vandenbulcke M, Dezutter J. Meaning in life matters for older adults with Alzheimer's disease in residential care: Associations with life satisfaction and depressive symptoms. *International Psychogeriatrics* 2019: 1–9.

103. Nolen-Hoeksema S, Davis CG. Positive responses to loss: Perceiving benefits and growth. In Snyder CR, Lopez S, eds. *Handbook of Positive Psychology*. New York, Oxford University Press, 2002; 598–606.

104. Dröes R-M, Boelens-Van Der Knoop ECC, Bos J, Meihuizen L, Ettema TP, Gerritsen DL, et al. Quality of life in dementia in perspective: An explorative study of variations in opinions among people with dementia and their professional caregivers, and in literature. *Dementia* 2006; 5(4): 533–58.

105. Van Vliet D, Persoon A, Bakker C, Koopmans RT, de Vugt ME, Bielderman A, et al. Feeling useful and engaged in daily life: Exploring the experiences of people with young-onset dementia. *International Psychogeriatrics* 2017; 29(11): 1889–98.

106. Aftab A, Jeste DV. Well-being in dementia and mild cognitive impairment. *International Psychogeriatrics* 2019; 31(5): 603–6.

107. Wolverson E, Clarke C, Moniz-Cook E. Living positively with dementia: A systematic review and synthesis of the qualitative literature. *Aging & Mental Health* 2016; 20(7): 676–99.

108. Lin S-Y, Lewis FM. Dementia friendly, dementia capable, and dementia positive: Concepts to prepare for the future. *The Gerontologist* 2015; 55(2): 237–44.

109. Harris PB, Keady J. Wisdom, resilience and successful aging: Changing public discourses on living with dementia. *Dementia* 2008; 7(1): 5–8.

110. Clarke C, Wolverson E. *Positive Psychology Approaches to Dementia*. Clarke C, Wolverson E, eds. London, Jessica Kingsley, 2016.

111. Lamont RA, Nelis SM, Quinn C, Martyr A, Rippon I, Kopelman MD, et al. Psychological predictors of 'living well' with dementia: Findings from the IDEAL study. *Aging & Mental Health* 2020; 24(6): 956–64.

112. Thorgrimsen L, Selwood A, Spector A, Royan L, de Madariaga Lopez M, Woods R, et al. Whose quality of life is it anyway? The validity and

reliability of the Quality of Life-Alzheimer's Disease (QoL-AD) scale. *Alzheimer Disease & Associated Disorders* 2003; 17(4): 201–8.

113. Schütz A, Baumeister RF. Positive illusions and the happy mind. In Robinson MD, Eid M, eds. *The Happy Mind: Cognitive Contributions to Well-Being.* Cham, Springer International, 2017; 177–93.

114. Taylor SE, Brown JD. Illusion and well-being: A social psychological perspective on mental health. *Psychological Bulletin* 1988; 103(2): 193.

115. Taylor SE, Kemeny ME, Reed GM, Bower JE, Gruenewald TL. Psychological resources, positive illusions, and health. *The American Psychologist* 2000; 55(1): 99–109.

116. Dunn DS. Positive meaning and illusions following disability: Reality negotiation, normative interpretation, and value change. *Journal of Social Behavior and Personality* 1994; 9(5): 123.

117. Post SG. The concept of Alzheimer disease in a hypercognitive society. In Whitehouse PJ, Maurer K, Ballenger JF, eds. *Concepts of Alzheimer Disease: Biological, Clinical and Cultural Perspectives.* Baltimore, MD, Johns Hopkins University Press, 2000; 245–56.

118. Post SG. Respectare: Moral respect for the lives of the deeply forgetful. In Hughes JC, Louw SJ, Sabat SR, eds. *Dementia: Mind, Meaning, and the Person.* Oxford, Oxford University Press, 2006, 223.

119. Post SG. *The Moral Challenge of Alzheimer Disease: Ethical Issues from Diagnosis to Dying.* Baltimore, MD, Johns Hopkins University Press, 2000.

120. Gendlin ET. *Experiencing and the Creation of Meaning: A Philosophical and Psychological Approach to the Subjective.* Evanston, IL, Northwestern University Press, 1962/97.

121. Gendlin ET. Experiential psychotherapy. In Corsini R, ed. *Current Psychotherapies.* Itasca, Peacock, 1973; 317–52.

122. Greenberg LS, Pascual-Leone J. A dialectical constructivist view of the creation of personal meaning. *Journal of Constructivist Psychology* 2001; 14(3): 165–86.

123. Hill CE. *Meaning in Life: A Therapist's Guide.* Washington, DC, American Psychological Association, 2018.

124. Hill CE, Kline KV, Miller M, Marks E, Pinto-Coelho K, Zetzer H. Development of the Meaning in Life measure. *Counselling Psychology Quarterly* 2019; 32(2): 205–26.

125. Heintzelman SJ, King LA. On knowing more than we can tell: Intuitive processes and the experience of meaning. *The Journal of Positive Psychology* 2013; 8(6): 471–82.

126. Heintzelman SJ, King LA. Meaning in life and intuition. *Journal of Personality and Social Psychology* 2016; 110(3): 477.

127. Vanhooren S. Struggling with meaninglessness: A case study from an experiential–existential perspective. *Person-Centered & Experiential Psychotherapies* 2019; 18(1): 1–21.

128. Salthouse TA. Consequences of age-related cognitive declines. *Annual Review of Psychology* 2012; 63: 201–26.

129. Sternberg RJ, Wagner RK. *Practical Intelligence: Nature and Origins of Competence in the Everyday World.* Cambridge, Cambridge University Press Archive, 1986.

130. Kunzmann U, Baltes PB. *Beyond the Traditional Scope of Intelligence: Wisdom in Action. Models of Intelligence: International Perspectives.* Washington, DC, American Psychological Association, 2003; 329–43.

131. Kontos P, Martin W. Embodiment and dementia: Exploring critical narratives of selfhood, surveillance, and dementia care. *Dementia* 2013; 12(3): 288–302.

132. Drayson Z, Clark A. Cognitive disability and embodied, extended minds. In Wasserman DT, Cureton A, eds. *The Oxford Handbook of Philosophy and Disability.* Oxford, Oxford University Press, 2020.

133. Matthews E. Dementia and the identity of the person. In Hughes JC, Louw SJ, Sabat SR, eds. *Dementia: Mind, Meaning, and the Person.* Oxford, Oxford University Press, 2006; 163.

134. Bellin ZJ. The meaning connection between mindfulness and happiness. *The Journal of Humanistic Counseling* 2015; 54(3): 221–35.

135. Kontos PC. Ethnographic reflections on selfhood, embodiment and Alzheimer's disease. *Ageing & Society* 2004; 24(6): 829–49.

136. Hughes JC, Louw SJ, Sabat SR. Seeing whole. In Hughes JC, Louw SJ, Sabat SR, eds. *Dementia: Mind, Meaning, and the Person.* Oxford, Oxford University Press, 2006; 1.

137. Nyman A, Josephsson S, Isaksson G. Being part of an enacted togetherness: Narratives of elderly people with depression. *Journal of Aging Studies* 2012; 26(4): 410–18.

138. Hydén LC, Örulv L. Narrative and identity in Alzheimer's disease: A case study. *Journal of Aging Studies* 2009; 23(4): 205–14.

139. Hydén L-C. Narrative collaboration and scaffolding in dementia. *Journal of Aging Studies* 2011; 25(4): 339–47.

140. Delle Fave A, Soosai-Nathan L. Meaning as inter-connectedness: Theoretical perspectives

and empirical evidence. *Journal of Psychology in Africa* 2014; 24(1): 53–68.

141. Drageset J, Haugan G, Tranvåg O. Crucial aspects promoting meaning and purpose in life: Perceptions of nursing home residents. *BMC Geriatrics* 2017; 17(1): 254.

142. Edvardsson D, Winblad B, Sandman P-O. Person-centred care of people with severe Alzheimer's disease: Current status and ways forward. *The Lancet Neurology* 2008; 7(4): 362–7.

143. Haugan G, Kuven BM, Eide WM, Taasen SE, Rinnan E, Xi Wu V, et al. Nurse–patient interaction and self-transcendence: Assets for a meaningful life in nursing home residents? *BMC Geriatrics* 2020; 20(1): 168.

144. Haugan G. The relationship between nurse–patient interaction and meaning-in-life in cognitively intact nursing home patients. *Journal of Advanced Nursing* 2014; 70(1): 107–20.

145. McGovern J. Couple meaning-making and dementia: Challenges to the deficit model. *Journal of Gerontological Social Work* 2011; 54(7): 678–90.

146. Quinn C, Clare L, Woods RT. What predicts whether caregivers of people with dementia find meaning in their role? *International Journal of Geriatric Psychiatry* 2012; 27(11): 1195–1202.

147. Shim B, Barroso J, Gilliss CL, Davis LL. Finding meaning in caring for a spouse with dementia. *Applied Nursing Research* 2013; 26(3): 121–6.

148. McLennon SM, Habermann B, Rice M. Finding meaning as a mediator of burden on the health of caregivers of spouses with dementia. *Aging & Mental Health* 2011; 15(4): 522–30.

149. Polenick CA, Sherman CW, Birditt KS, Zarit SH, Kales HC. Purpose in life among family care partners managing dementia: Links to caregiving gains. *The Gerontologist* 2019; 59(5): e424–e432.

150. Park CL, Pustejovsky JE, Trevino K, Sherman AC, Esposito C, Berendsen M, et al. Effects of psychosocial interventions on meaning and purpose in adults with cancer: A systematic review and meta-analysis. *Cancer* 2019; 125(14): 2383–93.

151. Ching-Teng Y, Ya-Ping Y, Chia-Ju L, Hsiu-Yueh L. Effect of group reminiscence therapy on depression and perceived meaning of life of veterans diagnosed with dementia at veteran homes. *Social Work in Health Care* 2020; 59(2): 75–90.

152. Wu LF, Koo M. Randomized controlled trial of a six-week spiritual reminiscence intervention on hope, life satisfaction, and spiritual well-being in elderly with mild and moderate dementia. *International Journal of Geriatric Psychiatry* 2016; 31(2): 120–7.

153. MacKinlay E, Trevitt C. Living in aged care: Using spiritual reminiscence to enhance meaning in life for those with dementia. *International Journal of Mental Health Nursing* 2010; 19(6): 394–401.

154. Ismail S, Christopher G, Dodd E, Wildschut T, Sedikides C, Ingram TA, et al. Psychological and mnemonic benefits of nostalgia for people with dementia. *Journal of Alzheimer's Disease* 2018; 65(4): 1327–44.

155. Kielsgaard K, Horghagen S, Nielsen D, Kristensen HK. Approaches to engaging people with dementia in meaningful occupations in institutional settings: A scoping review. *Scandinavian Journal of Occupational Therapy* 2020: 1–19.

156. Tierney L, Beattie E. Enjoyable, engaging and individualised: A concept analysis of meaningful activity for older adults with dementia. *International Journal of Older People Nursing* 2020: e12306.

157. Nyman SR, Szymczynska P. Meaningful activities for improving the wellbeing of people with dementia: Beyond mere pleasure to meeting fundamental psychological needs. *Perspectives in Public Health* 2016; 136(2): 99–107.

158. Han A, Radel J, McDowd JM, Sabata D. Perspectives of people with dementia about meaningful activities: A synthesis. *American Journal of Alzheimer's Disease & Other Dementias* 2016; 31(2): 115–23.

159. De Bruin SR, Buist Y, Hassink J, Vaandrager L. 'I want to make myself useful': The value of nature-based adult day services in urban areas for people with dementia and their family carers. *Ageing & Society* 2019: 1–23.

160. Haugan G. Nurse–patient interaction: A vital salutary factor and health promoting resource in nursing homes. In Haugan G, Eriksson M, eds. *Health Promotion in Health Care: Vital Salutogenic Theories and Research*. Berlin, Springer International, 2021; 117–35.

161. Dezutter J, Offenbaecher M, Vallejo MA, Vanhooren S, Thauvoye E, Toussaint L. Chronic pain care: The importance of a biopsychosocial-existential approach. *The International Journal of Psychiatry in Medicine* 2016; 51(6): 563–75.

162. Dezutter J. Het biopsychosociaal zorgmodel: Een integraal zorgmodel? *VIEWZ* 2016: 10–3.

163. Kitwood TM. *Dementia Reconsidered: The Person Comes First*. Buckingham, Open University Press, 1997.

164. Hutchinson TA. *Whole Person Care: A New Paradigm for the 21st Century*. New York, Springer, 2011.

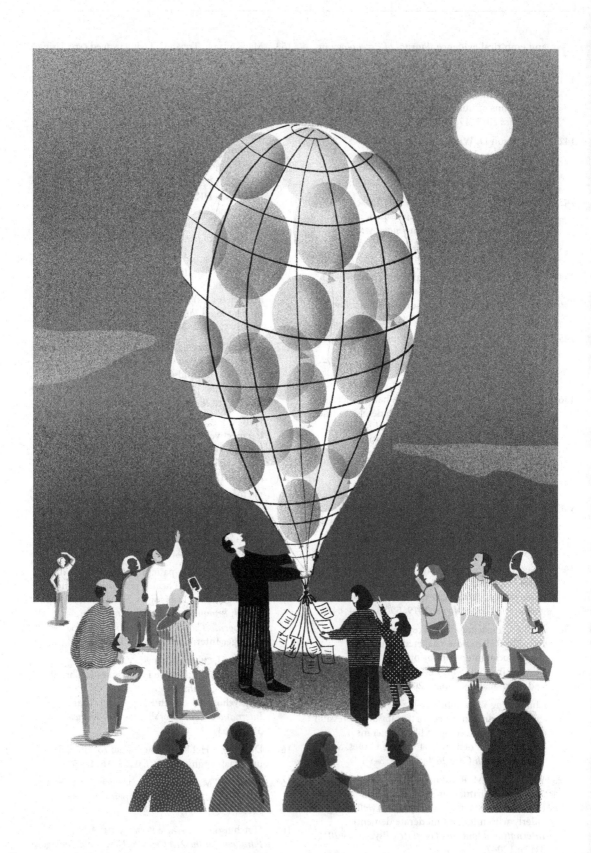

5

Quality of Life of Persons with Dementia
Different Disciplinary Perspectives

Rose-Marie Dröes, Teake Ettema, Martin Knapp
and Erik Schokkaert

1 Introduction

In a situation where dementia cannot be 'cured', care for persons with dementia becomes even more crucial. Care is important for supporting people to live with the consequences of dementia. The main objective of these care efforts is to maintain or optimize the quality of life (QoL). This QoL should be measured in terms of the integrated final outcome – that is, the dimensions of life that ultimately matter to the persons concerned.

The choice of a measure of QoL raises difficult normative questions. What is well-being? What makes a life good? Is it possible to narrow down well-being and formulate a kind of 'health-related QoL'? Is there a difference between QoL and happiness? Does QoL coincide with feeling well? How important are objective economic features (such as having a sufficient income) for well-being? There is a huge philosophical (and social science) literature on all these questions.

Many practitioners do not care very much about these fundamental questions because they aim at applying scales that are useful to answer specific care policy questions. As an example, economists want to implement an operational generic health-related QoL measure to evaluate and compare the cost-effectiveness of various therapies or care interventions. Yet even if this is not made explicit, the selected scales do take an implicit stance on these fundamental questions. In this chapter we focus on this basic question: what is QoL and how do we measure it? Starting from these questions allows us to get a better insight into the relationships between different specific measures that have been proposed in the literature by different disciplines, and informs us about the complementarity (or the conflicts) between them. It also suggests some important yet unanswered questions, and links the debate

about operational measures of QoL to the basic philosophical discussion on autonomy and identity in Chapter 3 of this book.

In Section 2 we discuss the different perspectives on well-being that have been developed in the philosophical literature. Sections 3 and 4 describe the two main applications of QoL measurement for persons with dementia: the psychological scales and the economic quality-adjusted life years (QALY)–type measures, respectively. We then return in Section 5 to the basic issues that come up when we compare the two types of approaches and confront them with the fundamental issues raised in Section 2. Section 6 concludes.

Psychometric properties of the scales and fundamental measurement issues are largely left aside. Another restriction is that we limit ourselves mainly to the QoL of persons with dementia themselves. The QoL of informal carers is mentioned only briefly in this chapter.

2 Different Perspectives on Well-Being

For centuries, philosophers have thought about what is a 'good life' or 'true happiness'. These questions about 'well-being' or a 'good life' go beyond the specific issue of measuring the QoL of persons with dementia. The subtle distinctions between different notions of well-being, as discussed by philosophers, are not always easy to translate into specific operational measures. Yet the basic questions raised in this philosophical debate are certainly relevant when examining the strengths and limitations of operational measures.

Most of the classifications of well-being found in the literature are variants of one initially proposed by Parfit [1]. In this tradition three broad approaches are distinguished (see [2] for a similar welfare economic perspective):

- Objective approaches use some external standard to define what is good in life and state that some life dimensions are important, even if they are not seen as such by the persons involved [3]. Typical examples of such 'objectively important dimensions of life' include cognitive performance and the number of close social contacts. The idea is not that the personal feelings or insights of the people concerned are irrelevant, but that some dimensions are important for everybody, even for individuals who personally do not care about them at all.

- Mental state approaches equate well-being with feeling well. This can be interpreted in different ways. A narrow hedonic approach, focussing on the balance of pleasures and pains, is exemplified in traditional Benthamite utilitarianism. Here the emphasis is on feelings – that is, on positive and negative affect. A broader interpretation equates feeling well with life satisfaction. This satisfaction view has a stronger cognitive component as it involves an overall evaluation of one's life. In some sense, mental state approaches can be called 'subjective' as they refer to a subjective state of mind. However, they can also (better?) be seen as a special case of the objective approach in which the balance of affects and feelings defines a good life, even if people themselves do not consider this specific balance an important component of their well-being. Of course, and as we see later in this chapter, 'feeling well' is an important item in almost all QoL scales. However, within the mental state approach, it is the *only* relevant dimension of life whereas other possible aspects of life (e.g. physical health) are important only insofar as they affect 'feeling well'.

- Desire-fulfilment approaches are the third broad group of theories. They are truly subjective in that they define well-being to be greater if the person better succeeds in satisfying their own desires, in reaching the goals they set for themself. Economists usually call this third group preferentialist approaches: to avoid any confusion, it must be emphasized that 'preferences' here go beyond narrow financial self-interest to cover all of the dimensions that are relevant in life. One could

wonder if the broader notion of life satisfaction coincides with desire fulfilment: it does not, and the difference is highly relevant. Consider a situation with two persons: Ann is in situation A and Bert is in situation B. Assume they agree situation A is better than situation B. It is then still possible that Bert is more satisfied with his life than Ann is with hers, because he has different aspirations. The point has been emphasized strongly by Sen [4] in the context of poverty measurement:

A person who has had a life of misfortune, with very limited opportunities, and rather little hope, may be more easily reconciled to deprivations than others reared in more fortunate and affluent circumstances. The metric of happiness may, therefore, distort the extent of deprivation, in a specific and biased way. The hopeless beggar, the precarious landless labourer, the dominated housewife, the hardened unemployed or the overexhausted coolie may all take pleasures in small mercies, and manage to suppress intense suffering for the necessity of continued survival, but it would be ethically deeply mistaken to attach a correspondingly small value to the loss of their well-being because of this survival strategy. *(pp. 45–6)*

Human beings can adapt their aspirations to their actual situation: this will make them more satisfied, but it does not mean that they are in a better situation. We discuss later in this chapter how this example is also relevant within the specific context of dementia.

Some specific proposals are rather difficult to classify in this scheme. The main example of this is the capability approach as originally proposed by Sen (see e.g. [5] for a recent overview). The capability approach focusses on the opportunities of people to choose from a set of attainable functionings (such as being healthy, well-fed, integrated into society, mobile etc.). This focus on opportunities or (positive) freedoms is an important original feature of the approach. Nussbaum [6] proposes a list of capabilities inspired by an Aristotelian view on human flourishing. She certainly belongs in the objective camp of well-being theorists. Sen himself, however, proposes to determine both the list of relevant capabilities and the relative weights to be given to them as the result of a deliberative process. While this is not a subjective approach, in that it does not work with individual desires or preferences (Sen explicitly rejects this subjective approach), it still gives an important role to the personal feelings and convictions of participants in the deliberative process. However, his proposal raises questions about the conditions that this deliberative process has to satisfy in order to yield ethically acceptable conclusions. This raises serious challenges in the context of dementia at an advanced stage.

In choosing between these different approaches, one can take (broadly summarized) two perspectives. One (common among philosophers) is to look for a 'deep' definition of what makes a human life really good. This raises deep questions about human flourishing, perhaps even about human nature. Another approach (more popular among social scientists of all sorts) is to start from the lived experiences of people or from the specific policy issues that have to be settled. One will then devise a measure of well-being that satisfies the normative requirements that are necessary in that specific situation. As an example: for the evaluation of economic policies we need a well-being measure that can function as a good measure of social progress and that can be used to evaluate redistribution in such a way that a transfer from someone with a higher to someone with a lower level of well-being (measured in that way) can be seen as a social improvement (see [2]). Applied to dementia policy, the pragmatic approach will prefer measures that respect the dignity and lived experience of the persons with dementia, that can be a reliable guide to evaluate the quality of care, and that ideally can identify the priorities when society has to decide about the allocation of scarce resources. The latter objective also necessitates a measure that can identify who is 'most' in need of care.

In our normative view, respect for the personal convictions and feelings of people with dementia is central. This almost unavoidably pushes us in the direction of the subjective approaches. The more one believes in the autonomy and dignity of persons with dementia, the larger the weight one wants to give to their own desires or preferences. In fact, one of the criticisms against the objective (including the mental state) views is that they are paternalistic. Paternalism certainly has to be avoided in the recent view on care for persons with dementia. This raises difficult issues for how long in the process it is possible for persons with dementia

to express their own desires, and how good the substitution is of their own answers by proxy assessments. We return to these issues in the following sections.

Until now we have interpreted well-being as related to the whole life of persons. This is indeed the dominant approach in the philosophical literature. However, in the health economic literature, many have proposed to work with a narrower concept – that is, 'health-related QoL'. This certainly holds for the popular notion of the QALY discussed further in this chapter. As we see herein, some dementia-specific scales also focus on 'health-related QoL'. Philosophers have expressed serious doubts about the theoretical meaning of this concept (see e.g. [7]). Surely restrictive assumptions are needed in order to claim that 'health-related QoL' per se is indicative of QoL without taking into account other life dimensions, or broader life projects of individuals. Losing the capacity to control very fine finger movements can be devastating for a professional pianist, but is much less of a restriction for a professional football player.

'Health-related QoL' is an attempt to narrow down a broad concept of well-being, influenced by many circumstances and policies, to something that should be easier to influence by (health) care. Starting from a similar inspiration, the notion of 'health' has been broadened to go beyond a purely physical interpretation of 'absence of disease'. Already in 1948, the World Health Organization (WHO) described health as 'a state of complete physical, mental and social well-being and not merely the absence of disease or infirmity'. With this definition, the boundary between health and well-being becomes blurred. In fact, the distinction between health so defined and 'health-related QoL' disappears almost completely. Recently, with the growing prevalence of chronic diseases, proposals have been made to reformulate the static WHO definition. This reformulation focusses on the ability to physically, mentally and socially adapt to one's situation ([8], operationalized for persons with dementia in [9]). This is an interesting move, but it also raises the deeper question of the relationship between overall well-being and health so defined.

Let us formulate a last caveat before we turn to the overview of measurement scales for the QoL of persons with dementia. Although it is very common for social scientists to evaluate policies on the basis of their effects on well-being (however defined), it has been argued that one should go beyond such a consequentialist approach and also introduce deontological considerations. As an example, one could say that it is necessary to respect the dignity of the persons with dementia because it is their right to be respected, even if such respect for dignity did not increase their well-being. We do not follow this track in this chapter, but rather try to present an attractive normative approach to well-being. This means that respect for dignity and lived experiences will be one of the criteria used to evaluate specific operational scales.

3 The Measurement of Quality of Life in Persons with Dementia

In the past 25 years there has been growth in the development of instruments to measure QoL as one of the main outcomes of treatments and care for people with chronic and incurable diseases. This includes psychological and psychosocial treatments for people living with dementia. Dementia-specific QoL instruments can be divided into two categories: self-report instruments and proxy-based instruments. Self-report instruments are administered directly to the person with dementia by means of an interview, reflecting the person's opinion on their own QoL. If we see QoL as a subjective construct, this is the preferred way of measuring it [10]. Proxy-based instruments rely on proxy report, either by asking the opinion of a proxy, such as the informal carer or a professional caregiver, directly or by means of an interview on QoL aspects of the person with dementia, or by using standardized behaviour observation scales. These scales can be used when the person with dementia cannot understand or reply to the questions of the self-report instruments or, for example, for longitudinal research purposes covering longer time periods. Standardized behaviour observation scales are generally meant to be used by professional caregivers. The self-report instruments can be applied in people with mild to moderate dementia and in all types of settings, while the proxy-based and observational instruments are meant specifically for use in care facilities throughout the dementia career or in late-stage dementia. It must be said that from the list of QoL domains mentioned as relevant by people with dementia – that is, affect, self-esteem, attachment, social contact, enjoyment of activities, sense of aesthetics in living environment, physical and mental health, financial situation, security and privacy, self-determination and freedom, being useful and spirituality [74] – all of the mentioned instruments assess only part of these, which also characterizes their difference ([43]; see also Table 5.1).

3.1 Self-Report Instruments

The Alzheimer's Disease–Related Quality of Life (QOL-AD [11]) scale is a popular, widely used brief scale for assessing QoL [12–17] which can be administered in 10–15 minutes. It covers the domains of physical health, mood, energy, living situation, memory, interpersonal relations, ability to do chores, fun, money, self and life as a whole. It has been extensively validated, and it can be completed by the person with dementia or carer until severe dementia (Mini-Mental State Examination (MMSE) score 3; [18]). Patient as well as proxy versions are available. It has demonstrated sensitivity to psychosocial intervention and correlates with health utility measures [17]. The QOL-AD can therefore be applied in both intervention and longitudinal research, but is also very useful for quick evaluation in clinical practice [19–21]. Edelman and colleagues adapted the QOL-AD to the QOL-AD NH for the nursing home setting [22] through deleting two original items, adding four new ones and changing the wording of three others. The psychometric properties were considered sufficient for use in this setting [16].

The Dementia Quality of Life (DQoL [23]) instrument can be administered in people with mild to moderate dementia (MMSE score >12). It has an advantage over the QOL-AD when more in-depth evaluation on quality of life is required [24, 25]. Ten domains on five subscales (self esteem, positive and negative affect, feelings of belonging and sense of aesthetics) are assessed on a five-point Likert scale, providing a profile of scores. The scale is available in many languages. It is widely used in both intervention and longitudinal research [17, 26–28].

The Bath Assessment of Subjective Quality of Life in Dementia (BASQID [29, 30]) is a measure for people with mild to moderate dementia and

Table 5.1 Characteristics of the most frequently used dementia-specific and general quality of life scales

Stage of dementia	QOL-AD	DQoL	BASQID	DEMQOL	SEIQoL	QUALID	QUALIDEM	DS-DAT
	Mild-moderate	Mild-moderate	Mild-moderate	All stages	Mild	Late stage dementia	Mild-severe	Severe
QoL domains	Physical health, mood, energy, living situation, memory, interpersonal relations, ability to do chores, fun, money, self and life as a whole	Positive affect, negative affect, self-esteem, feelings of belonging, sense of aesthetics	Health, social interaction, function, mobility, being occupied, energy, psychological well-being	Daily activities, health and well-being, cognitive functioning, social relationships, self-concept	Personalized: 5 most important life areas for the individual are assessed	Positive and negative dimensions of observable mood and performance: affective state in daily life, signs of comfort and engagement in basic activities	Care relationship, positive affect, negative affect, restless tense behaviour Positive self image, social relations, feeling at home, social isolation, having something to do	(Discomfort scale) Content – sad mood Agitation – calm Engagement – apathy Discomfort, including pain
Included QoL domains based on	Literature and reviewed by people with dementia, caregivers, older people, dementia experts	Three focus groups of caregivers, healthcare providers, persons with mild dementia	Qualitative interviews with 30 people with mild to moderate dementia	Literature, qualitative interviews with people with dementia and carers, expert opinion, team discussion	Interviewed individual person him/ herself; and if needed a prompt list of domains	A group of clinicians with an extensive experience in dealing with people with dementia	Literature, focus groups with people with mild to moderate dementia, participant observation in nursing homes and two expert panels of dementia care professionals	Empirically generated from the perspectives of nursing staff practicing on special care Alzheimer units
Number of items	12	29	14	28	5	11	37 (18 for very severe dementia)	9
Setting	Community, institution	Community, institution	Community institution	Community, institution	Community, institution	Institution	Institution	Institution
Data collection	Interview with PwD	Interview with PwD	Interview with PwD	Interview with PwD	Interview with PwD	Interview with proxy	Observation	Observation
Rating by	O	O	N/NA/O	Ph, N	O	N/NA	2 N/NA	O, N

Table 5.1 (cont.)

	QOL-AD	DQoL	BASQID	DEMQOL	SEIQoL	QUALID	QUALIDEM	DS-DAT
Stage of dementia	Mild-moderate	Mild-moderate	Mild-moderate	All stages	Mild	Late stage dementia	Mild-severe	Severe
Proxy version available	Yes (CQOL)	No	No	Yes	Yes	Yes	Yes	Yes
Difficulty of application	No training required	No training required	No training required	No training required	Trained interviewer	No training required	No training required	Trained interviewer
Language	C,E,ES,F,G	C,D,E,ES,F,G,	E	E,ES,G,J	E,D,I,G,S	C,CZ,D,E,ES,I,N,S	D,E,G,DA	E,D
Reliability	good	good	moderate	Moderate for mild/moderate dementia	good	Weak to good	Weak to good	good
Validated in	C,E,ES,F,G	E,ES,F,G,	E	E,ES,G,J	E,D	C,CZ,E,ES,N,S	D,G	E,D

E = English; C = Chinese; CZ = Czech; D = Dutch; DA = Danish; ES = Spanish; G = German; I = Italian; J = Japanese; N = Norwegian; S = Swedish; PwD = person with dementia; N = nurse; NA = nurse assistant; Ph = physician; O = other investigators assesses a range of QoL aspects (related to health, social interaction, function, mobility, being occupied, energy and psychological well-being) and is administered via interview. Each question is presented visually on an individual card and orally. Five-point Likert response scales ('not at all satisfied' to 'extremely satisfied', and 'not at all' to 'a great deal') are also printed on individual cards. The scale is based on a conceptual framework generated from in-depth interviews with people with mild to moderate dementia, exploring issues that were important to their QoL and the ways in which dementia impacted these areas. It is considered a robust clinical instrument [17]. The internal consistency, test-retest reliability and construct validity, as well as responsiveness to change, were investigated with sufficient results [16, 31–33].

The Dementia Quality of Life (DEMQOL [34–36]) scale is aimed to measure health-related QoL and consists of the following five subscales: daily activities, health and well-being, cognitive functioning, social relationships and self-concept. It is suitable for use at all stages of dementia and across care settings and is available in several languages. It only takes 10 minutes to administer and requires no specific training. It is administered directly to the person with dementia by means of interview, reflecting the person's opinion on their own QoL.

A proxy version (31 items) is available for people with more advanced dementia. The DEMQOL has good psychometric properties and has been used in Europe in both intervention and cost-effectiveness studies [14, 37]. There is also an algorithm to convert DEMQOL into QALY scores ([38]; see later in this chapter).

These four self-report scales all work with a predefined set of life dimensions. If these dimensions are weighted, this is also done on the basis of weights that are identical for all individuals. Therefore these scales are not really 'subjective' in the sense defined in the previous section, although they are based on self-reports. A personalizable, health-related QoL scale, which asks individuals to indicate the five areas of life they consider most important to their overall QoL, is the Schedule for the Evaluation of Individual Quality of Life (SEIQoL [39]). The scale, which is administered by a trained interviewer, was originally developed for oncology research, but has been used in patients with different diseases, including people with mild (SEIQoL [40, 41]) and moderate dementia (SEIQoL-DW [42, 43]). The psychometric properties of the instrument when used in people with dementia were good in the first small sample studies, but need further investigation. Although the SEIQoL is not widely used in dementia research and clinical practice, we believe that assessment of personalized QoL is a route that needs further investigation. A recent attempt to personalize QoL measurement is described by Hendriks et al. (2021), who calculated personalized QOL-AD and DQoL scores by giving weights to individual QoL domains depending on their importance reported by the individual person with dementia.

3.2 Proxy-Based Instruments

Proxy-based instruments can make use of interviews or of behavioural observation.

i Self-Report/Interview

As mentioned, the QOL-AD and the DEMQOL also have proxy versions which can be used for people with more severe dementia who cannot understand the self-report questions anymore.

Another instrument is the Quality of Life in Late-Stage Dementia (QUALID [44]) scale. This is a short (approximately 5 minutes) interview with a proxy (generally a nurse or nurse aide) on the person's affective state in daily life, signs of comfort and engagement in basic activities, especially geared towards late-stage dementia in long-term care settings. It has good psychometric properties and is widely used in European intervention studies [14, 16, 45, 46]. The scale is available in many languages.

ii Behaviour Observation Instruments

The Quality of Life for People with Dementia (QUALIDEM [47, 48]) instrument is a behaviour observation scale meant for use throughout the dementia 'career' (mild to very severe dementia) for people living in different care settings. The QUALIDEM has nine subscales (care relationship, positive and negative affect, restless/tense behaviour, positive self image, social relations, social isolation, feeling at home and having something to do) which provide a QoL profile. For people with very severe dementia a shortened version is used. The observation scale is easy to administer in 10–15 minutes (preferably by two professional carers) and requires no specific training [49]. The scale is available in Dutch, English, Danish and German [50, 16] and has been increasingly used throughout Europe in the past 10 years.

The fact that the QUALIDEM can be used throughout the dementia 'career' and in different care facilities (including small-scale homelike care settings [49]) makes it useful both for intervention studies in different long-term care settings and for longitudinal studies. The scale has proven sensitive for change in both types of studies [51, 52]. Its psychometric properties have been reported in several studies [47, 48] and reliability and validity of the different subscales are found to be good or acceptable in different stages of the disease [50, 53–55].

The Discomfort Scale Dementia of Alzheimer Type (DS-DAT [56, 57]), an observation-based proxy measure focussing on mood, psychomotor behaviour and discomfort, has been rated as a qualitative good measure, especially useful in palliative and late-stage dementia to assess discomfort, including pain [17]. As such it is used in the context of QoL measurement. Several studies on end-of-life and palliative care successfully applied the scale in nursing home settings [58–60]. In the past decade it has not been used often in dementia care research across Europe.

3.3 Experienced Quality of Life in People with Dementia and Psychosocial Interventions

With the availability of these QoL measures, a growing amount of research has been done in the past decades on factors related to QoL and interventions aimed at improving QoL of people with dementia. Contrary to the widely felt belief in the general public, QoL, as measured by these scales, does not necessarily decline when the dementia progresses [18, 33]. However, awareness of memory deficit in people with dementia does affect their rating of QoL negatively [31] as does increased dependency [32].

In a review of 198 studies Martyr et al. [61] found that greater social engagement, better quality of the current relationship with the carer and religious beliefs/spirituality were moderately associated with better QoL. Another review of 20 studies, however, showed that there is currently no strong or consistent evidence on the effects of elements of the relationship quality between the person with dementia and their main informal carer on institutionalization, hospitalization, death or QoL of people with dementia [62]. For people in residential settings, being cared for in a specialized dementia unit and receiving more person-centred care had small or mainly small positive associations with better QoL. Depression and neuropsychiatric symptoms were moderately associated with poorer QoL.

Many studies into person-centred and psychosocial care interventions for people with dementia showed (some) improved QoL [63]. Kim and Park [64] concluded in their review of 19 interventional studies that, in comparison to regular care, person-centred care in clinical practice for people with dementia reduced agitation, neuropsychiatric symptoms, and depression and improved their QoL. Based on his review of 14 studies into psychological interventions for people with dementia and carers, Poon [65] advises clinicians to routinely involve dyads of people with dementia and their informal caregivers when they aim to improve their QoL. This is in line with the studies into the combined Meeting Centres Support Programme (MCSP) for community-dwelling people with dementia and their carers, which showed that compared to regular day care the combined MCSP had positive effects on QoL such as self-esteem, positive affect and feeling of belonging [28, 66, 67].

Two reviews on the effect of occupational therapy on QoL for people with dementia showed mixed results. Ojagbemi and Owolabi [68] found no conclusive evidence for improved QoL in the 10 studies on occupational therapy interventions they reviewed, whereas Bennett et al. [69] concluded in their review of 15 trials that occupational therapy provided at home may improve the QoL of people with dementia, in addition to better performance of activities of daily living (ADL) and reduction of behavioural and psychological symptoms.

A recent systematic review of 12 studies evaluating cognitive stimulation therapy (CST) showed improvements in cognition, quality of life, depression and impact on caregivers [70, 71]. Ojagbemi and Akin-Ojagbemi [72] found small positive effects of exercise interventions, especially aerobic exercise, on QoL. However, because of inconsistent results in their meta-analysis of (13) trials which included QoL as an outcome measure, they concluded that the evidence on the beneficial effect of exercise interventions on the QoL of people with dementia is yet inconclusive. Positive effects of music therapy on QoL were found in a recent systematic review in addition to effects on depressive symptoms and behaviour problems [59].

Finally, a recent review into 22 randomized controlled trials on reminiscence therapy found some evidence that it can improve QoL in people with dementia [73], although the benefits were small. Further research is suggested to understand who may benefit from what type of reminiscence therapy.

As we have seen before, domains of life included in one instrument to measure QoL are sometimes lacking in other instruments. It would therefore be interesting to investigate whether the different results in different studies are related to the use of different QoL measures.

3.4 Quality of Life and the Concept of Well-Being

When one considers the QoL measures in the previous sections, two observations are striking. First, the measures are targeted at (experienced) QoL, and not at subjective well-being or life satisfaction.[1] At the same time, QoL in dementia is interpreted broadly, including dimensions such as 'being valued by others' or 'having a meaningful life' that are closely related to the eudemonic aspects of life satisfaction. On the other hand, however, it is also narrower than one might expect, since more objective features of life are often not included. An obvious example is the financial situation of persons with dementia (see Chapter 14). The personal economic costs related to dementia may cause economic trouble for many persons with dementia, and income is an important prerequisite to buy enjoyable things (going out, travel, holidays etc.). It is difficult to imagine that having to give up such activities for economic reasons would not have an effect on QoL. This suggests that most scales measure

a kind of 'health-related QoL' (with a broad interpretation of health, including the physical, mental and social domain). Yet, as mentioned before, 'health-related QoL' is a blurred concept, as it cannot be seen independently from other important life dimensions.

Second, in the mild to moderate stage of dementia, self-reporting by persons with dementia is possible and, within the subjective approach, preferable. However, there are only few examples where the selection of life dimensions and the importance attached to them are determined by the persons with dementia themselves. In this sense the most popular scales are not preferentialist. In more severe stages, self-reported measures are generally no longer feasible. The QOL-AD is the only instrument that can be used as a self-report scale until severe dementia (MMSE score of 3). When one resorts to reporting by others (informal carers or health professionals), it is important to distinguish between 'informant ratings', reflecting the informant's appraisal of the person with dementia or based on observations of the behaviour of the person (QUALIDEM [47, 48]), and 'proxy ratings', reflecting the appraisal that the proxy thinks the person with dementia would make [61]. If one takes the subjective approach seriously, proxy ratings should be preferred. Of course, proxy rating is difficult, and empirical research has shown that informal carers or healthcare professionals may take into account a different set of life dimensions than the persons with dementia themselves [74].

4 Quality of Life in Economic Evaluation

4.1 Policy Evaluation

Outcome measurement plays an essential role in all economic (consequentialist) policy evaluations. In cost-effectiveness analysis the costs are usually measured in monetary terms, although this is not always straightforward. Costs can be measured narrowly – focussing just on the immediate policy itself – or more broadly to consider resource impacts across all areas of public and private activity, and including resources that are not bought and sold in any market, such as the time commitments of family and other carers (see

---

[1] Martyr et al. [61] mention in their meta-study that they found data on QoL reported in 205 studies, on well-being in 5 studies and on life satisfaction in 3 studies.

Chapter 14). In this chapter we do not focus on the costs, but only on the measurement of outcomes for people with dementia, more specifically quality of life.

It is important to distinguish different levels of policy evaluation requiring different outcome measures:

- If one aims at comparing and evaluating different treatments and care options for dementia, the outcome measures can be taken from the list of dementia-specific QoL measures we referred to in the previous section. Some studies have focussed on narrow indicators – for example, of cognitive impairment – but many have also made use of existing generic instruments to measure QoL.

- A key ambition of cost-effectiveness analysis is to inform choices within the healthcare budget – for example, what is the share of the healthcare budget that should go to dementia care relative to the share that should go to the reimbursement of expensive cancer drugs? Or how should an increase in the healthcare budget be allocated across different interventions and diagnostic areas? To tackle this kind of issue, one needs an outcome measure that can be applied to the various domains in healthcare – that is, across different diseases and conditions. Measures of dementia-specific QoL or dementia symptoms are then no longer adequate, and one has to use a generic measure. The most widely used of these generic measures is the QALY, but other broader measures of well-being have also been proposed, such as the disability-adjusted life year (DALY) and, more recently, measures of subjective well-being. Our focus in this section is on these generic health measures.

- An important broader policy question is the optimal size of the healthcare budget compared to other uses of economic resources. This requires a comparison of the outcomes obtained with healthcare to the outcomes obtained with other policies (e.g. educational or environmental policies). Health-related QoL measures are then not adequate because they are too narrowly conceived. An overall measure of well-being is needed. It has been common practice historically to use cost-benefit analysis for this

purpose, which means that one also aims to express the value of the outcomes in monetary terms. We do not go into this issue in this chapter, as the discussion about the optimal size of the dementia care budget is taken up in Chapter 14. Suffice it to say that it is rare to see a cost-benefit analysis conducted in the health domain because it is very difficult to convert a clinical measure of outcome (e.g. symptom alleviation, cognition or quality of life) into a monetary value. Comparing costs expended with savings achieved is *not* a cost-benefit analysis.

There is a huge debate on whether it is necessary to include considerations of distributive justice in these economic evaluation exercises, and many specific proposals have been made for how to do this [75]. We do not explicitly discuss that issue in this chapter, except insofar as it has implications for the measurement of QoL in persons with dementia. Indeed, if one wants to differentiate policies or investment of resources between individuals at different levels of well-being, or QoL – for example, by focussing more efforts on those who are worse off – one needs a measure of QoL that is suitable for interpersonal comparisons – that is, that makes it possible to relate the severity of states of dementia to the resulting QoL of those persons.

4.2 Quality-Adjusted Life Years

As noted earlier, decision makers in healthcare systems need to compare outcomes across a range of conditions or diagnostic groups – for example, for the purposes of resource allocation across medical specialty budgets within a hospital, or when taking high-level strategic decisions about which conditions should be prioritized for treatment or support. In these circumstances, condition-specific measures are inadequate and a generic measure is needed.

The QALY is the most widely used such construct: it is a unidimensional measure which captures both life expectancy and the health-related quality of those life years. The QALY is a preference-based measure that belongs in the 'desire-fulfilment' category introduced earlier. Quality scores are conventionally fixed to run from 1, representing perfect health, to 0, representing death. Each year (or part year) of additional life resulting from a healthcare intervention is weighted by this score (often called a 'utility score' in genuflection to utilitarianism) in order to generate a measure of the total number of QALYs gained, and – in economic evaluation – then compared with QALYs gained from an alternative use of the resources used up to deliver the intervention. An example is given in what follows.

The most commonly used tool for generating QALYs is the EuroQoL or EQ-5D. In its original construction, the tool had five dimensions (mobility, self-care, usual activity, pain/discomfort and anxiety/depression), each rated on one of three levels (no problem, some problems and major problems). A later version had five levels for each dimension (bad, rather bad, satisfying, good and very good). These versions are now referred to as EQ-5D-3L and EQ-5D-5L. This particular tool has been used in tens of thousands of evaluations and other studies worldwide. Another long-standing generic QALY–generating tool is the Health Utilities Index (HUI [76]). Both the EQ-5D and the HUI have been used in dementia studies, but may not perform as sensitively as needed given the symptoms typically experienced, and this has led to the development of condition-specific utility-generating measures such as the DEMQOL-U [38]. In a study of a frail older population in the post-hospitalization phase following hip fracture, the EQ-5D-5L and its proxy-completed version (CEQ-5D-5L) were more responsive to the physical recovery trajectory following surgery, whilst the DEMQOL-U and its proxy-completed version (DEMQOL-Proxy-U) were more responsive to changes in delirium and dementia symptoms [77].

If we return to the EQ-5D, we can illustrate a key debating point, which is how to combine the five domains into a unidimensional measure. With the original three-level version there are 245 possible combinations or health states, and with the newer five-level version there are 3,125 possible states. Health economists have sought to assign values to each of these states (i.e. each of these different combinations of mobility, self-care, pain and so on) by conducting exercises which ask samples of people for their preference, using methods such as time trade-off and standard gamble [78]. The resulting values represent the relative importance of different health states. For example, societal weights derived through large field surveys include:

Score = 1.000 was assigned to perfect health-related quality of life: Mobility – no problems, Self-care – no problems, Usual activities – no problems, Pain/discomfort – no problems, Anxiety depression – no problems

Score = 0.727 was obtained from preference ratings of this combination: Mobility – some problems, Self-care – no problems, Usual activities – no problems, Pain/discomfort – some problems, Anxiety depression – no problems

Score = 0.255 was obtained from preference ratings from the field survey for this combination: Mobility – no problems, Self-care – no problems, Usual activities – some problems, Pain/discomfort – some problems, Anxiety depression – major problems

These are the utility scores derived from the EQ-5D-3 L [79], which then can be used to generate QALY measures (see later in this chapter).

How then is the QALY used in resource allocation decisions? Decision makers first need evidence on how different interventions might generate different gains in QALYs, and what it costs to achieve those gains. Resource allocation decisions at a strategic level within the healthcare system will then be based (partly) upon evidence from clinical trials and other studies. The question usually posed is: which available resources (i.e. which patterns of spending on candidate interventions) would be likely to generate the greatest outcome gains from those resources? Trials therefore use measures such as the EQ-5D and the DEMQOL, alongside condition-specific measures (e.g. of cognition, agitation etc.) and tools to measure costs.

The evidence that such an approach would generate is then often summarized by calculating an incremental cost-effectiveness ratio (ICER) for each comparison between interventions. This ratio is equal to the extra (or incremental) cost associated with one intervention compared to another, divided by the extra effect or outcome. The latter could be a measure of cognition or agitation, or it could be a measure of QALY gain. It is important to emphasize that decisions are informed by incremental differences, not by some absolute health-related quality of life. From this efficiency standpoint, the decision-making focus is on how to achieve the greatest impact from the resources that are managed (sometimes crudely referred to as 'biggest bang for the buck'), and not on comparisons of how different conditions are associated with higher or lower quality of life. It is also important to emphasize that decisions are not solely based on ICER values, as other considerations such as human rights and distributional justice also play a part [80].

In some countries, resource allocation decisions are informed (but not determined) by formalized approaches: health technology assessment bodies may employ cost-utility thresholds. In England, for example, the National Institute for Health and Care Excellence (NICE) employs a threshold of between £20,000 and £30,000 per QALY: if an intervention costs less than this threshold, it is more likely to be recommended for use across the public healthcare system, whereas an intervention costing more than £30,000 to achieve one additional QALY is unlikely to be recommended. However, as noted earlier, other considerations also influence decisions, such as fairness and evaluation findings in relation to outcomes that are not adequately reflected in the more reductionist QALY measure: the threshold is always a guide and not a rigid rule [81]. There are also ongoing arguments about the value at which any such threshold should be set [82]. A number of countries also now employ similar health technology appraisal procedures.

A couple of examples can be offered. The DOMINO study looked at pharmacotherapy for treating people with Alzheimer's disease when their symptoms become severe: the evaluation question was whether continuing donepezil treatment (which is used in the earlier stages of the disease) or commencing memantine (a medication with a different mechanism of action) was more effective and cost-effective for patients with moderate to severe Alzheimer's disease. A 52-week trial conducted in the UK randomized patients who had consented to participate to one of four groups: continue donepezil, discontinue donepezil, discontinue donepezil and start memantine, or continue donepezil and start memantine. Both donepezil and memantine are generic medications, and the trial was funded by the UK Medical Research Council and UK Alzheimer's Society, not by pharmaceutical companies.

To capture as many effects as feasible in a trial of this nature, the DOMINO research team measured cognition, functioning in ADL, behavioural and psychological symptoms, dementia-specific health-related QoL (DEMQOL-Proxy, rated by carers); generic health-related QoL (EQ-5D-3L, again rated by carers) and the health status of family or other unpaid carers. The economic evaluation was therefore able to look at a range of dementia-specific symptoms, as well as QALY scores generated from both generic and condition-specific instruments. The EQ-5D-3L was completed at five time points: at baseline (when a patient was randomized to a particular drug option) and then 6, 18, 30 and 52 weeks later. Utility scores were assigned to each observed combination of scores on the five dimensions using societal weights [79]. For patients getting donepezil alone, the mean utility scores were 0.57 at baseline, 0.56 at 6 weeks, 0.52 at 18 weeks, 0.51 at 30 weeks and 0.48 at 52 weeks. For the placebo group, the respective scores were 0.55, 0.48, 0.40, 0.37 and 0.26 [83]. Using what is called the area-under-curve method (what mathematicians call integration), it is then possible to calculate the difference in QALYs between the two patient groups over the full 52-week period of the trial. For example, between baseline and 6 weeks the utility score for the donepezil group fell 0.01 whilst the score for the placebo group fell by 0.07. This represents a difference in QALYs of 0.0069 (= difference in utility fall of 0.06, multiplied by 6/52 of a year). In the next period (from 6 to 18 weeks) the respective reductions were 0.04 for donepezil and 0.08 for placebo, representing a difference of 0.0092 QALYs. Over the course of each of the time intervals between data collection points, the health of both groups of patients got worse, but the decline was noticeably greater for the placebo group. By the end of the trial, the placebo group had lost 0.11 of a QALY more than the donepezil group, which was statistically significant. It would also be noticeably different for any person experiencing such a difference in health-related QoL.

It was found in the DOMINO trial that continuing donepezil for 52 weeks was more cost-effective than discontinuation, based on indicators of cognition, ADL and health-related QoL. Starting memantine was more cost-effective than discontinuing donepezil. Donepezil and memantine combined was not more cost-effective than donepezil alone [83, 84]. The trial also found that stopping donepezil treatment increased the risk of nursing home placement during the 52-week trial period, but not subsequently [85]. Findings from the study, including the cost-per-QALY estimates, influenced new NICE [86] recommendations for medication use in treating Alzheimer's disease in England.

A second example is a study of family carers of people with dementia, where the EQ-5D-3L was used to assess the impact of a manual-based coping strategy on those carers. Again, a randomized trial design was used, comparing the new intervention (called START) with usual forms of carer support, with follow-up for as long as 6 years [87]. Carers in the intervention group were found to have significantly better outcomes as measured in terms of symptoms of mental illness linked to the stress of caring, as well as QALY gains [88]. Costs were actually slightly higher for the carers who received the coping strategy intervention, compared to those who were supported as usual, but the incremental cost-effectiveness ratio was only £6,000 per QALY gained, considerably below the usual NICE threshold.

By way of illustration, the figures in Table 5.2 show utility scores from four measures: the DEMQOL and the EQ-5D completed by older people with dementia, and the DEMQOL-Proxy and the EQ-5D proxy completed about those same people by their main carers. Data come originally from the Study of the Use of Antidepressants for Depression in Dementia (SADD) study [89] and were reanalysed by Mulhern et al. [38]. Mean values for these four measures are reported for people with dementia grouped by severity of cognitive impairment, measured by the MMSE [90]. The table shows a number of things: mean scores vary with severity of cognitive impairment, but not greatly; scores differ quite noticeably between instruments

(compare the EQ-5D with the DEMQOL); and scores differ between self-report and proxy report, especially for the EQ-5D.

It is important to remember that dementia symptoms extend beyond cognitive impairment, and it may be other symptoms that drive QoL differences [91]. Classifying dementia in terms of severity of cognitive impairment alone is therefore rather coarse. This also illustrates the unavoidable trade-off between specific and generic scales, to which we return in Section 5. Of course, in decision-making contexts about, for example, which drug to use for a particular condition, or which of two interventions for different diseases should be prioritized, it is incremental rather than absolute values of health-related QoL (utility) that would be compared.

There is another important issue with respect to QALY measurement: who is to set the values for the different health states? To answer this question, one can take two different perspectives. If the aim is to set priorities between interventions in different health domains, use should be made of a generic scale (like the EQ-5D), and it is natural to assume that the health values corresponding to the different states should be set by the (average) citizen. In deciding about the allocation of the overall healthcare budget, the preferences of all citizens should count, since they ultimately have to pay the bill. If the aim is to focus specifically on (different treatments for) dementia, this is less

Table 5.2 Utility values generated from the EQ-5D and the DEMQOL, and their proxy versions, for people with different severities of cognitive impairment

	Cognitive impairment		
	Mild (MMSE score > 20)	Moderate (MMSE 20–10)	Severe (MMSE < 10)
EQ-5D			
N	101	114	25
Mean (SD)	0.71 (0.26)	0.69 (0.27)	0.67 (0.33)
CEQ-5D			
N	101	118	30
Mean (SD)	0.57 (0.28)	0.47 (0.33)	0.43 (0.31)
DEMQOL-U			
N	100	113	22
Mean (SD)	0.82 (0.09)	0.80 (0.11)	0.79 (0.12)
DEMQOL-U-Proxy			
N	99	118	30
Mean (SD)	0.79 (0.09)	0.78 (0.10)	0.79 (0.11)

straightforward. Surely, the average citizen has an imperfect and biased idea of what it means to live with dementia – and if (s)he is sufficiently rational, (s)he will be aware of this imperfect knowledge. Why would (s)he not trust the evaluation of this situation by the experience experts – that is, the persons with dementia themselves?[2] Since the 'broad' and the 'narrow' perspectives are complementary, it would be good practice to give policymakers information on both.

4.3 Broader Generic Well-Being Scales

Many economists accept the limitations of the QALY as a health-related QoL measure. Some newly proposed well-being measures that are growing in popularity are inspired by the capability approach ([93] gives an overview). The best known of these measures is the ICEpop CAPability (ICECAP) measure, with a specific version, the ICECAP-O, for older people [94]. The ICECAP-O measures five attributes: attachment (love and friendship), security (thinking about the future without concern), role (doing things that make you feel valued), enjoyment (pleasure) and control (independence) [95].

The ICECAP-O scale is generic and can therefore be used to compare the (cost-)effectiveness of different types of healthcare interventions for older patients. At the same time, the list of included attributes immediately shows that it is closely related to the dementia-specific scales of QoL as described in the previous section. In fact, the ICECAP-O has been validated for nursing home residents with dementia [96]. Of course, being a generic scale, it offers less detailed information that is specifically relevant for measuring the QoL of persons with dementia.

There has been discussion about how well the ICECAP measures (and similar instruments) indeed capture the basic intuitions of the capability approach (see e.g. [93]). Crucial in this respect is the distinction between the attained level of functioning – and the ability to reach the various functionings. For a true capability approach, the latter should be the main focus of attention. The questionnaires try to make this operational through the specific formulation of the questions

('I am able to . . . ', 'I can . . . '), but one can doubt whether this is sufficient to make a credible distinction between attainments and opportunities.

Another broad outcome measure that is quite widely used is the Adult Social Care Outcomes Toolkit (ASCOT [97]), built on a slightly different conceptual basis from the ICECAP, but with shared roots in capability theory and with an emphasis on choice and control. The ASCOT has eight domains linked to aspects of QoL relevant to social care needs (control over daily life, personal cleanliness and comfort, food and drink, personal safety, social participation and involvement, occupation, accommodation cleanliness and comfort and dignity). Given its social care focus, it is certainly relevant to people living with dementia. There is also a version for measuring carers' social care-related quality of life [98]. It is possible to convert ASCOT scores into QALY-like measures.

5 Specificity and Coherence: Back to the Fundamental Questions

Let us start from a striking observation: there are only very few links between researchers working in the different domains discussed in the previous sections. Most philosophers have a primitive idea about the empirical literature on well-being scales; most social scientists are too pragmatic to be very much interested in the fundamental philosophical questions. Apart from some important work on cross-validation, the literature on generic outcomes in economic evaluation has developed largely independently of the work on the construction of dementia-specific QoL scales. And even within this domain of specific QoL scales, there is a long list of different scales. What to make of this list of different approaches?

Of course, one can claim that there is no problem, as these different scales and approaches serve different purposes – and that in each specific case one has to select the instrument that best matches the specific objectives one wants to reach with specific interventions [43]. From this perspective, it is not a problem to use QALYs for economic evaluation, other specific scales to evaluate the effectiveness of different psychological and psychosocial interventions, and yet other scales to compare the QoL of different groups of persons with dementia or the relative success of different care settings in promoting QoL.

---

[2] A balanced overview of the literature advocating this position can be found in [92].

It is indeed obvious that some scales are better suited for some purposes and other scales for other purposes and that the analyst has to choose the best for each situation. However, this should not be used as an easy excuse to remain within one's own disciplinary boundaries and to avoid looking at the alternatives. First, in restricting oneself to a narrow perspective, one misses the opportunity to learn from other perspectives. Philosophical reasoning is needed to better understand the implicit value judgements underlying the operational scales. The experience with the specific detailed scales to measure the QoL of persons with dementia can improve the coarse classifications used in the QALY approach to dementia. Philosophers can get a better grip on well-being by studying in detail the experiences of persons with dementia, as measured by social scientists.

Second, and more important from a policy point of view, to get at coherent policies, one should at least aim at using scales that are consistent with each other. Assume one analysis uses the dementia-specific scale A to evaluate the cost-effectiveness of different interventions x and y in the context of dementia. Another scale B is used for a cost-effectiveness analysis of x and y in a context of priority setting within the healthcare budget. Scale B is a generic scale of health-related QoL with a coarse two-category classification. It is then possible that x is preferred to y according to scale A while at the same time based on scale B x is below the bar and y above the bar when compared to interventions in other healthcare domains. What should the policymaker then decide?

Basic questions have to be answered if we aim at a more coherent set of scales. Some of these questions are methodological, while some are basically normative.

5.1 Specific versus Generic

There is obviously a relationship between the specificity of QoL scales on one hand and the practical feasibility of implementing them in different contexts on the other. Dementia-specific scales can give detailed information on QoL in dementia, but they are not useful if we want to go beyond the dementia domain and compare the effectiveness of interventions in different healthcare sectors. On the other hand, generic scales do not capture the specific information needed for

disease-specific analyses and evaluation of interventions. All of these statements are trivial. Yet, as shown by the example given previously, if the generic and the disease-specific scales are not consistent, it is possible that they result in conflicting policy advice. More work is needed to cross-validate the two types of scales. One should check, for example, whether the ordinal ranking of the QoL of different individuals is the same with both types of scales (taking into account that there may be large indifference classes with some simple generic scales).

Even more challenging issues arise when one wants to broaden the concept of well-being beyond 'health-related QoL'. In some policy settings such a broader concept is certainly needed. Take the example of the economic situation of persons with dementia living at home. Suppose one could use a given budget either to provide people with dementia with an income, which would allow them to have better material conditions (a better house, a richer use of leisure time), or to give them better professional care, or to support their informal carers both psychologically and economically. To compare the effects of these three policies on the lives of the persons with dementia, one needs a notion of well-being that goes beyond health-related dimensions. This raises immediately the difficult issue of how these various dimensions then can be aggregated to arrive at one overall measure. We return to this issue.

In fact, the previous example also draws our attention to the position of the informal carers. Carers will be affected by many policies in the context of dementia. The effects on their own QoL should therefore be taken into account. We know that health effects are an important part of the burden of carers (see Chapter 7), but for them also other aspects certainly are crucial, such as income loss or effects on job satisfaction and social integration as a consequence of having had to give up their labour market position. If we want to evaluate policy measures or interventions that have effects on the persons with dementia and on their carers, and we want to take into account potential trade-offs between the QoL outcomes for both groups, we need a measure that can capture the relevant life domains for both. This is an additional argument to think about how to devise broader measures of well-being.

Specific scales are likely to be sufficient in many contexts – for example, when one wants to evaluate the effectiveness of different psychological and psychosocial interventions. From an analytical point of view, however, a challenging question is how they can be integrated into such a broader concept of well-being.

5.2 Subjective versus Objective

The most fundamental choice to be made is about the basic philosophical foundation of the QoL concept to be implemented. As suggested before, this choice will be motivated by a mixture of conceptual and normative considerations. Throughout this chapter (and this book) we have opted for an approach to dementia emphasizing the dignity of persons with dementia, respect for their own objectives, and the capacities they have to give meaning to their life and to be socially integrated. As mentioned before, this suggests an a priori position in favour of the more subjective (preferentialist) scales.

We certainly see this shift in the development of the dementia-specific QoL scales that have been developed in the literature (see Section 3). Yet it remains to some extent ambiguous whether these scales are really 'subjective', in the sense that they respect the wishes and desires (the preferences) of the persons with dementia, or that they are more closely linked to what we called 'mental state' approaches.

The issue can be illustrated with the treatment of adaptive and coping strategies. There is no doubt that adaptation to the new situation and coping with deteriorating cognitive possibilities and the practical, emotional and social consequences are essential strategies for persons with dementia to maintain well-being. Helping persons with dementia to cope better with their growing cognitive and functional problems as well as the emotional and social consequences of these problems is an important element in any successful care strategy. Coping and adaptation may explain to some extent why self-ratings of QoL by persons with dementia are often higher than the ratings by carers – and certainly higher than the expectations in the general population. Yet they also raise a difficult problem for interpersonal comparisons of QoL. This is closely related to Sen's criticism on the use of mental state measures of well-being introduced in Section 2.

We can make this more specific in the context of dementia (see [99] for a more general application to successful ageing). Consider a person moving through different stages of severity of the disease. Certainly, if one asked him in the beginning whether he would like to stop that process of cognitive deterioration, he is very likely to say yes. He is likely to prefer a less severe state of dementia to a more severe state. In a preferentialist approach more severe states of dementia are valued less. Yet, if he manages to cope well with the process, it is possible that his self-reported QoL does not decline very much or even remains the same. Evaluating QoL on the basis of wishes and desires (in which the less severe state would be better) then comes into conflict with evaluation on the basis of reported QoL (in which there is no decline). This is not only a theoretical curiosity. It may have deep implications for the optimal care strategy, if this strategy aims at improving the measured QoL. To put it very provocatively: if persons with dementia can adapt almost fully to the worsening of their physical condition, and we take this up in our measure of QoL, then there is no reason anymore to worry about the whole process of moving into more severe stages of dementia. Of course, this does not detract from the basic message that many people need support in the adaptation and coping process, also because of the deteriorating cognitive appraisal of situations, and that they can really suffer if this support is inadequate as shown by behavioural and mood symptoms and people being emotionally out of balance.

The example illustrates that the choice of a measure of QoL has strong normative implications. It relates to the view we have on well-being, on what is a good life and on the identity of human beings. Humans could not survive if they were not able to adapt to and cope with deteriorating circumstances, and they certainly should be helped (and learnt) to adapt and to cope. But striving for adaptation should not hamper the ambition to improve the circumstances themselves.

5.3 Multidimensional Standard versus Weighted

Everybody agrees that QoL of persons with dementia (as of all other human beings) consists of different dimensions. In principle, in a subjective approach, one should first check which dimensions matter for the persons themselves, but it can reasonably be assumed that the relevant dimensions will be very similar for different persons. In fact, as we have seen, while different scales include different dimensions, in general there is much overlap. Positive and negative affect, the quality of social interactions and the feeling of having a meaningful life and of remaining 'useful for others' are essential elements in most dementia specific scales. It is less clear, however, that all persons attach the same weight to these dimensions: it is even very likely that they have different ideas about what is more or less important to have a good life. How should this issue of weighting the dimensions be tackled?

One possible route to escape this thorny issue is not weighting at all and remaining contented with a profile of indicators that together describe the QoL of the person with dementia. This profile approach may indeed be sufficient for a purely descriptive exercise. Yet it is not useful if we want to rank the QoL of different individuals, to evaluate the effectiveness of different interventions or to compare the impact of quality care in different institutions. We then need one aggregate measure of QoL, and ultimately this means that we need to apply a set of weights to the different dimensions.

Economists tend to claim that the QALY measure is a 'preference-based' aggregate measure and to use this as a criterion to differentiate it from the psychological scales. Yet we discussed some of the problems with the interpretation of the QALYs in Section 4. Surely, if the QALY for persons with dementia is based on the average (or median) answer of a representative sample of the population, it does not at all capture inter-individual differences.

In the psychological scaling literature it is common to use either simple summation or statistical techniques to aggregate. This practice clashes with the inherently evaluative nature of the weighing system. Taking a simple sum means that all dimensions get the same weight – yet there is no good reason to assume that they are all equally important for QoL. Statistical techniques usually derive the weighing system on the basis of the correlation between the different measures, often in terms of the fraction of the common variation that is explained by the different dimensions. However, fixing the weights to aggregate different life dimensions is an evaluative and not a statistical exercise. This question cannot be answered by statistical techniques.

In fact, one can reasonably argue that all weighting schemes that apply the same set of weights to calculate the QoL for different individuals are difficult to square with the existence of individual differences in ideas about what is a good life. If such a uniform weighting scheme boils down to a kind of group average of individual opinions, it can perhaps give some idea about average QoL at the group level, but 'average' scores will not give a reliable image of the variation of QoL *within* the group – that is, at the level of the persons involved. Really respecting the personal opinions on QoL of the persons with dementia would mean also taking serious the heterogeneity in their life perspectives (what economists would call preference heterogeneity). The weights of the dimensions should then be based on the individual evaluations of the importance of each dimension, as proposed by Hendriks et al. [100] (see 3.1).

This is obviously crucial when we want to evaluate the effectiveness of different psychological and psychosocial interventions. Suppose that an intervention affects one dimension positively for all persons (let us say the feeling of social integration) but another dimension negatively (let us say feelings of security). Depending on the preferences of the individual person with dementia, the net effect on QoL may be negative for some and positive for others. Just using the same scale with an identical weighting scheme may then be misleading – in fact, the estimated average QoL will depend on the composition of the perspectives on QoL within the group and is therefore likely to be unstable over time and over different settings.

Taking interpersonal preference heterogeneity into account is not only important for measuring the 'average' effectiveness of different interventions. It is also crucial to respect the differences between different persons with dementia. From a broader perspective, it is essential to take account of distributional considerations. While this may seem less relevant at the micro level, where all persons with dementia should count equally, it becomes very important at the macro level, if decisions have to be taken about the allocation of resources to the treatment and the care of different (sub)groups of persons with dementia. If we want these macro decisions to take account of the QoL of these different (sub)groups, we need a measure that respects their own opinions about what is important in life.

We think the elaboration of individual-specific measures of QoL is an important domain for further research. Different methodological tracks can be followed. One possibility is to ask directly for the relevant weights (see e.g. [100]). Another is to ask individuals to indicate, for instance, the five areas of life they consider most important to their overall QoL, as done with the SEIQoL (see e.g. [41]). A third option is the use of discrete choice models. Inspiration can also be found in the growing economic literature on measuring well-being with due respect for individual preferences (for an overview see [2] and [101]).

Note that the distinction between measuring the 'performance' on different life dimensions and devising a set of weights to construct an aggregate indicator may influence the reliability of proxy reporting. Proxies may have a good idea of the value of the different life dimensions for a person with dementia (How well is the person socially integrated? Does he/she feel safe in their environment?), but it is much more difficult for them as external observers to evaluate the relative importance of these different dimensions for the individual person with dementia. (How important are social integration and feelings of safety for the person concerned?)

While we have emphasized the difficulties related to taking into account interpersonal preference heterogeneity, introducing flexible weights has the convenient side effect that it makes the choice of the relevant dimensions easier for designers of QoL measures. In fact, one can start from a broad all-encompassing list of dimensions and apply this list to everybody. If a given dimension is irrelevant for a person, this will be reflected in a zero weight given to this dimension.

The difficult issue of devising an individual-specific weighting system for the dimensions of life is only relevant within a subjective, preferentialist approach. For an objectivist, a uniform set of weights is perfectly acceptable, if it captures the objectively given ideal of a good life or of human flourishing. For a utilitarian mental state approach, the different dimensions only matter insofar as they contribute to happiness or life satisfaction. A direct one-dimensional measure of life satisfaction would therefore be a sufficient measure of individual QoL or well-being, and there would then in fact be no need to consider the different dimensions separately. We have seen, however, that this mental state approach does not necessarily reflect individual opinions about the good life.

6 Conclusion

To evaluate psychological and psychosocial interventions or to decide whether it is cost-effective to reimburse specific therapies or medicines, one needs a measure of the QoL of the persons with dementia and their carers. A large battery of specific dementia scales is available that can be used to evaluate psychological and psychosocial interventions, while cost-effectiveness is usually analysed with generic QALY–type health measures. While there are certainly attempts to cross-validate some of these measures, more and better interdisciplinary communication between analysts in the different fields could lead to useful cross-fertilization. Of even greater importance, different measures of QoL reflect different fundamental perspectives on what makes a good life. The choice between various measures cannot be made only on statistical or technical grounds because it has crucial ethical implications. From an ethical perspective that emphasizes the dignity and the lived experience of persons with dementia themselves, more attention should be given to the construction of scales that sufficiently take into account that different persons with dementia may have widely different views on the importance of the various life domains.

References

1. Parfit D. *Reasons and Persons*. Oxford, Clarendon, 1984.

2. Decancq K, Fleurbaey M, Schokkaert, E. Inequality, income and well-being. In Atkinson A, Bourguignon F, eds. *Handbook of Income Distribution, Vol. 2A*. New York, Elsevier, 2015; 67–140.

3. Hurka T. Objective goods. In Adler M, Fleurbaey M, eds. *Oxford Handbook of Well-Being and Public Policy*. Oxford, Oxford University Press, 2016; 379–402.

4. Sen A. *On Ethics and Economics*. Oxford, Oxford University Press, 1987.

5. Robeyns I. *Wellbeing, Freedom and Social Justice*. Cambridge, Open Book, 2017.

6. Nussbaum M. *Women and Human Development: The Capabilities Approach*. Cambridge, Cambridge University Press, 2000.

7. Hausman D. *Valuing Health: Well-Being, Freedom, and Suffering.* Oxford, Oxford University Press, 2015.

8. Huber M, Knottnerus JA, Green L, Van der Horst H, Jadad A, et al. How should we define health? *British Medical Journal* 2011; **343**: d4163.

9. Dröes RM, INTERDEM Social Health Taskforce. Social health and dementia: A European consensus on the operationalization of the concept and directions for research and practice. *Aging and Mental Health* 2017; **21**: 4–17.

10. Thorgrimson L, Selwood A, Spector A, Royan L, Madariaga Lopez M, et al. Whose quality of life is it anyway? The validity and reliability of the Quality of Life-Alzheimer's Disease (QOL-AD). *Alzheimer's Disease & Associated Disorders* 2003; **17**, 201–8.

11. Logsdon RG, Gibbons LE, McCurry SM, Teri L. Assessing quality of life in older adults with cognitive impairment. *Psychosomatic Medicine* 2002 May–Jun; **64**(3): 510–19.

12. Moniz-Cook E, Vernooij-Dassen M, Woods R, Verhey F, Chattat R, et al. For the Interdem group A European Consensus on outcome measures for psychosocial intervention research in dementia care. *Aging & Mental Health* 2008; **12**(1): 14–29.

13. Sheehan B. Assessment scales in dementia. *Therapeutic Advances in Neurological Disorders* 2005; **5**(6): 349–58.

14. Bowling A, Rowe G, Adams S, Sands P, Samsi, K, et al. Quality of life in dementia: A systematically conducted narrative review of dementia-specific measurement scales. *Aging & Mental Health* 2015; **19**(1): 13–31.

15. Nehen H-G, Hermann DM. Supporting dementia patients and their caregivers in daily life challenges: Review of physical, cognitive and psychosocial intervention studies. *European Journal of Neurology* 2015; **22**(2): 246–e20.

16. Dichter MN, Schwab CG, Meyer G, Bartholomeyczik S, Halek M. Linguistic validation and reliability properties are weak investigated of most dementia-specific quality of life measurements: A systematic review. *Journal of Clinical Epidemiology* 2016 Feb; **70**: 233–45.

17. Missotten P, Dupuis G, Adam S. Dementia-specific quality of life instruments: A conceptual analysis. *International Psychogeriatrics* 2016; **28**(8): 1245–62.

18. Hoe J, Hancock G, Livingston G, Woods B, Challis D, Orrell M. Changes in the quality of life of people with dementia living in care homes. *Alzheimer Disease and Associated Disorders* 2009; **23**(3): 285–90.

19. Vogel A, Bhattacharya S, Waldorff FB, Waldemar G. Proxy-rated quality of life in Alzheimer's disease: a three-year longitudinal study. *International Psychogeriatrics* 2012 Jan; **24**(1): 82–9.

20. Orrell M, Aguirre E, Spector A, Hoare Z, Woods RT, et al. Maintenance cognitive stimulation therapy for dementia: Single-blind, multicentre, pragmatic randomised controlled trial. *British Journal of Psychiatry* 2014 Jun; **204**(6): 454–61.

21. Bosboom PR, Almeida OP. Do changes in specific cognitive functions predict changes in health-related quality of life in people with Alzheimer's disease? *International Journal of Geriatric Psychiatry* 2014 Jul; **29**(7): 694–703.

22. Edelman P, Fulton BR, Kuhn D, Chang CH. A comparison of three methods of measuring dementia-specific quality of life: Perspectives of residents, staff, and observers. *Gerontologist* 2005; 45 Spec No. 1 (1):27e36.

23. Brod M, Stewart AL, Sands L, Walton P. Conceptualization and measurement of quality of life in dementia: The dementia quality of life instrument (DQoL). *Gerontologist* 1999 Feb; **39**(1): 25–35.

24. Moyle W, Gracia N, Murfield JE, Griffiths SG, Venturato L. Assessing quality of life of older people with dementia in long-term care: A comparison of two self-report measures. *Journal of Clinical Nursing* 2012; **21**(11–12): 1632–40.

25. Wolak-Thierry A, Novella JL, Barbe C, Morrone I, Mahmoudi R, Jolly D. Comparison of QOL-AD and DQoL in elderly with Alzheimer's disease. *Aging and Mental Health* 2015; **19**(3): 274–8.

26. Graff MJ, Vernooij-Dassen MJ, Thijssen M, Dekker J, Hoefnagels WH, Olderikkert MG. Effects of community occupational therapy on quality of life, mood, and health status in dementia patients and their caregivers: A randomized controlled trial. *Journals of Gerontology, Series A: Biological Sciences and Medical Sciences* 2007; **62**(9): 1002–9.

27. Te Boekhorst S, Depla MF, De Lange J, Pot AM, Eefsting JA. The effects of group living homes on older people with dementia: A comparison with traditional nursing home care. *International Journal of Geriatric Psychiatry* 2009 Sep; **24**(9): 970–8.

28. Brooker D, Evans SC, Evans SB, Bray J, Saibene FL, et al. Evaluation of the implementation of the Meeting Centres Support Program in Italy, Poland, and the UK: Exploration of the effects on people with dementia. *International Journal of Geriatric Psychiatry* 2018 Jul; **33**(7): 883–92.

29. Trigg R, Skevington SM, Jones RW. How can we best assess the quality of life of people with dementia? The Bath assessment of subjective

quality of life in dementia (BASQID). *Gerontologist* 2007; **47**: 789–97.

30. Trigg R, Jones RW, Skevington SM. Can people with mild to moderate dementia provide reliable answers about their quality of life? *Age & Ageing* 2007; **36**: 663–9.

31. Trigg R, Watts S, Jones R, Tod A. Predictors of quality of life ratings from persons with dementia: The role of insight. *International Journal of Geriatric Psychiatry* 2011 Jan; **26**(1): 83–91.

32. Trigg R, Jones R, Lacey L, Niecko T. Relationship between patient self-assessed and proxy-assessed quality of life (QoL) and patient dependence on others as illness progresses in Alzheimer's disease: Results from the Dependence in Alzheimer's Disease in England (DADE) study. *Alzheimer's and Dementia* 2012; **8**(4): Suppl., P250–P251.

33. Trigg R, Jones RW, Knapp M, King D, Lacey LA, DADE-2 Investigator Groups. The relationship between changes in quality of life outcomes and progression of Alzheimer's disease: Results from the dependence in AD in England 2 longitudinal study. *International Journal of Geriatric Psychiatry* 2015; **30**(4): 400–8.

34. Smith SC, Lamping DL, Banerjee S, Harwood RH, Foley B, et al. Measurement of health-related quality of life for people with dementia: Development of a new instrument (DEMQOL) and an evaluation of current methodology. *Health Technology Assessment* 2005; **9**(193): III–IV.

35. Smith SC, Murray J, Banerjee S, Foley B, Cook JC, Lamping DL, et al. What constitutes health-related quality of life in dementia? Development of a conceptual framework for people with dementia and their carers. *International Journal of Geriatric Psychiatry* 2005; **20**: 889–95.

36. Banerjee S, Smith SC, Lamping DL, et al. Quality of life in dementia: More than just cognition. An analysis of associations with quality of life in dementia. *Journal of Neurology, Neurosurgery and Psychiatry* 2006; **77**: 146–8.

37. Voigt-Radloff S, Leonhart R, Schützwohl M, Jurjanz L, Reuster T, et al. Dementia quality of life instrument: Construct and concurrent validity in patients with mild to moderate dementia. *European Journal of Neurology* 2012; **19**(3): 376–84.

38. Mulhern B, Rowen D, Brazier J, Smith S, Romeo R, et al. Development of DEMQOL-U and DEMQOL-PROXY-U: Generation of preference-based indices from DEMQOL and DEMQOL-PROXY for use in economic evaluation. *Health Technology Assessment* 2013; **17**: 5.

39. McGee HM, O'Boyle CA, Hickey A et al. Assessing the quality of life of the individual: The SEIQoL with a healthy and a gastroenterology unit population. *Psychological Medicine* 1991; **21**: 749–59.

40. Coen R, O'Mahony D, O'Boyle C, et al. Measuring the quality of life of dementia patients using the Schedule for the Evaluation of Individual Quality of Life. *Irish Journal of Psychology* 1993; **14**: 154–63.

41. Schölzel-Dorenbos CJ [Measurement of quality of life in patients with dementia of Alzheimer type and their caregivers: Schedule for the Evaluation of Individual Quality of Life (SEIQoL)]. *Tijdschrift voor Gerontologie en Geriatrie* 2000 Feb; **31**(1): 23–6.

42. Hickey AM, Bury G, O'Boyle CA, Bradley F, O'Kelly FD, Shannon W. A new short form individual quality of life measure (SEIQoL-DW): Application in a cohort of individuals with HIV/AIDS. *British Medical Journal* 1996 Jul 6; **313** (7048): 29–33.

43. Schölzel-Dorenbos CJM, Ettema TP, Boelens-Van der Knoop ECC, Bos J, Gerritsen DL, Hoogeveen F, et al. Evaluating the outcome of psychosocial and pharmacological interventions on quality of life of people with dementia: When to use what QoL instrument? *International Journal of Geriatric Psychiatry* 2007; **22**: 511–19.

44. Weiner MF, Martin-Cook K, Svetlik DA, Saine K, Foster B, Fontain CS. The quality of life in late-stage dementia (QUALID) scale. *Journal of the American Medical Directors' Association* 2000; **1**: 114–16.

45. Schalkwijk D, Verlare LR, Muller MT, Knol DL, Van der Steen JT. [Measuring quality of life in nursing home residents with severe dementia: Psychometric properties of the QUALID scale] [Article in Dutch]. *Tijdschrift voor Gerontologie en Geriatrie* 2009 Oct; **40**(5): 184–92.

46. Perales J, Cosco TD, Stephan B, Haro JM, Brayne C. Health-related quality-of-life instruments for Alzheimer's disease and mixed dementia. *International Psychogeriatrics* 2013; **25**(5): 691–706.

47. Ettema TP, Dröes RM, De Lange J, Ooms ME, Mellenbergh GJ, Ribbe MW. The QUALIDEM: Development and evaluation of a dementia specific quality of life instrument. Part I: scalability, reliability and internal structure. *International Journal of Geriatric Psychiatry* 2007; **22**(6): 549–56.

48. Ettema TP, Dröes RM, De Lange J, Ooms ME, Mellenbergh GJ, Ribbe MW. The QUALIDEM: Development and evaluation of a dementia specific Quality of Life instrument. Part II: Validation. *International Journal of Geriatric Psychiatry* 2007; **22**(5): 424–30.

49. Gräske J, Verbeek H, Gellert P, Fischer T, Kuhlmey A, Wolf-Ostermann K. How to measure quality of life in shared-housing arrangements? A comparison of dementia-specific instruments. *Quality of Life Research* 2014; 23(2): 549–59.

50. Dichter MN, Dortmann O, Halek M, Meyer G, Holle D, et al. Scalability and internal consistency of the German version of the dementia-specific quality of life instrument QUALIDEM in nursing homes: A secondary data analysis. *Health and Quality of Life Outcomes* 2013 Jun; 5(11): 91.

51. Van de Ven-Vakhteeva J, Bor H, Wetzels RB, Koopmans RT, Zuidema SU. The impact of antipsychotics and neuropsychiatric symptoms on the quality of life of people with dementia living in nursing homes. *International Journal of Geriatric Psychiatry* 2013 May; 28(5): 530–8.

52. Oudman E, Veurink B. Quality of life in nursing home residents with advanced dementia: A 2-year follow-up. *Psychogeriatrics* 2014 Dec; 14(4): 235–40.

53. Aspden T, Bradshaw SA, Playford ED, Riazi A. Quality-of-life measures for use within care homes: A systematic review of their measurement properties. *Age and Ageing* 2014; 43(5): 596–603.

54. Dichter MN, Schwab CG, Meyer G, Bartholomeyczik S, Dortmann O, Halek M. Measuring the quality of life in mild to very severe dementia: Testing the inter-rater and intra-rater reliability of the German version of the QUALIDEM. *International Psychogeriatrics* 2014; 26(5): 825–36.

55. Bouman AIE, Ettema TP, Wetzels RB, Van Beek APA, De Lange J, Dröes RM. Evaluation of QUALIDEM: A dementia-specific quality of life instrument for persons with dementia in residential settings. Scalability and reliability of subscales in four Dutch field surveys. *International Journal of Geriatric Psychiatry* 2011; 26(7): 711–22.

56. Hurley AC, Volicer B, Hanrahan PA, Houde S, Volicer L. Assessment of discomfort in advanced Alzheimer patients. *Research in Nursing & Health* 1992; 15, 369–77.

57. Volicer L, Hurley A, Canberg L. A model of psychological well-being in advanced dementia. *Journal of Mental Health & Aging* 1999; 5: 83–94.

58. Van der Steen JT, Pasman HR, Ribbe MW, Van der Wal G, Onwuteaka-Philipsen BD. Discomfort in dementia patients dying from pneumonia and its relief by antibiotics. *Scandinavian Journal of Infectious Diseases* 2009; 41(2): 143–51.

59. Van der Steen JT, Di Giulio P, Giunco F, Monti M, Gentile S, et al. End of Life Observatory. Prospective Study on Dementia Patients Care (EoLO-PSODEC) Research Group. Pneumonia in nursing home patients with advanced dementia:

Decisions, intravenous rehydration therapy, and discomfort. *American Journal of Hospice and Palliative Care* 2018 Mar; 35(3): 423–30.

60. Klapwijk MS, Caljouw MA, Van Soest-Poortvliet MC, Van der Steen JT, Achterberg WP. Symptoms and treatment when death is expected in dementia patients in long-term care facilities. *BMC Geriatrics* 2014 Sep 2; 14: 99.

61. Martyr A, Nelis S, Quinn C, Wu Y, Lamont R, et al. Living well with dementia: A systematic review and correlational meta-analysis of factors associated with quality of life, well-being and life satisfaction in people with dementia. *Psychological Medicine* 2018; 48(13): 2130–9.

62. Edwards HB, Ijaz S, Whiting PF, et al. Quality of family relationships and outcomes of dementia: A systematic review, *BMJ Open* 2018; 8: e015538. doi: 10.1136/bmjopen-2016-015538

63. Sikkes Sietske AM, Tang Y, Jutten RJ, Wesselman L, Turkstra LS, et al. Toward a theory-based specification of non-pharmacological treatments in aging and dementia: Focused reviews and methodological recommendations. *Alzheimer's & Dementia* (2020). https://alz-journals.onlinelibrary.wiley.com/doi/full/10.1002/alz.12188

64. Kim SK, Park M. Effectiveness of person-centered care on people with dementia: A systematic review and meta-analysis. *Clinical Interventions in Aging* 2017; 12: 381–97. doi: 10.2147/CIA.S117637

65. Poon E. A systematic review and meta-analysis of dyadic psychological interventions for BPSD, quality of life and/or caregiver burden in dementia or MCI. *Clinical Gerontologist* 2019. doi: 10.1080/07317115.2019.1694117

66. Dröes RM, Breebaart E, Van Tilburg W, Mellenbergh GJ. The effect of integrated family support versus day care only on behavior and mood of patients with dementia. *International Psychogeriatrics* 2000; 12(1): 99–116.

67. Dröes RM, Meiland FJM, Schmitz M, Van Tilburg W. Effect of combined support for people with dementia and carers versus regular day care on behaviour and mood of persons with dementia: Results from a multi-centre implementation study. *International Journal of Geriatric Psychiatry* 2004; 19: 673–84.

68. Ojagbemi A, Owolabi, M. Do occupational therapy interventions improve quality of life in persons with dementia? A meta-analysis with implications for future directions. *Psychogeriatrics* 2017; 17: 133–41.

69. Bennett S, Laver K, Voigt-Radloff S, et al. Occupational therapy for people with dementia and their family carers provided at home: A systematic

review and meta-analysis. *BMJ Open* 2019; **9**: e026308. doi: 10.1136/bmjopen-2018-026308

70. Lobbia A, Carbone E, Faggia S, et al. The efficacy of cognitive stimulation therapy (CST) for people with mild-to-moderate dementia: A review. *European Psychologist* 2019; **24**(3): 257–77.

71. Woods B, Aguirre E, Spector AE, Orrell M. Cognitive stimulation to improve cognitive functioning in people with dementia. *Cochrane Database of Systematic Reviews* 2012, Issue 2. Art. No.: CD005562. doi: 10.1002/14651858. CD005562.pub2

72. Ojagbemi A, Akin-Ojagbemi N. Exercise and quality of life in dementia: A systematic review and meta-analysis of randomized controlled trials. *Journal of Applied Gerontology* 2019; **38**(1): 27–48.

73. Redulla R. Reminiscence therapy for dementia. *Issues in Mental Health Nursing* 2019. doi: 10.1080/01612840.2019.1654572

74. Dröes RM, Boelens-Van der Knoop ECC, Bos J, Meihuizen L, Ettema TP, et al. Quality of life in dementia in perspective: An explorative study of variations in opinions among people with dementia and their professional caregivers, and in literature. *Dementia: The International Journal of Social Research and Practice* 2006; **5**(4): 533–58.

75. Cookson R, Griffin S, Norheim OF, Culyer AJ, eds. *Distributional Cost-Effectiveness Analysis: Quantifying Health Equity Impacts and Trade-offs.* Oxford, Oxford University Press, 2020.

76. Feeny D, Furlong W, Torrance G, et al. Multiattribute and single-attribute utility functions for the Health Utilities Index Mark 3 system. *Medical Care* 2002; **40**: 113–28.

77. Ratcliffe J, Flint T, Easton T, et al. An empirical comparison of the EQ-5D-5 L, DEMQOL-U and DEMQOL-Proxy-U in a post-hospitalisation population of frail older people living in residential aged care. *Applied Health Economics and Health Policy* 2017; **15**: 399–412.

78. Drummond M, Sculpher M, Torrance G, O'Brien B, Stoddart G. *Methods for the Economic Evaluation of Health Care Programmes.* 3rd ed. Oxford, Oxford University Press, 2005.

79. Dolan P, Gudex C, Kind P, et al. A social tariff for EuroQoL: Results from a UK population survey. Discussion Paper 138. University of York. 1995.

80. Schokkaert E. How to introduce more (or better) ethical arguments in HTA? *International Journal of Technology Assessment in Health Care* 2015; **31**: 111–12.

81. Appleby J, Devlin N, Parkin D. NICE's cost effectiveness threshold. *British Medical Journal* 2007; **335**(7616): 358–9.

82. Claxton K, Martin S, Soares M. Methods for the estimation of the National Institute for Health and Care Excellence cost-effectiveness threshold. *Health Technology Assessment* 2015; **19**: 1–503, v–vi.

83. Knapp M, King D, Romeo R, et al. Cost-effectiveness of donepezil and memantine in moderate to severe Alzheimer's disease (the DOMINO-AD trial). *International Journal of Geriatric Psychiatry* 2017; **32**(12): 1205–16.

84. Howard R, McShane R, Lindesay J, et al. Donepezil and memantine in moderate to severe Alzheimer's disease: The DOMINO trial. *New England Journal of Medicine* 2012; **366**: 893–903.

85. Howard R, McShane R, Lindesay J, Ritchie C, Baldwin A, et al. Nursing home placement in the donepezil and memantine in moderate to severe Alzheimer's disease (DOMINO-AD) trial: Secondary and post-hoc analyses. *Lancet Neurology* 2015; **14**(12): 1171–81.

86. NICE. *Dementia: Assessment, Management and Support for People Living with Dementia and Their Carers.* London, NICE, 2018.

87. Livingston G, Manela M, O'Keeffe, A et al. Clinical effectiveness of START (STrAtegies for RelaTives) psychological intervention for family carers and the effects on cost of care for people with dementia: Six year follow-up of a randomised controlled trial. *British Journal of Psychiatry* 2019; **216**(1): 35–42.

88. Knapp M, King D, Romeo R, et al. The START study (STrAtegies for RelaTives). Cost-effectiveness of a manual-based coping strategy programme in promoting the mental health of family carers of people with dementia: A pragmatic randomised controlled trial. *British Medical Journal*; 2013; **347**: f6342.

89. Banerjee S, Hellier J, Dewey M, et al. Sertraline or mirtazapine for depression in dementia (HTA-SADD): A randomised, multicentre, double-blind, placebo-controlled trial. *The Lancet* 2011; **378**(9789): 403–11.

90. Folstein MF, Folstein SE, McHugh PR. Mini-mental state: A practical method for grading the cognitive state of patients for the clinician. *Journal of Psychiatric Research* 1975; **12**: 189–98.

91. Farina N, King D, Burgon C. Disease severity accounts for minimal variance of quality of life in people with dementia and their carers: Analyses of cross-sectional data from the MODEM study. *BMC Geriatrics* 2020; **20**: 232.

92. Helgesson G, Erntsson O, Aström M, Burström K. Whom should we ask? A systematic literature review of the arguments regarding the most accurate source of information for valuation of health states. *Quality of Life Research* 2020; **29**: 1465–82.

93. Karimi M, Brazier J, Basarir H. The capability approach: A critical review of its application in health economics. *Value in Health* 2016; **19**: 795–9.

94. Grewal I, Lewis J, Flynn T, Brown J, Bond J, Coast J. Developing attributes for a generic quality of life measure for older people: Preferences or capabilities? *Social Science and Medicine* 2006; **62**: 1891–1901.

95. Coast J, Flynn T, Natarajan L, Sproston K, Lewis J, et al. Valuing the ICECAP capability index for older people. *Social Science and Medicine* 2008; **67**: 874–82.

96. Makai P, Beckebans F, Van Exel J, Brouwer W. Quality of life of nursing home residents with dementia: Validation of the German version of the ICECAP-O. *PLOS One* 2014; **9**: e92016.

97. Netten A, Burge P, Malley J, et al. Outcomes of social care for adults: Developing a preference-weighted measure. *Health Technology Assessment* 2012; **16**: 16.

98. Rand S, Malley J, Netten A, Forder J. Factor structure and construct validity of the Adult Social Care Outcomes Toolkit for Carers (ASCOT-Carer). *Quality of Life Research* 2015; **24**: 2601–14.

99. Decancq K, Michiels A. Measuring successful aging with respect for preferences of older persons. *Journal of Gerontology: Social Sciences* 2019; **74**: 364–73.

100. Hendriks I, Demetrio R, Meiland FJM, Chattat R, Szcześniak D, Rymaszewska J, et al. Value of personalized dementia-specific quality of life scales: An explorative study in 3 European countries. *American Journal of Alzheimer's Disease and Other Dementias* 2021 Jan–Dec; 36: 15333175211033721. doi: 10.1177/15333175211033721. PMID: 34424058

101. Decancq K, Neumann D. Does the choice of well-being measure matter empirically? An illustration with German data. In Adler M, Fleurbaey M, eds. *Oxford Handbook of Well-Being and Public Policy*. Oxford, Oxford University Press, 2016; 553–87.

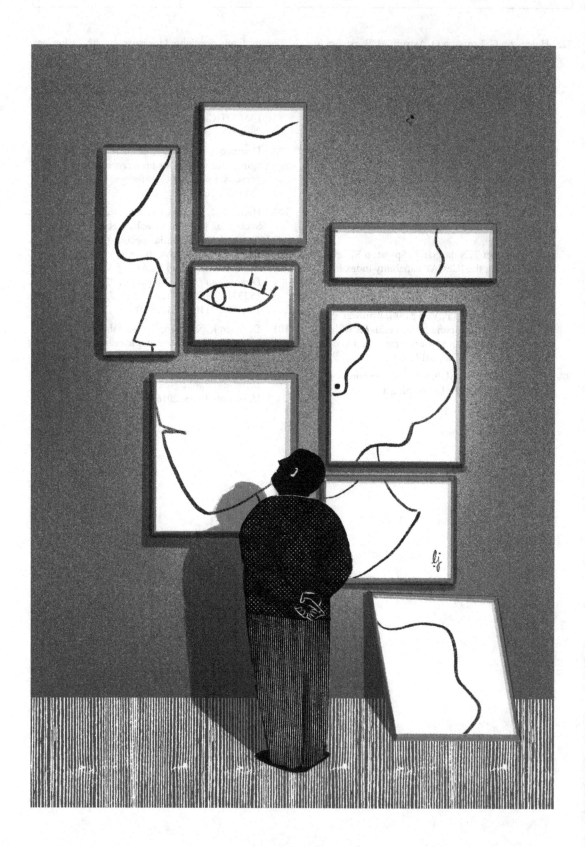

Living with Dementia
Relationships, Intimacy, Sexuality and Care

Frauke Claes, Nelle Frederix and Paul Enzlin

Dementia changed my partner, but not my love for her.

1 Introduction

Worldwide, the ageing population presents societies with various political, economic and ethical challenges that all have to be resolved in order to realize one important aim – that is, helping the elderly to reach a good quality of life (QoL). For 'modern' elderly, a good QoL means a long, happy and healthy life in which well-being is central. In this context, intimacy and sexuality are increasingly recognized as part of healthy and successful ageing. Intimacy and sexuality, however, often remain unaddressed in research and policy focussing on the QoL of the elderly. This lack of attention for sexuality can probably be explained by the culturally held belief that older people are asexual, but nothing is less true. There is growing evidence that a considerable number of elderly people continue to have an interest in sexuality into old age, long for it, fantasize about it, reflect on it, talk about it and above all remain sexually active. That is not surprising. After all, should people who have a satisfying sex life suddenly stop being sexually active because they happen to reach a certain age or become in ill health? Should people stop longing for or having sex because others – that is, family members, healthcare providers, administrators and policymakers – minimize, ignore or deny their sexual needs?

The answer to both questions is clearly negative, and it is time that we as a society stop forcing the elderly to hide or push aside their sexuality, because for the elderly too sexuality contributes to their QoL. While many are willing to follow this argumentation for healthy elderly, there is probably less openness to think about the importance of sexuality for people with dementia and their partners. They are probably even more discouraged and hindered by the environment to continue their 'inappropriate' sexual expressions.

This chapter focusses on the impact of dementia on the partner and sexual relationships of couples living with dementia. First, we describe the impact of dementia on a partner relationship from the perspectives of both the person with dementia and the partner and present the most common relational changes in couples confronted with a diagnosis of dementia. Second, we focus on the impact of dementia on the sexual relationship during both the phase of home care and the phase after admission to a residential care facility (RCF). In that context, we discuss ethical aspects of sexuality of people with dementia and how these can be addressed in RCFs.

2 Dementia and Partner Relationships

Dementia clearly has an impact on persons with dementia and on their partners, and on how patients as well as partners experience their relationship. The relational impact of dementia varies between different types and stages of dementia and between couples, and couples may use diverse strategies to cope with the impact of the disease. It is important to discuss the relational impact of dementia from both partners' perspectives because it is highly relevant for healthcare providers to know what persons with dementia as well as their partners find important and what can help them to improve their lives (e.g. maximizing their QoL) [1].

This section covers how patients and partners perceive the impact of dementia on partner relationships. While the first part focusses on the perception of patients with dementia, the second part focusses on how the partners perceive and experience the impact of dementia on the relationship. Third, the importance of differentiating between the impact of early- and late-onset dementia on a partner relationship is highlighted. Finally, we advocate a systemic approach and make a plea to include the network in coping with these (relational) changes.

2.1 Patients' Perspective

Literature about patients' views on the partner relationship is scarce because patients with dementia are (perceived as) a difficult-to-reach population, and, moreover, this kind of research raises many ethical questions. There is, for example, doubt whether patients with dementia can voluntarily consent to participate in studies and whether they can inform us correctly about their perceptions. However, it is necessary to investigate patients in order to gain knowledge about their own beliefs about dementia and its impact on relationships that might be inspiring to develop tailored care.

Few studies that have included persons with dementia show that persons with dementia – despite sometimes feeling useless and as if they are a burden to their partners [2] – have more positive perceptions about the impact of dementia on their partner relationships and report a higher QoL compared to their partners [3, 4]. This shows the need to also include the partners' perspective in studies on dementia.

2.2 Partners' Perspective

Partners of persons with dementia are also challenged by the disease, but their experiences (as caregivers) are also often neglected in care, in research and in our society. In this section, the many losses and feelings of grief that partners experience and partners' experiences with the most common relational changes are presented. As dementia is a progressive disease, it is important to keep in mind that partners' experiences with the impact of dementia on their partner relationships are likely to vary over different stages of the disease.

2.2.1 Loss and Pre-death Grief

A diagnosis of dementia entails many losses for persons with dementia as well as their partners. Partners go through an actual grieving process as they need to recognize the finiteness of their (normal) relationship [5–8]. This experience is described as a 'pre-death grieving process' due to the 'social death' of the patient with dementia and

the personal sacrifices partners have to make [8]. It is a gradual process of letting go and losing the patient mentally (e.g. personality changes) and physically (e.g. due to admission to an RCF). Many partners start to see the patient as a stranger and therefore feel like they are 'married-widow(er)s' [1, 5, 9]. The patient becomes 'absent present', meaning that their essence is missing [1].

Well-intentioned comments such as 'at least your partner is still alive' testify to a limited understanding of the grieving process partners of people with dementia go through. Moreover, loved ones and the broader network of partners of people with dementia are possibly not fully aware of these feelings of grief as the couple might pretend to be and do better when other people are around. Feelings of grief in partners of people with dementia are as real and as intense as post-death grief and can end in depression [8]. This shows the need to pay attention to these feelings and raise awareness about the existence of pre-death grief in partners of persons living with dementia [10, 11].

Feelings of loss occurring at various levels are an overwhelming theme in literature about dementia. Apart from losing their partners [8], partners of people with dementia also experience losses (e.g. communication, support) in their relationship [12]. These relational losses may result in lower happiness, lower relationship quality, a decrease in emotional connection and an increase in emotional distress [12, 13]. Nevertheless, many couples put effort in adapting to these losses in order to preserve the (quality of the) relationship using strategies to search for a balance between facing these losses and distancing from them [12]. In short, partners experience loss of the patient ('is (s)he still present?') and loss of the marriage or relationship ('are we still a couple?') [9].

2.2.2 Relational Changes

Partners of people with dementia report that these feelings of grief and loss are accompanied by many changes in the relationship. Dementia results in gradual transitions in the relationship with partners reporting relational deterioration and deprivation and a decrease in relationship quality, possibly leading to feelings of depression [3]. As mentioned before, partners report a lower QoL and a greater negative relational impact of dementia than patients [3, 4]. In addition, female partners report more stress, more depression and lower intimacy scores compared to male partners [3, 7]. In what follows, common relational changes experienced by partners of people with dementia are discussed. These changes are likely more prominent in certain stages of the disease and must therefore be viewed as fluid.

2.2.2.1 Loneliness and Social Isolation

Partners of persons with dementia frequently mention loneliness and social isolation due to a reduction in social support (e.g. friends who withdraw themselves) [1, 5, 14, 19]. These feelings of loneliness can trace back to the network (e.g. loss of friendships), but also to their own partner (e.g. behavioural changes of the patient leading to disconnection) [5]. With decreasing companionship in the relationship, partners can feel increasingly lonely in their own marriage [9]. Fortunately, some couples remain close as a couple, maintain close friendships and find sources of social support (e.g. fellow sufferers). Investing in and using the social network seems valuable to counter loneliness (see Section 1.4).

2.2.2.2 Shifting Roles

One of the most frequently reported changes described by partners of people with dementia is a shift in roles with a consequent loss in equality in their relationship [3, 5, 15, 20]. Partners report feeling more like a parent or a caregiver than a partner and that this changes the nature of the relationship. This shift in roles causes the partner to have more responsibilities and creates the need of both partners to help each other adjust to these new roles [9]. As the disease progresses, the relationship often shifts from a symmetrical, equal relationship to an asymmetrical relationship in which the patient becomes dependent on the partner – a relational dynamic that often leads to tension and feelings of distance [9]. However, people with dementia remain individuals with agency who – at least to a certain stage of the disease – can still make their own decisions and take responsibilities [16]. This implies that the shifting roles can be minimalized if the patient wants to, is allowed to and is still able to take these responsibilities.

Nevertheless, for most partners the changing roles are an extremely challenging part of a dementia diagnosis, with intimate care (e.g. washing the patient) being the most challenging

new role in most cases [14]. A consequence of the shift in roles is that partners need to develop a new kind of relationship with the patient, and this implies that new types of intimacy and closeness need to be explored [7]. Moreover, both patients and partners will have to learn new skills and shift roles due to changes in responsibilities [7, 9]. If a couple manages to meet these challenges, the impact of the shifting roles can be overcome.

2.2.2.3 Communication

Cognitive impairment of a person with dementia can lead to changes in and difficulties with communication on the patient's side [2]. As communication plays a critical role in how partners rate the quality of and satisfaction with their relationship, these changes are of great importance [3]. Changes in communication due to dementia are often negative because people with dementia become less expressive and receptive, which leads partners to report a lower quality and/or a loss of reciprocity in communication that may result in annoyance in partners [1, 7, 9, 17, 20]. While in people with Alzheimer's disease and Lewy body dementia non-verbal communication is mostly preserved, it is often impaired in people with frontotemporal dementia (FTD) [18].

Frontotemporal dementia patients also have more difficulties with verbal communication and with participation in communication [18]. This suggests that FTD – especially the semantic variant of FTD – is likely to have the greatest impact on communication. Furthermore, as cognitive decline of the patient continues over the course of the disease, the further stages of dementia are likely to impact the communication skills the most. It is clear that communication within the relationship becomes more complex after a diagnosis of dementia, but partners generally invest a lot of time and effort to maintain and maximize the relational communication as they do not want to lose their conversation partner [6]. Partners can motivate the patient to engage in verbal communication as much as possible and can try and learn to communicate more non-verbally.

2.2.2.4 Reciprocity

Similar to the lack of reciprocity in communication, another important aspect in the perception of the relationship by partners is that persons with dementia become increasingly indifferent and take less initiative [20]. This lack of initiative applies to everyday life and decision-making as well as to intimacy and sexuality and is related to certain symptoms of dementia such as apathy [20]. Some partners state that they need to remind the patient to respond to the (intimate) activities that they themselves need to initiate [20]. Indecisiveness and loss of reciprocity can be an obstacle in the partner relationship in general and in experiencing intimacy and sexuality specifically.

2.2.2.5 Couplehood and Personhood

Dementia often causes the shared feeling of being a couple to diminish [6] as well as an identity crisis in both partners [7] (see also Chapter 3). This means that both a shared identity – that is, the extent to which the couple feels as if they are 'one' – and the individual identities of both partners are being challenged by, for example, changes in equality and power in the relationship [14]. This is, however, stage, person and couple dependent. Some couples preserve a shared identity and if they do so, they rate the quality of their relationship as higher than couples that do not have a preserved sense of being a couple [12].

As to individual identities, almost all partners of people with dementia (96.4%) report a change in the identity of the patient and that this negatively affects his or her own mental and physical health [17]. This association is mediated by the perceived quality of the current relationship [17]. The change in identity of the patient can be seen as a process in which the patient (gradually) becomes a stranger, leading to distress in the partner and a decrease in intimacy within the couple [17]. However, personhood of patient and partner can also change for the better, having positive effects on the relationship [16]. Imagine, for example, a person with dementia who used to be very dominant becoming less bossy due to Alzheimer's disease. Strikingly, patients themselves often feel like they are still themselves or even feel like dementia led to personal growth and better self-understanding [16].

2.2.2.6 Positive Perspective

Generally, partners perceive the relationship as different after a dementia diagnosis, but this difference does not necessarily imply negative changes. While relational problems often are present [15], positive influences on the partner relationship are also commonly reported. Partners report, for instance, feeling useful and proud of how they are handling the situation, leading to feelings of self-fulfilment [1, 3]. Partners sometimes perceive their relationship as deeper and closer than before the diagnosis as both partners have empathy for and want to protect each other [1, 3, 14]. This means that the patient, for example, hides certain difficulties and that the partner, for example, promotes the agency of the patient [14].

Couples often see the 'dementia journey' as a journey they are taking together with mutual support [14]. Many couples show resilience and step away from feelings such as uncertainty and hopelessness by accepting the diagnosis, leading to a new perspective in which the little things are more appreciated, forgiveness is central and the couple tries to make the best of it [14]. If a couple continues to share love, humour, respect and warmth, they report higher relationship quality [12]. However, the previously described – mostly negative – influences of dementia on a partner relationship prove that this positive perspective is not always accessible and that there may be many obstacles to overcome to reach it. Nevertheless, many couples put in a lot of effort to be positive and to accept a life with dementia.

2.3 Early- versus Late-Onset Dementia

For all of the aforementioned changes, it is important to differentiate between early-onset dementia (EOD), also referred to as young-onset dementia (YOD), and late-onset dementia (LOD) when considering the relational impact of dementia. Early-onset dementia is any type of dementia with symptoms occurring before the age of 65, whereas in LOD symptoms commence after the age of 65 [19]. Given that EOD sometimes arises at very early ages (e.g. at 40 years old), EOD will often have a different impact on a partner relationship than LOD.

In their reviews, Holdsworth and McCabe described the impact of EOD [19] and LOD [20] on relationships, intimacy and sexuality. They found that the relational impact of EOD and LOD partly overlapped – with recurring themes such as a shift in responsibilities and roles and changes in identity and self-esteem of both patients with dementia and their partners (see Section 2.2.2) – but also described important differences between EOD and LOD. First, the shifting roles and responsibilities can have a bigger impact in EOD couples than in LOD couples, as EOD couples often need to retire early. As a result, financial problems – which put extra strain on the relationship – often arise.

Furthermore, aspects related to identity (e.g. work, family and sexuality) are often more heavily influenced by EOD than by LOD. People with EOD are younger, have younger children to care for and attach greater value to sexuality. This means that the identity of people with EOD is often more heavily disrupted. Moreover, couples confronted with EOD lack age-appropriate information and services and often have to deal with an extensive and long process before receiving a (correct) diagnosis [19]. These additional stress factors possibly make it more difficult to adjust to the challenges of a life with dementia for EOD couples compared to LOD couples.

2.4 Importance of the Network: A Systemic Approach

As becomes clear from this section, both the patient and the partner as well as their relationship deserve attention in care. This means that it is important that healthcare providers also focus on the relational impact of dementia. However, addressing the (broader) network of couples confronted with dementia is equally important [21]. Therefore, we advocate a systemic perspective that highlights the importance of the (broader) network (of the family and friends) in home care since a supporting network can mean that (partners of) persons with dementia feel less lonely, less socially isolated and better understood and supported [21].

Besides, including the network in therapy is an effective way to enhance the care for the person with dementia [21]. It can, for example, initiate beneficial changes in the interaction patterns within the system. We believe that during the phase of home care engaging the broader system (in treatment) is likely to make the impact of dementia more manageable for the patient and the partner, but also that when a patient is no longer living at home and residing in an RCF it is important to involve and engage the broader supporting network.

3 Dementia and Sexuality

As dementia greatly affects partner relationships with changing roles and responsibilities between partners, it will also affect the (meaning of) sexual experiences of both partners. It is striking that although sexuality is everywhere in today's society, the link between dementia and sexuality is only scantly addressed in studies and literature on dementia [22]. In this section, we explore that link by focussing on the sociocultural context, stages of change in sexual relationships, sexuality during home care, sexuality after admission to an RCF, the broader system, inappropriate sexual behaviour and ethical issues.

3.1 The Sociocultural Context

In general, the perception of sexuality in the elderly suffers from an ageist tendency that 'desexualizes' older people and portrays them as 'sexless' [23], which results in a 'delegitimization' of sexuality in later life, implying that elderly people are no longer expected to be sexually active. As a consequence, the sexual needs of older people are invisible, inaudible and concealed in our society. This 'social concealment' of sexuality of the elderly, combined with a lack of role models in media and movies, results in some older men and women feeling embarrassed, ashamed or guilty about their 'persisting' sexual needs. Some elderly might even have the impression that they have to hide their sexuality.

This cultural repudiation of sexuality of the elderly stands in stark contrast to recent findings showing that intimacy and sexuality are part of successful ageing [24–26]. Considering how aging is associated with factors that may affect sexual behaviour (e.g. changes in physical functioning, disease, medication use) or may account for a decline in frequency of sexual activity (e.g. partner in an RCF), successful ageing also depends on the willingness to explore new sexual scripts. Nevertheless, for a lot of men and women interest in sexuality remains high [22, 25, 26] and it is even becoming more important to successive cohorts of older people [24] because sexual life impacts psychological and relational well-being [27]. However, in these representations of the new 'sexy oldies', persons with dementia are not included [28]. That is striking because paying attention to intimacy and sexuality of persons with dementia may not only contribute to their QoL, but may also be helpful for their partner, broader family network and formal carers to cope with this (challenging) aspect of life [27].

3.2 Stages of Change in the Sexual Relation of Couples Confronted with Dementia

We believe that couples living with dementia go through five stages of change in their sexual relationship while being confronted with the progression of the disease (Figure 6.1). The first phase is the phase (long) before the dementia diagnosis in which two partners create their own sexual relationship that is more or less satisfying for each partner. This sexual relationship is shaped by both partners' attitudes about sexuality. The next phase refers to the preclinical stage in which both partners already experience changes in their intimate and sexual relationship that they do not understand and cannot explain. This phase often causes stress, uncertainty and frustration about what is going on. The sexual relationship is based on both partners' attitudes about sexuality and uncertainty, which may weigh on the intimate and sexual relationship that may suffer from the incomprehensibly changed behaviour of the partner. Partners will be challenged to renegotiate and reshape their sexual relationship.

The third phase starts with the dementia diagnosis, which can be experienced as reassuring for both partners as it gives an explanation for these changes. In this third phase, not only both partners', but also healthcare professionals' attitudes about sexuality and dementia impact how sexuality is shaped in the relationship. Here again,

a renegotiation and reshaping of their sexual relationship will be needed and the couple living with dementia will maybe consult a healthcare provider to discuss eventual difficulties regarding intimacy and sexuality.

The next two phases are related to an admission to an RCF of the partner with dementia, which will hinder the possibility to give shape to the sexual relationship as a couple due to new rules of the new environment including privacy issues. Moreover, the involvement of the RCF will become bigger in these last two stages and will depend on whether the RCF adheres to a holistic person-centred or a problem-oriented vision about sexuality and dementia. In the last phase, the 'absent presence' of the patient with end-stage dementia will hamper positive sexual relationships even more. This situation can be aggravated when the partner with dementia starts a 'new relationship' with another resident or when the partner starts a new (extramarital) relationship with a new partner in order to satisfy needs that the partner no longer can fulfil.

3.3 Sexuality during Home Care

A lot of partners care for their partner with dementia at home and the relational changes imposed by dementia will change partners' ideas and experiences about feeling as or being a couple with the 'changing'/'new' partner with dementia. While the vast majority of research on couples living with dementia has focussed on spousal care, partner relationships in dementia are not

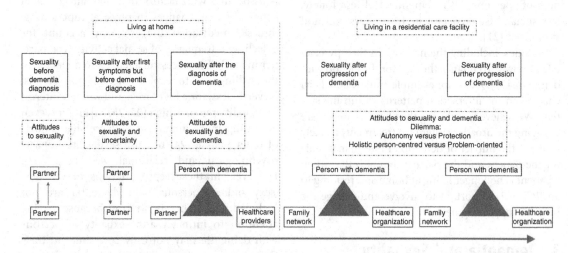

Figure 6.1 The reiterating discussion of sexuality of persons with dementia

merely about care. Partner relations of couples living with dementia need to be understood in the broader relational history of the couple, with a recognition that intimacy and sexuality are key in relational histories [29]. This means that experiences of intimacy and sexuality of couples living with dementia are shaped by the overall quality of the relationship in the past and present [30]. In other words, the level of sexual satisfaction before the diagnosis is probably the best predictor for both the emotional loss of satisfying sexuality and the positive recreation of satisfying sexuality after the diagnosis.

Dementia is a gradually developing brain disease causing symptoms such as mental decline, decreased physical fitness, fatigue, incoordination and difficulties with performing daily activities. These changes occur gradually, and patients will gradually become aware of them and will try to hide them. All of the physical and emotional changes that persons with dementia experience may affect how they and their partners feel about sexuality and intimate relationships. Initially, both partners often do not understand the changes they experience in their sexual or intimate relationships, which means that a diagnosis of dementia can be reassuring for partners and helpful to understand (better) what was and is happening.

A variety of changes can occur in the expression of intimacy and sexuality of persons living with dementia. They may experience changes in interest in sex (no, less or more interest), in the ability to perform sexually (no, less or more ability), in sexual responses (e.g. react less sensitively to the needs of the partner) and in levels of inhibition (e.g. doing or saying 'inappropriate' things), and they may even become sexually aggressive [31]. On the one hand, it is possible that at any stage of the condition, a person with dementia loses (all) interest in sex, which can be either relieving or frustrating for the partner. While it is as partner important to respect this reduced interest, it might be possible to find other – for the patient – acceptable ways (e.g. caressing, hugging, kissing) to express feelings. After the onset of dementia any form of preserved sexual relationship can be an important dimension in the partner relationship and may also be important to maintain the feeling of being a couple [15, 17, 32].

On the other hand, there are accounts of persons with dementia showing an increased interest in sex, which can again be a positive or a negative change for a partner. Partners may feel unable to adapt to an increased desire for sex, and this could be difficult for both partners in the relationship. Consequently, some partners have reported feeling uneasy at showing any affection at all – while missing it heavily – because their partner with dementia always mistakes such initiative for a sexual advance. It is also possible that a person with increased desire repeatedly demands sex, but it could be that this is a person's (new) way of expressing a need for intimacy, rather than a need for sex. Some people with dementia become aggressive if turned down for sex because they feel rejected. Therefore it could be difficult for partners to try to turn down requests for sex and if they do so, they should try to do it in such a way that patients still feel acknowledged in their sexual needs. Partners could try to find an alternative way of meeting their partner with dementia's need for intimacy either alone (e.g. masturbation), together (e.g. kissing, touching or other forms of physical intimacy) or by other non-sexual activities which might help meet the person's need for intimacy or social interaction (e.g. activity groups) [31].

It is clear that with the onset of a dementing illness, sexual interest and activity do not disappear [33]; neither does the basic need for skin hunger, close human contact, to belong, to be desired, to share oneself with another end with dementia. Moreover, sexuality is not so much about what we do. It is more about who we are. We are all gendered and sexual beings who profit from the many health benefits of sex, such as lower stress levels, improved self-esteem and positive emotional bonding with your partner.

As there is a differential impact of EOD and LOD on partner relationships (see Section 2.1), there is also a difference in the changes occurring in the expression of intimacy and sexuality between couples confronted with EOD and LOD. These changes seem related to differences in expectations about sexual activity between older and younger couples and with the timing of dementia in a person's life course. Older couples regarded the sexual changes as 'timely' and in accordance with their life course and fitting in their (already changing) sexual scripts.

Harris [34] found that the narratives of both partners were very consistent and that both partners mentioned having an overall positive relationship earlier and now, related changes to embodied ageing, and understood intimacy and touch as being more important today. However, younger couples understood these changes as 'premature' and at odds with their life course and sexual scripts [30]. Younger couples living with dementia stated that dementia had caused a breakdown in their intimate sexual relationships, resulting in a loss of sexual intimacy, which they experienced as damaging their intimate and sexual relationship and resulting in relational dissatisfaction [35]. Older couples learned to cope with changes in their sexual relationships before the onset of dementia, implying that these changes were attributed more to normal ageing than to dementia [30]. Moreover, in older couples, both partners agreed on and confirmed their relationship whereas in younger couples, there were significant differences between the views of persons with dementia and their partner [30].

3.3.1 Patients' Perspective

In a study on patients with Alzheimer's disease, Nogueira et al. [36] found that 63.5% reported sexual activity and that of this group 67.3% noticed a change in sexual activity and reported overall moderate sexual dissatisfaction. Patients who mentioned no change in their sexual activity reported higher sexual satisfaction – but also more dementia symptoms with lower functionality and cognition. Patients who reported a change in sexual activity showed higher rates of sexual dissatisfaction. Patients who reported no sexual activity were moderately to severely dissatisfied. Overall, 18.9% of patients reported a high level of sexual satisfaction, 44.6% a mild to moderate level of dissatisfaction and 36.5% a moderate to severe level of dissatisfaction. A higher level of sexual dissatisfaction was associated with a mild severity of dementia, which was independent from a patient's gender.

In another survey study, Tsatali and Tsolaki [37] observed changes in general sexual function in the dementia group in the previous month as well as during the previous year. They concluded that cognitive decline can be linked with lower sexual activity and willingness, but they did find a gender difference – that is, men reported higher levels of deterioration than women.

While age-related sexual dysfunctions (e.g. hypoactive sexual desire disorder (HSDD), menopause-induced genito-pelvic pain and penetration disorder (GPPPD), erectile dysfunction (ED), anorgasmia, delayed ejaculation) are probably also frequent in men and women and may – apart from dementia – impact sexual functioning, these are often overlooked and undertreated disorders in people with dementia. The same may be true for changes in sexual preference (paraphilic-related disorder) that are also omitted from the literature on sexuality of patients with dementia [38].

While these findings are interesting, they do not shed light on how the sexual and intimate relationship is experienced by people with dementia themselves [some exceptions: 23, 34, 39, 40]. That is striking because in the early stages, persons with dementia are probably well able to provide valuable, valid and truthful information about their need for and the meaning they attach to intimacy and sexual behaviour [22]. Moreover, research on people in the early stages of dementia shows that they continue to regard themselves as sexual beings [34]. That is not unexpected because sexuality is often an important aspect of a person's subjectivity even when being confronted with illness and disability.

Apart from these changes in sexual feelings, some studies suggested that some patients show sexual indifference – that is, a complete loss of sexual interest [15, 41], others found a decrease in sexual activity, interest and sexual satisfaction [15, 36, 37, 42], and some reported an increased sexual desire or even hyper-sexuality [33]. When the impact of dementia is increasing, couples confronted with dementia may have to renegotiate their sexual scripts. This renegotiation can result in sexual scripts away from penetrative intercourse towards non-genital sexual practices and intimacy (e.g. kissing, hugging, cuddling, tenderness, lying naked next to each other), but can also be hampered by relational factors.

In Sandberg's study, a man reported that he was 'no longer attracted to his wife who was interfering and depriving him of this independence which made him angry and frustrated' [30]. It seems that the narratives of patients with dementia on their decrease of sexuality and intimacy are linked to disappointment about changes in themselves, to disappointment about how their partners recognized their (dis)abilities, to conflicts and feelings of anger and frustration and to an overall sense of dissatisfaction with their situation [30, 34].

3.3.2 Partners' Perspective

As mentioned before, partners often take responsibility for the increasingly dependent partner with dementia, which means that partners need to rethink and renegotiate their relationship [2, 3]. These negotiations also include the sexual relationship because the care burden of spouses has a negative impact on their well-being and not seldom results in a decrease in sexual desire and affection (particularly for women) [17, 30, 34, 42, 43] for different reasons. Some partners argued that dementia caused their partner to change (e.g. no longer able to have long, full, intellectual conversations; that they no longer take responsibility for everyday tasks such as cleaning and shopping) and that this affected their sexual relationships with them [30]. Other partners reported how their partner with dementia became different (e.g. no longer offering emotional support) and even unrecognizable (e.g. the experience of living with a stranger who is no longer helping in making plans and taking decisions), as if the 'body remained but the person disappeared' [30]. Other partners confirmed the experience of dementia as a loss of self and stated that their relationship changed from one between equal adult lovers to a relationship that was more like that between a parent and a child [17, 32, 44].

This change from a 'partner to love' to a 'partner to care for' had a clear impact on partners' sexual desire for their partner with dementia [17, 44], and for some it even led to rejecting all kinds of physical intimacy [30]. Similarly, Youell and Callaghan [29] showed how carers' experiences of the partner with dementia as 'absent present' contributed to ambivalent feelings about sex [44]. Apart from affecting their sexual desire for their partners, the experience of having 'lost' their partners due to dementia also affected their personal experiences as sexual and gendered beings [30]. Caring partners revealed that growing into the role of spouse of a partner with dementia instigated a transformation from being a sexual partner into becoming a(n) (asexual) carer [30] – that is, a transformation that goes with a loss of sexual intimacy resulting in a kind of sexual grief [45].

Nilsson [46] found that partners felt sad about the inability to evoke memories of past intimacies and that they could no longer share these past pleasures, which highlights how conversations about sex and intimacy can be another sphere of everyday life where couples may lose common ground [30]. Apart from changes in the relational meaning of sexuality between partners, sexual desire may also decrease due to changes in sexual behaviour of partners with dementia and consequent sexual experiences of partners.

Eloniemi-Sulkava et al. [13] described several sexual behavioural changes that spousal carers experienced during sexual activity with their partners and that negatively affected their sexual experiences and desire. These negative sexual behavioural changes included the inability to recognize the partners' sexual feelings – that is, being more focussed on one's own needs [30] – constantly expressing a need for making love, inability to recall recent intercourse, indifference during intercourse, aggressive behaviour during intercourse, inability to recognize the partner after intercourse, demanding intercourse in an aggressive way and other inappropriate sexual behaviour. In their study, Eloniemi-Sulkava et al. [13] found that 60% of the partners reported at least one negative sexual behaviour change, but that these changes had little impact on whether the couple continued to have intercourse.

In the same study, 10% of spouse caregivers reported at least one positive sexual behaviour change. These positive behavioural changes included increased tenderness, increased ability to recognize his/her partner's needs, general improvement in marital sexual behaviour and positive improvement in sexual willingness [15]. Harris [34] found that some participants had become less sexually active but more intimate in other ways, and that this was linked to an 'appreciation of (the) smaller things in life' after the onset of Alzheimer's disease [30]. Older participants also questioned the importance of sexuality that was often made 'too big a deal of' and stressed more the importance of a committed, positive relationship overall [30]. This is in line with qualitative research suggesting that in the context of dementia a committed relationship is important for partners' continued feelings of intimacy, love and togetherness, which may be maintained by increased touch [29, 32, 44, 47]. For older partners, an increase in touching often fits with changes to move away from sex with penetration, a movement that may have begun earlier due to age- or illness-related factors affecting sexual functioning.

Simonelli [42] found that the perception of burden by spouse caregivers is higher in women than in men and that it is related to the severity of dementia of their partners. Other scholars found differences between female and male carers. Women carers have expressed difficulties in combining their roles as wives and sexual partners with that of carers [17, 32, 44]. Hayes et al. [44], for example, highlight the significance of gender differences for spouses' experiences of sexual intimacy when living with Alzheimer's disease. The women in their study cited a loss of emotional and social intimacy as leading to a decline in physical intimacy and that seeing their husbands as child-like decreased their sexual desire. The men, in contrast, were mostly concerned with knowing whether their female partners with dementia consented to sex, and they still regarded their partners as wives. Male caregivers also desired and had more sexual intercourse than female caregivers [30].

3.3.3 Recreating Sexuality

In summary, when a couple is living with dementia, the sexual behaviour, needs and desires of both the patient and the partner may change over time and with advancing stages of dementia. While many partners still enjoy sex and intimacy in their relationship, a diagnosis of dementia may change the way partners express affection for each other and may challenge partners to search for new ways of sharing closeness, comfort and intimacy. It may be that intimacy and sexuality become more or less important for either or both partners. There may also come change in what partners consider 'sex' and in how partners prefer to be physically intimate. It is helpful that partners can keep an open mind about what 'sex' and 'intimacy' is and what it means for both partners. It might be that the sex life of couples needs to change (too) dramatically and that couples might need advice on how to cope with these changes. Such advice might especially be needed when the impact of dementia is increasing due to the progress of the disease and/or the impact of the medication prescribed for the disease. Thus, over time dementia challenges couples to renegotiate and recreate their sexuality in such way

that it fulfils both partners' physical and emotional needs. This renegotiation often needs to be redone when a person with dementia moves to an RCF [31].

3.4 Sexuality after Admission to a Residential Care Facility

Most people with dementia live in the community and are often looked after and cared for by their partner. The responsibility to care for a partner may provoke distress in caregivers (see Chapter 7) due to a progressive accumulation of the attendance load linked with dementia-related behavioural and cognitive disturbances [48]. However, when care burden increases and care needs exceed the capacity of the spouse and the informal care network (e.g. due to progressing cognitive and physical disabilities, declining ability to care for oneself, death of the spouse), admission to an RCF often becomes inevitable [32, 49]. Such an admission mostly results in a decline of QoL in people with dementia (residents) as well as their partners. That is understandable because an admission separates older partners who often have been together for most of their lives [49], and this separation challenges them to retain the feeling of being a couple, including the feeling of being intimate and sexual partners.

Elias and Ryan [50] found that interest in sex does not necessarily decrease on admission to care homes, but that the opportunities to engage in sexual behaviour do. These opportunities decrease due to several reasons such as progression of the disease, lack of privacy and staff attitudes, and because more people (i.e. partners, family, other residents, nursing and clinical staff, administrators and directors) get involved in the discussion about the appropriateness of sexuality in the context of the organization. This brings up a question: 'Who decides about what is appropriate sexual behaviour in the context of an RCF?' In general, the culture of the environment or the RCF defines the range of what is 'appropriate' – that is, 'normal' or 'acceptable' – sexual behaviour [51].

3.4.1 Inappropriate Sexual Behaviour

Although the frequency of inappropriate sexual behaviour (ISB) is (rather) low – about 4–5% to 25% [22, 52] – it is highly emotionally laden problem behaviour that represents a considerable source of stress to patients, families and care-givers. Partners, families and medical practitioners often perceive ISB as difficult, distressing and embarrassing, and it has been rated as the most difficult to manage symptom of the behavioural and psychological symptoms of dementia (BPSD) [51]. Although several authors have developed classifications of ISB, there is still little consensus on what terminology to use or how to classify it. This may be due to the diversity of how ISB manifests in excessive sexual comments, hugging/kissing, preoccupation with sex, increased libido, grabbing at the breasts or genitals of residents or staff, masturbation in public, sexual hallucinations, delusions of spousal infidelity, attempting to seduce and even chasing residents or staff for sexual purposes, exposing one's genitals, disrobing in public and changes in sexual preference [38].

Alagiakrishnan et al. [53] suggested a distinction between verbally inappropriate behaviours (e.g. excessive sexual comments, preoccupation with sex), physically inappropriate behaviours (e.g. sexual touching, fondling, disrobing, masturbation, sexual advances) or both, and labelled some behaviour as 'sexually ambiguous' (e.g. appearing naked or incompletely dressed). Other scholars use the term 'hypersexual behaviour', defined as 'persistent, uninhibited sexual behaviours directed at oneself or at others' [54], and make a distinction between sex talk, sex acts and implied sexual acts (e.g. requesting unnecessary genital care) [38, 54].

Another classification started from the interpretations of the behaviours and used the expression 'improper sexual behaviours' [55]. This classification distinguishes between intimacy seeking (e.g. misdirected affection to another resident who is not the partner), disinhibited behaviour (e.g. longing for closeness/intimacy) and non-sexual behaviours (e.g. taking off one's clothes in severe dementia, which may be mistakenly regarded as sexual).

Benbow and Beeston [27] argued that a more descriptive classification would seem more appropriate and that the categories of sex talk, sex acts (involving self or others) and implied sexual acts are probably simplest to use in practice as these avoid too much interpretation. Chapman and Spitznagel [56] identified five distinct domains of inappropriate sexual behaviour that are assessed in current available measures – hyper-sexuality, lewd/aberrant sexual behaviour, inappropriate sexual advances, inappropriate sexual comments and socially disruptive behaviour – and suggested developing a new measure that could address all these content domains. This is in line with Abdo's suggestion that there is a need for standardization of definitions and terminology so as to focus on improvement of both assessment and treatment [38].

3.4.2 Inappropriate Sexual Behaviour for Whom?

In general, in scientific as well as in everyday discourses, intimate and sexual behaviours of people with dementia are often classified as 'problematic'. Again, an important difficulty here is who decides about the 'problematic character' of that 'disturbing' behaviour. Consequently, sexual expression of the elderly living in RCFs is restricted because it is often evaluated based on the predominantly medical model of care focussing on providing physical care and ensuring safety and protection. This (paternalistic) protective reflex often causes an overreaction on the part of the administration, nursing staff, patients and their families when residents (start to) 'behave sexually' – whether or not in an 'appropriate' way [57].

This negative perspective on sexualities of persons with dementia is part of a wider 'halo effect of dementia' which implies that individuals with dementia are – irrespective of their actual capacity – regarded as lacking capacity for any responsibility due to the dementia diagnosis [58]. This means that sexualities of residents with dementia are mostly considered pathological, challenging behaviours 'due to' dementia and that they are seldom discussed as an expression of a normal and healthy need for intimacy and sex [39].

Could the 'inappropriate' expression of a 'normal' and human need for intimacy and sex be a normal reaction to an abnormal environment? [52]. Persons with dementia living in RCFs are clearly hindered in the expression of their (normal) need for intimacy and sexuality by several practical challenges. These challenges include the loss of their partner, the relative lack of men, physical health problems, lack of environmental privacy, lack of informational privacy and the attitudes of other residents, healthcare providers and family members, notably adult children.

Abdo [38] suggested that the lack of physical closeness in an RCF may enhance the psychological need for intimacy in patients with dementia, and that sex may compensate for cognitive and/or functional losses, which lower patient's self-esteem. Similarly, masturbation can be a sign of boredom in certain patients. In short, 'sexual' behaviour in patients with dementia should not always be considered sexual, but rather a non-intentional behavioural problem because sexual (mis)behaviour is often a display of other, non-sexual needs [22].

While the World Health Organization (WHO) recognizes sexuality as an important, lifelong aspect of human life, there is a lack of first-hand evidence from people with dementia living in an RCF of their experience of this deeply personal and private aspect of life [49]. Only qualitative, individual-based studies will be helpful to explore the residents' perspective, but this is currently neglected in the literature [49]. More insight into the residents' perspective would be helpful to address the misconceptions about intimacy and sexuality in people with dementia.

Mahieu and Gastmans [59] argued that in the ethical debate about sexuality of adults living in RCFs, respect for autonomy should always be privileged. However, as dementia is a progressive disease, more advanced stages of the disease, including decline in cognition, raise important considerations related to sexual behaviour and especially the ability to give consent [52]. When residents with dementia become incapable of appreciating or respecting moral or legal boundaries (in specific environments [52]), ethical dilemmas arise about finding the right balance between granting residents freedom to express their sexual needs versus guaranteeing residents' safety. This kind of ethical dilemma often results in anxiety, embarrassment or unease in healthcare providers [54].

After admission to an RCF, sexuality is no longer a private activity between two partners/persons. In RCFs, sexuality becomes an activity that is also felt, interpreted and controlled by the (rules of the) new 'environment' in which people with different roles are involved. Research has shown discrepancies between the views of people with dementia and those of partners, carers and significant others [34, 36].

3.5 The Broader System: Family

While it has been argued that in RCFs the autonomy of the residents should always be privileged [59], it has been shown that in reality the wishes of family members are often privileged [27]. For a person with dementia living in an RCF, the term 'family' is by necessity broad and encompasses a wide range of relationships, including parent/child, spouse/partner, grandparent/grandchild or close 'family like' friends, which makes determining attitudes difficult [23]. All family members involved with an admission of a family member with dementia to an RCF are often concerned. They hope that the resident will be well cared for, be protected and spared from harm, including sexual harm. Family members may perceive tolerance from staff towards sexual expression as putting the resident at unnecessary risk [23].

3.6 The Broader System: Healthcare Providers

In general, healthcare providers do not regard sexual health as a legitimate topic to raise with older adults [e.g. 60]. Healthcare providers' beliefs often reflect stereotypical views and myths regarding sexuality that result in healthcare providers feeling uncomfortable and untrained to address this area of health. It is likely that attitudes towards the sexual lives of people living with dementia will be even more influenced, and that this might affect aspects of their care [27].

It has been suggested that nursing homes exist merely to meet the needs of basic body care and that sexuality does not play a vital role in the maintenance of bodily functions. This means that creating an environment conducive towards fulfilment of sexual needs is not seen as part of the primary caregiving role of RCFs [57]. Also, the expression of sexuality of residents can be hampered because some nursing staff report feeling troubled or anxious when confronted with sexual expressions of residents, whereas others merely ignore such expressions [57].

3.7 Inappropriate Sexual Behaviour and Types of Dementia

Sexually inappropriate behaviours are seen in mild cognitive impairment as well as in severe dementia [53]. Moreover, it seems that different types of dementia, which all affect the brain differently, are related to different types of sexual behavioural problems that depend on which parts of the person's brain are affected and what medication they are taking. Inappropriate sexual behaviour is mostly an expression of the interaction of brain, physical, psychological and environmental factors and is usually caused by damage to neuroanatomical structures – that is, the frontal lobes, the temporolimbic system, the striatum and the hypothalamus – implicated in sexual motivation and behaviour [52]. Specifically, frontal lobe dysfunction may lead to alterations of the inhibitory mechanisms of sexual behaviour, while temporal lobe dysfunctions may involve problems regarding the emotional and intellectual interpretation of sexual arousal [52].

De Medeiros et al. [55] found that Alzheimer's disease was associated with intimacy-seeking behaviours. Based on case reports of patients with Alzheimer's disease, Davies et al. [61] described that dementia patients can experience various problems such as impaired cognitive sequencing during lovemaking, forgetfulness of previous lovemaking and declines in decision-making capacity. Hartmans et al. [22] added the inability to take into account the feelings of others, the inability to understand the meaning of these behaviours in the contextual environment and disinhibition.

It is important to note that these behaviours are often new and not necessarily related to the way the sexual relationships or preferences were before the illness. It has been suggested that non–Alzheimer's disease dementias are associated with more 'disinhibited behaviours' [51]. One study compared sexual changes in patients with Alzheimer's and FTD and found the same frequency of increased sex drive in both conditions (8%) [62]. However, Mendez and Shapira [63] posited that FTD involves greater disinhibition and lower sexual drive than Alzheimer's disease and that this may pose different problems in sexual and intimate relationships. Several studies [e.g. 53] have found that vascular dementia is most commonly associated with inappropriate sexual behaviours with a higher frequency of provocative behaviour and more intentional sexual behaviour [39].

In persons with dementia the appearance of ISB has also been linked to certain psychoactive drugs (e.g. levodopa, benzodiazepine and alcohol) [54] as well as to psychosocial factors (e.g. lack of privacy, restrictive attitudes, mistaking someone – including opposite-gender carers – for his or her partner and trying to make sexual advances).

Thus ISB should be interpreted in a broader perspective as a part of the symptom cluster of behavioural disturbances associated with dementia and is more prevalent in men [e.g. 53].

3.8 Management of Inappropriate Sexual Behaviour

With an estimated prevalence range from 4–5% to 25% [52], ISB is not the most common behavioural change among dementia patients, but it may have harmful, particularly intense outcomes affecting patients as well as those around them. This means that management of ISB in both home care and RCFs is often an important challenge. Therefore, it is striking that the evidence about the effectiveness of non-pharmacological as well as pharmacological treatments is still limited and mainly consists of case reports, case series and expert opinion. Hitherto, there are no randomized controlled trials for any treatment of sexual disinhibition in dementia available.

While several drug classes – that is, antipsychotics, antidepressants, cholinesterase inhibitors, anti-epileptics, hormonal and non-hormonal anti-androgens and beta-blockers – are considered efficacious, there are different opinions about which pharmacotherapies to use first to 'treat' ISB [51]. The suggestion to base the choice of the initial agent on other clinical features is interesting but founded on expert opinion only. Clearly, more research is needed to clarify the indications and effectiveness of these medications [51].

Similarly, more research is required on the effectiveness of non-pharmacological approaches (e.g. environmental approaches such as clothing modification and distraction techniques to avoid unnecessary use of medications that can have harmful side effects, environmental manipulation, same-sex caregivers) [51]. Apart from these specific behaviour-targeted treatments, RCFs should also develop a management approach of sexuality and ISB at the level of the organization (e.g. policy development, staff education and support, clear communication with and involvement of relatives) [27].

Tucker presented an interesting comprehensive approach to assessment and management of 'inappropriate' sexual behaviour in patients with dementia [51]. Apart from the practical aspects of such an approach, ISBs are viewed as posing diffuse and difficult ethical questions about assessment and treatment in RCFs. These ethical concerns mostly refer to finding a balance between a resident's need for sexual expression and the needs, feelings, expectations and beliefs of healthcare providers, other residents, partners and family members, which may be based on ageist ideas reflecting that sexuality is deemed inappropriate, dysfunctional or non-existent in elderly people (with dementia) (see Section 2.1). Management of ISB in vulnerable cognitively impaired people with (hormonal) medications is still ethically contentious. In RCFs, these ethical concerns arise even stronger when two cognitively impaired residents engage in an intimate and sexual relationship. In such cases, residential care staff should assess both individuals' capacity to consent to this relationship and use that as a criterion to determine if this relationship could be continued. This brings us to the question of how care staff could do so.

3.9 Ethical Issues

Sexuality of persons living with dementia clearly shows that sexuality involves more than physical (inter)actions, and that sexuality is also related to psychological, emotional and social processes, including ethical issues. That sexuality and ethics often go hand in hand is reflected in concepts as 'capacity', 'sexual consent' and 'privacy'. When and how does someone give his or her consent to have sex? When is someone able to give consent to certain sexual activities? How do we guarantee physical, social and psychological privacy? In this section, we explore how 'capacity', 'sexual consent' and 'privacy' relate to people with dementia and how RCFs, healthcare professionals, the partner and the broader family network can use these in their appreciation of the sexual behaviour of persons with dementia.

3.9.1 Definition of Capacity and Sexual Consent

In the literature on the sexuality of people living with dementia, their capacity to consent to intimate or sexual acts is often questioned. Wilkins [64] proposed six criteria to judge whether a person has capacity to give sexual consent: voluntariness, safety (person is protected or recognizes dangerous situations), no exploitation, no physical or psychological abuse, ability to say 'no' (verbally or non-verbally) and social appropriateness (time and place). Wilkins [64] stated

that a capacity assessment based on these six criteria can be a useful tool in the initial evaluation of the ability to consent to sexual activities.

Kennedy and Niederbuhl [65] described sexual consent as an informed, competent and voluntary commitment to a particular sexual activity. The American Bar Association (ABA) and the American Psychological Association (APA) [66] posited that there are no universal or uniform criteria to define sexual consent and confirmed that the most important criteria are knowledge (*informed*), understanding or reasoning (*competent*) and voluntariness (*voluntary*). In the context of sexuality, this means that a person must: (a) know what is happening and know the risks and benefits of certain sexual behaviour, (b) understand what the sexual behaviour will entail and that it is consistent with one's personal values and (c) be able to give consent free from undue influence or coercion [66]. While these criteria formulated for capacity and consent seem very logical and should be pursued by all women and men in all situations, they challenge partners as well as healthcare providers working with patients and residents with dementia. How do partners and caregivers know these criteria are met if persons with dementia have difficulties with verbal communication and if their decision-making is difficult to understand?

3.9.1.1 Sexual Consent and Dementia

This attempt to develop a capacity assessment (see Chapter 11) for sexual consent demonstrates that we are dealing with a complex phenomenon. This complexity seems even bigger in the context of care for people with dementia as we must consider their capabilities and limitations while respecting their autonomy. In this context, we have to be aware of several issues.

First, everyone – including people with dementia – has a right to take risks. In their duty to provide good care, healthcare providers, however, often tend to avoid, remove or eliminate all risks. In care, it is of course crucial that vulnerable people are protected and that their safety is guaranteed, but human life entails risk. Especially in the world of love, romance and sexuality, people get hurt, rejected or dumped, which may cause emotional stress, but that is also a part of life. By not allowing people with dementia to express their sexual needs and take sexual risks, healthcare providers violate their autonomy and personhood. We should not confuse the 'possibility to make a bad or unwise decision' with 'incompetence to engage in sexual interaction' [67].

Second, in our society, the dominant discourse about (heterosexual) couples, sex and romance is strongly reinforced by how ('good') sex is depicted in literature, art and film. Reynolds uses an ethical social angle to point to the complexity of sexual consent. This discourse entails a fixed gender-based scenario about an idealized notion of the sexual encounter in which neither power nor permission is problematized [68]. In the life of real people, (sexual) relationships are not always 'a rose garden', but that does not preclude people from having relationships – and this may also apply to people with dementia.

Reynolds [68] also signals the cultural importance of verbal and non-verbal communication in the context of sexuality. People often find it hard to express their sexual desires in words. But they may find it even more difficult to interpret non-verbal sexual communication (e.g. the person who permits sex with a good friend hoping it will turn into a romantic relationship, the person who passionately kisses back but is unwilling to take further steps, leaving the other confused), and this may weigh on the ability to give or understand sexual consent from someone else. In sum, we all, not just people with dementia, have the challenge to improve our communication about sexuality. In addition, practical situations demonstrate that sexual consent is not always visible or may change during a sexual interaction.

Reynolds [68] further discusses the gender characteristics of sexual context. The dominant idea of an active man and a more passive woman is still present and influences sexual expectations and behaviour. Healthcare providers often assume that if a man is involved, he will take the initiative (i.e. is the perpetrator) and that a woman is passive (i.e. is the victim). In real life, this is not always true: a man (with dementia) may only need some human warmth or intimacy or can be overwhelmed by the actions of a woman.

The network of people caring for persons with dementia should support them in their (non-verbal) quest for sexuality starting from an open mind, and they should in their caring not be stricter for their patients than for themselves. Reynolds [68] concludes that although sexual consent is a very important concept, it is only a part of the broader picture of sex and should

not only be used to combat the frequent occurrence of non-consensual sex.

3.9.1.2 Approaches to Assess Capacity and Sexual Consent

Currently, there is no generic rule or principle that fits for all persons with dementia, a progressive disease evolving in stages (e.g. mild symptoms, severe memory loss and loss of other cognitive functions). This implies that there is not a single 'one-size-fits-all' approach for all people with dementia in all stages of the disease. Tarzia et al. [67] argue that 'there is plenty of support within the literature to suggest that people with dementia can and do continue to make decisions about various aspects of their daily lives, even if they are unable to decide how their finances are to be managed' (p. 611). They continue: 'individuals with moderate, or even advanced, dementia who may have lost the ability to communicate verbally … convey preferences and choices including body language and facial expressions' (p. 611). This viewpoint implies that even when it is difficult or no longer possible to have a verbal conversation with a person with dementia, partners and caregivers should observe their non-verbal communication in order to evaluate whether the person gets a good or bad feeling about the sexual experience.

This means that healthcare providers should not limit or even eliminate sexual needs and behaviours or (hide themselves behind the) tussle with complex ethical dilemmas about the definition of capacity and sexual consent [67]. Healthcare providers should recognize the sexual needs and expressions of patients with dementia and ask themselves, 'How can we make (informed, competent, voluntary and safe) sex possible for people with dementia?' Healthcare providers can find inspiration in a framework developed by the ABA/APA [66].

This framework is a helpful method to determine whether a person with dementia is capable to give sexual consent. This framework is presented as a balance in which several categories of evidence can be measured, with 'more objective factors' on one side of the scale and 'more subjective factors' on the other. The tipping point of the scale is clinical judgement of the care providers who must weigh the different factors while taking into account the benefit to the patient with dementia. The objective measures that can be taken into account are: (a) functional assessment (e.g. knowledge, understanding, reasoning), (b) diagnoses that may affect capacity (e.g. disinhibition due to FTD), (c) cognitive underpinnings of cognitive, emotional and everyday functioning (e.g. memory, attention) and (d) emotional or psychiatric factors (e.g. depression or anxiety). The subjective measures refer to: (a) values and preferences of the individual, (b) the risk of harm in the activity for which capacity is assessed and (c) possible interventions to enhance capacity. This framework may be helpful for healthcare providers to determine whether a person with dementia can give (sexual) consent.

In some cases, this complex framework may not give enough support and guidance. Wilkins [64] therefore presented two alternatives. First, he proposed advocacy by family or caregivers. They should represent the person with dementia and advocate their autonomy, dignity and right to sexual expression while minimizing harm. However, healthcare providers should be aware of the prejudices and biases of the representatives (e.g. conflict of interest by family members or caregivers who favour the opinion of the family).

Second, Wilkins [64] pled for a committee approach meaning that the person with dementia, family members and care providers assemble to discuss the matter based on the best interest standard. In this committee, the balance between benefit and harm is explored openly and sexual expression of the patient is allowed if the potential benefits exceed the risks [64].

A third option is a living will in which a person records wishes in advance. That will can be used as a support as dementia advances. Tarzia et al. [67] questioned this option because 'it negates the right of the resident to change his or her mind, and also ignores the effect that dementia can have on an individual's personality' (p. 610).

Finally, Frederix et al. [69] present a '10 shades of grey' approach to evaluate sexual consent in persons with dementia. This approach uses the notion of 'limited capacity' [71] and different types of relationships with associated sexual activities [59]. White [71] emphasizes avoiding looking at capacity as an all-or-nothing phenomenon – that is, a person with dementia is either capable or not to give consent for a specific sexual behaviour. 'Alternatively, a limited capacity system acknowledges shades of grey … an individual could be deemed to have capacity to consent to certain intimate behaviours but not to others or to

have capacity to consent to a certain sexual partner but not to others' (p. 152). As a result, caregivers 'need to provide sufficient supervision and monitoring to ensure that individuals do not engage in behaviours that are outside of their recognized capacities' (p. 152).

On a similar note, Mahieu et al. [59] recognize different types of relationships with associated sexual activities – that is, loving and caring, romantic and erotic relationships. A loving and caring relationship is based on a strong friendship. The partners show great affection for each other, seek each other's company regularly, give hugs and hold hands. A romantic relationship entails more sexual intimacy including behaviours such as kissing, hugging, caressing each other and laying in the same bed together. Finally, the erotic relationship is filled with sexual desires, excitement, activities and satisfaction. This typology of relationships with associated sexual activities can serve as a practical guideline for the 'limited capacity' approach. This practical tool provides in a more person-centred approach in which different characteristics (e.g. personality, values, abilities and limitations) of those who express a sexual need can be taken into account. This tool aims to find answers and interventions that can promote the sexual health and well-being of persons with dementia.

In conclusion, capacity and sexual consent are clearly important but complex aspects of sexual health and sexual well-being of persons with dementia. Sexual consent can, however, only be understood as a part of a broad perspective on sexuality and caregivers should not only limit their focus on the (in)ability or capacity to give sexual consent. Healthcare providers should be aware that there are different perspectives to approach sexuality in persons with dementia and that a person-centred approach presupposes that all (in)abilities, (im)possibilities and the autonomy of a person with dementia should be taken into account.

3.9.2 Privacy

Privacy is another essential aspect of sexuality that is related to ethics, but it is also connected to sexual rights, patients' rights and human rights.

3.9.2.1 Sexual Rights

The International Planned Parenthood Federation (IPPF) advocates for sexual and reproductive health and rights for all and described the right to privacy based on international human rights as follows [72; Article 4]:

> All persons have the right not to be subjected to arbitrary interference with their privacy, family, home, papers or correspondence and the right to privacy which is essential to the exercise of sexual autonomy. All persons are entitled to sexual autonomy and shall be able to make decisions about their sexuality, sexual behaviour and intimacy without arbitrary interference. All persons have the right to confidentiality regarding equal health services and care, medical records, and in general to protect information concerning their HIV status and to be protected from arbitrary disclosures or threats of arbitrary disclosures, within the framework of permissible limitations and without discrimination. All persons have the right to control the disclosure of information regarding their sexual choices, sexual history, sexual partners and behaviours and other matters related to sexuality.

In our society, most people who are independent and do not need assistance for personal care can monitor and manage these rights. However, for people with dementia who depend on others for personal care or who are not able to express or speak for themselves, it is less evident to preserve their right to privacy. As dementia can affect people's decorum, they might also need guidance in assessing a situation to safeguard their own and/or other persons' privacy. In these situations, healthcare providers are even more challenged to act consciously and pay attention to respect a person with dementia's privacy and sexual autonomy.

3.9.2.2 Dementia Care and Privacy

Swinnen [73] distinguished physical privacy from social privacy. Physical privacy refers to several aspects of the environment that are helpful to protect privacy (e.g. doors that can be locked, curtains that can be closed, individual rooms, personal bathroom). Social privacy refers to how healthcare professionals handle privacy in a social environment (e.g. the attitudes of other residents in RCFs, attitudes about closing doors and curtains during washing, exchanging information about a resident in a meeting room instead of the hallway).

In care practice, this means that to guarantee social privacy healthcare providers should take into account the following points. They should begin with asking for permission to enter the client's home or room. Even if a caregiver has a key, he or she knocks on the door and waits for an answer. Healthcare providers should at least announce their presence and wait for an answer if the person has hearing or mobility disabilities. During care moments, curtains and doors are closed, bodies are covered, physical contact is announced and granted and there are no unnecessary interruptions from outsiders.

Some RCFs use 'do not disturb' signs on doors or provide a room specifically dedicated to sexual experiences for inhabitants. The purpose of these 'tools' is to enable persons to experience sexuality while granting and guaranteeing privacy, but to achieve this purpose, these tools must be properly integrated and used in daily care. Residential care facilities should deliberately think about the use of door signs and consider multiple reasons for using the sign (e.g. a consultation with the general practitioner, a conversation with family, an hour's rest in bed, masturbation, watching pornography, hugging with a partner in bed). In that way, it will not be clear for an outsider why someone wishes not to be disturbed. Residential care facilities must carefully consider the location and ways of implementing a 'private' room. They should reflect on when and by whom the room can be used. The broader the aims and reasons for using the room (e.g. to have a massage, to relax, to rest, to be intimate as a couple, to masturbate in private while using porn, to have sex with a sex (care) worker), the better the privacy of the users is guaranteed.

Residential care facilities should also reflect on the accessibility of the room. Can patients access the room freely (e.g. how can one guarantee privacy if residents need to ask the key first)? Can residents visit the room discreetly without having to pass too many inmates or employees? Of course, some people with dementia will need assistance to use these 'tools'. In these cases, caregivers should act vicariously with respect for the individual needs and privacy of the person with dementia. These guidelines apply to caregivers in home care and in residential care [69].

Another aspect of privacy is confidentiality and disclosure of information – that is, social and psychological aspects of privacy. To highly value privacy in home care as well as in residential care there should be a clear policy about sharing information about the persons who are cared for, including information about intimate and sexual issues. Where are data of persons kept and who has access to them? Who should inform whom in case of needs or problems? What about informing family and externals? Bauer et al. [23] found that families of persons with dementia wished to be kept informed about the sexual behaviour of their relatives. While it has been suggested that family members have the right to be informed about the well-being of their beloved ones, including sexual well-being [69], it is important to consider the capacity of residents with dementia and whether they can give consent.

Bauer et al. [23] also found that families often place great liability on the organization and great responsibility on the care providers to supervise, adjust or even prevent certain sexual behaviours. For organizations and healthcare providers that want to provide high-quality care, this implies that they have to find a good balance between family members' right to information and the person with dementia's right to privacy [69]. In ethical advice for Care Network Flanders, Mahieu et al. [74] states:

> A proportional consideration must be made between the involvement of a family member on the one hand, and the nature, meaning, and potential consequences of the behaviour on the other … owning information about the older person's initial behaviour gives the person with whom the information is shared (e.g., the children) a certain authority. However, this does not mean that this person automatically has the authority for making certain decisions. Moreover, sharing information also involves a certain degree of objectification of the older person. We must always guard against reducing people to the information we have about them.

This argument does not only apply to family members, but also to other team members.

In conclusion, in both home and residential care, healthcare providers need useable tools and a clear policy to guarantee the sexual rights including the right to privacy of persons with dementia. This policy should provide support and backup and inform healthcare providers to act professionally with respect for multiple aspects of the privacy of the person with dementia they care for.

3.10 Vision and Policy in Healthcare

Bauer et al. [75] stated that sexuality 'is a key component of quality of life and well-being and a need to express one's sexuality continues into old age' (p. 1). This idea of continuity is not new and not different for persons with dementia. In order to do justice to this wish for continuity, it is necessary that healthcare professionals can rely on a clear vision and a manageable policy that is supported by the administrators, managers and directors of healthcare organizations.

3.10.1 Vision and Mission

Healthcare organizations best embed their vision about (the importance of) sexuality in their general mission (statement) and vision. Both the mission and vision of an organization give direction and support to the daily working and workers of an organization. A mission defines the field of action of an organization and stands for its (ethical) unique identity. A vision defines the desired future of an organization and takes on the evolution in a changing environment bearing in mind the mission [69]. Ideally, a vision about sexuality includes the different target groups (i.e. elderly or persons with dementia, family, care providers and third parties or outsiders) as well as embraces diversity within sexuality. It is important to be aware that we still live in a heteronormative society in which sexuality is viewed as 'penetrative sex between a woman and a man', marginalizing lesbian, gay, bisexual and transgender (LGBT) identities and other expressions of sexuality (e.g. solo sex, masturbation or 'skin hunger' – i.e. the need of human beings to be touched from skin to skin).

For organizations, there are two possible methods to formulate a vision. An organization can choose to appoint one person to lead the development of a vision or appoint a team. In recent years, the team approach has gained more interest because of its positive effects (e.g. better connection with practice and from the beginning useful input from the workplace), but it also challenges teams (e.g. finding compromises) that have to keep in mind that a vision should be helpful and clarifying.

Teams should take into account the following points for successful development of a vision. A team should: (a) take enough time to do it right from the first time, (b) be open to unpredictability as this may result in unexpected but valuable input, (c) be ambitious and not confine itself to formulate vague, obvious or general goals, (d) formulate clearly both the ethical codes and the codes of conduct and (e) invest in a broad perspective on sexuality and do not focus on a single (negative or challenging) item [69].

3.10.2 Policy: Vision Translated into Practice

To translate a vision into daily practice, RCFs need to formulate a policy on sexuality care. Residential care facilities can find inspiration in the 'Sexuality and Policy Framework' [76]. This framework consists of three parts: a concept vision for policy, instruments that make the policy applicable in practice and background information. The concept of vision for policy formulates three levels of policy – quality, prevention and reaction. First, quality means that a policy reflects a wide perspective on sexuality – that is, it includes positive aspects of sexuality and is not restricted to a procedure to prevent and sanction 'inappropriate' sexual behaviour. Second, prevention builds on quality with awareness of possible risks. Third, reaction builds on prevention and determines how to deal with an incident.

In the next step, these three levels must be translated in specific targets for four policy domains: care and education, house rules and accommodation, expertise and screening employees, and communication. An organization can combine these three policy levels and four policy domains and create its own, unique policy matrix [76]. The Framework provides nine instruments to support the implementation of the policy [76]. The last part that the Framework presents is background information. This part aims to foresee useful background information that is helpful in the development of an informed and reasoned policy on sexuality and physical integrity. It contains helpful information such as the framework of rights, a legal and judicial framework, an ethical framework and information and actual legislation about concepts such as professional confidentiality [76].

This Framework is quite extensive and can therefore be overwhelming. Not everything has to be addressed immediately or simultaneously. These points are, however, helpful to develop a vision and policy about sexuality and it will be important to keep this interest in sexuality vivid as part of QoL of residents with dementia. Change takes time, which means that changing attitudes and actions related to sexuality will also take time. For those who are looking for support with this transformation process in their RCF, Kotter has developed a change model with eight steps [69, 70]. In conclusion, the availability of a clear vision and a manageable policy helps healthcare professionals to feel confident to include this topic in their daily practice and deal with questions about sexual care or sexual situations of people with dementia.

4 Conclusion

In this chapter, we have provided an overview of the impact of living with dementia on the partner relationship and on intimacy and sexuality between partners. A dementia diagnosis has a clear and huge impact on the patient as well as on the partner and causes important relational changes partners have to learn to cope with. Many changes and losses occur for both partners, but they can create a new balance or a new 'normal' (e.g. new roles, responsibilities, coping mechanisms) by adjusting and renegotiating their relationship [16, 17]. This renegotiation in couples with dementia develops gradually and has to be repeated as a function of progression of dementia. Surely, not all couples will reach a positive outcome, and this should urge healthcare professionals and researchers to pay more attention to the partner relationship thereby involving the broader social network as a source of support. These relational changes may also have an impact on the need for, feelings about, meaning of and experience with intimacy and sexuality.

This chapter provides a description of the complex dialogue and relations between all parties involved and their different viewpoints on sexuality of persons with dementia (see Figure 6.2). While the sexuality of patients with dementia is often interpreted as a 'problem', it is for them probably just a *human need* that will be reshaped by age-related, health-related, dementia-related and medication-related changes that challenge couples living with dementia. For the partner (and the broader family network), dementia often raises *concerns* about several domains of life both in the home care phase and after admission to an RCF.

One of the domains that often raises huge concern is the (changing) sexuality of the (changing) partner with dementia. Concerns about (inappropriate) sexual behaviour often cause

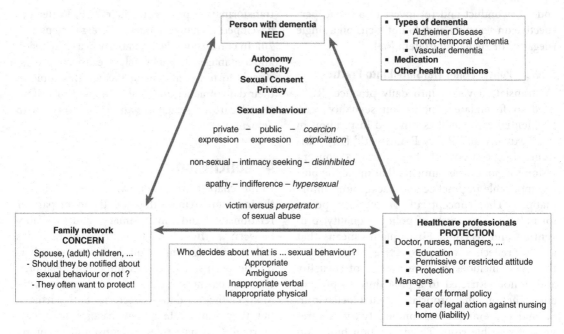

Figure 6.2 The complex triangle of discussing the sexuality of persons with dementia

shame and result in a willingness to protect family members or other residents from its negative consequences. Family members often want to be informed about problem behaviour. Healthcare professionals and personnel of RCFs are the third party that is involved and co-creates the dialogue about the sexual needs of patients from a protection perspective. In this dialogue, the autonomy of the patient should be central, but decisions will be informed by a judgement of the capacity of a patient to give sexual consent to certain intimate or sexual behaviour that the patient should be able to experience in privacy. In this judgement, healthcare professionals will not only consider the autonomy and needs of the patient, but will also probably try to find a balance between the 'needs' and possibilities of all parties involved.

In this balance, certain organizations may provide sexual assistance to elderly and persons with disabilities including dementia. Although ethical questions have been posed about this form of care, it has proven valuable for some patients with dementia as these sexual assistance workers provide professional, patient-tailored care. This means that the starting point of the professionals is mutual respect, privacy and equality while fulfilling the intimate and/or sexual needs of the patient with dementia. As privacy and consent are guaranteed, sexual assistance from a well-informed professional is an ethical way of helping patients with dementia to experience intimacy and sex.

Although this chapter contains interesting information about the impact of dementia on partner relations, intimacy and sexuality, the scientific literature on this topic remains very limited. Moreover, this small number of studies had a range of methodological limitations including small sample sizes, inclusion of only the patient, the partner or caregiver. Studies did not give good information about the establishment of the dementia diagnosis or about the stage of the dementia. Participants were often recruited via memory clinics, hospitals, local Alzheimer's associations or universities, hampering the generalizability, and most data were collected at one point in time only.

Nevertheless, all of this information should be helpful to better 'manage' sexual behaviour of individuals with dementia living at home as well as in RCFs and to prevent caregivers to react passively rather than promoting it. As more caregivers become aware and convinced about the sexual needs of persons with dementia and have more tools to decide about the 'appropriateness' of sexual behaviour, they might be less anxious to be involved in legal situations. Better education, clear guidelines, policy and vision development of RCFs will help caregivers to manage specific sexual situations in a more objective and respectful way. Information on the importance of sexuality for individuals with dementia – including positive aspects as well as 'problematic' sexual behaviour – should become a part of nursing and medical school curricula and continuing educational programmes that should be easily accessible for caregivers as well as residents and family members [77]. Only in this way can we provide in a care context in which the sexual needs of all patients with dementia can be fully respected – maybe including ours in the future.

References

1. Benbow SM, Tsaroucha A, Sharman V. 'It is not the same': Relationships and dementia. *Educ Gerontol* 2019; **45**(7): 454–68.

2. De Boer ME, Hertogh CM, Dröes R, Riphagen II, Jonker C, Eefsting JA. Suffering from dementia: The patient's perspective. A review of the literature. *Int Psychogeriatr* 2007; **19**(6): 1021–39.

3. Braun M, Scholz U, Bailey B, Perren S, Hornung R, Martin M. Dementia caregiving in spousal relationships: A dyadic perspective. *Aging Ment Health* 2009; **13**(3): 426–36.

4. Ablitt A, Jones GV, Muers J. Living with dementia: A systematic review of the influence of relationship factors. *Aging Ment Health* 2009; **13**(4): 497–511.

5. Pozzebon M, Douglas J, Ames D. Spouses' experience of living with a partner diagnosed with a dementia: A synthesis of the qualitative research. *Int Psychogeriatr* 2016; **28**(4): 537–56.

6. Youell J, Callaghan JE, Buchanan K. 'I don't know if you want to know this': Carers' understandings of intimacy in long-term relationships when one partner has dementia. *Ageing Soc* 2016; **36**: 946–67.

7. Sanders S, Power J. Roles, responsibilities, and relationships among older husbands caring for wives with progressive dementia and other chronic conditions. *Health Soc Work* 2009; **34**(1): 41–51.

8. Meuser TM, Marwit SJ. A comprehensive, stage-sensitive model of grief in dementia caregiving. *Gerontologist* 2001; **41**(5): 658–70.

9. Evans D, Lee E. Impact of dementia on marriage: A qualitative systematic review. *Dementia* 2014; **13**(3): 330–49.

10. Lindauer A, Harvath TA. Pre-death grief in the context of dementia caregiving: A concept analysis. *J Adv Nurs* 2014; **70**: 2196–2207.

11. Herbert R, Schulz R, Copeland VC, Arnold RM. Preparing family caregivers for death and bereavement. Insights from caregivers of terminally ill patients. *J Pain Symptom Manage* 2009; **37**(1): 3–12.

12. Colquhoun A, Moses J, Offord R. Experiences of loss and relationship quality in couples living with dementia. *Dementia* 2019; **18**(6): 2158–72.

13. Eloniemi-Sulkava U, Notkola IL, Hämäläinen K, Rahkonen T, Viramo P, Hentinen M, et al. Spouse caregivers' perceptions of influence of dementia on marriage. *Int Psychogeriatr* 2002; **14**(1): 47–58.

14. Wadham O, Simpson J, Rust J, Murray C. Couples' shared experiences of dementia: A meta-synthesis of the impact upon relationships and couplehood. *Aging Ment Health* 2016; **20**(5): 463–73.

15. Davies HD, Newkirk LA, Pitts CB, Coughlin CA, Sridhar SB, Zeiss LM, Zeiss AM. The impact of dementia and mild memory impairment (MMI) on intimacy and sexuality in spousal relationships. *Int Psychogeriatr* 2010; **22**(4): 618–28.

16. Wolverson E, Clarke C, Moniz-Cook E. Living positively with dementia: A systematic review and synthesis of the qualitative literature. *Aging Ment Health* 2016; **20**: 676–99.

17. Enright J, O'Connell ME, Branger C, Kirk A, Morgan D. Identity, relationship quality, and subjective burden in caregivers of persons with dementia. *Dementia* 2018; **0**: 1–17.

18. Rousseaux M, Sève A, Vallet M, Pasquier F, Mackowiak-Cordoliani MA. An analysis of communication in conversation in patients with dementia. *Neuropsychologia* 2010; **48**(13): 3884–90.

19. Holdsworth K, McCabe M. The impact of younger-onset dementia on relationships, intimacy, and sexuality in midlife couples: A systematic review. *Int Psychogeriatr* 2018a; **30**(1): 15–29.

20. Holdsworth K, McCabe M. The impact of dementia on relationships, intimacy, and sexuality in later life couples: An integrative qualitative analysis of existing literature. *Clin Gerontol* 2018b; **41**(1): 3–19.

21. Mitrani VB, Czaja SJ. Family-based therapy for dementia caregivers: Clinical observations. *Aging Ment Health* 2008; **4**(3): 200–9.

22. Hartmans C, Comijs H, Jonker C. Cognitive functioning and its influence on sexual behavior in normal aging and dementia. *Int J Geriatr Psychiatry* 2014; **29**(5), 441–6.

23. Bauer M, Nay R, Fetherstonhaugh D, Wellman D, Beattie E. We need to know what's going on: Views of family members toward the sexual expressions of people with dementia in residential aged care. *Dementia* 2013; **13**(5): 571–85.

24. Scherrer KS. Images of sexuality and aging in gerontological literature. *Sex Res Soc Policy* 2009; **6**: 5–12.

25. Traeen B, Hald G, Graham C, Enzlin P, Janssen E, Lundin Kvalem I, et al. Sexuality in older adults (65+) – an overview of the literature, part 1: Sexual function and its difficulties. *Int J Sex Health* 2017; **29**(1): 1–10.

26. Traeen B, Carvalheira A, Lundin Kvalem I, Štulhofer A, Janssen E, Graham C, et al. Sexuality in older adults (65+) – an overview of the recent literature, part 2: Body image and sexual satisfaction. *Int J Sex Health* 2017; **29**(1): 11–21.

27. Benbow SM, Beeston D. Sexuality, aging, and dementia. *Int Psychogeriatr* 2012; **24**(7): 1026–33.

28. Gott M. *Sexuality, Sexual Health and Ageing.* Berkshire, Open University Press, 2005; 176.

29. Youell J, Callaghan J. An investigation into the changes in intimacy in long-term relationships when one partner has dementia. *Ageing Soc* 2016; **35**(5): 946–67.

30. Sandberg LJ. Too late for love? Sexuality and intimacy in heterosexual couples living with an Alzheimer's disease diagnosis. *Sex Relatsh Ther* 2020; 1–22.

31. Alzheimer's Society. How can dementia affect a person's sexual behaviour? (Internet). UK: Alzheimer's Society; (date unknown). Consulted on 1 April 2021, available from www .alzheimers.org.uk/get-support/daily-living/how-dementia-affects-sexual-behaviour.

32. Baikie E. The impact of dementia on marital relationships. *Sex and Relatsh Ther* 2002; **17**(3): 289–99.

33. Rheaume C, Mitty E. Sexuality and intimacy in older adults. *Geriatr Nurs* 2008; **29**(5): 342–9.

34. Harris PB. Intimacy, sexuality, and early-stage dementia. The changing marital relationship. *Alzheimer's Care Today* 2009; **10**(2): 63–77.

35. Ballard CG, Solis M, Gahir M, Cullen P, Georges S, Oyebode R, Wilcock G. Sexual relationships in married dementia sufferers. *Int J Geriat Psychiatry* 1997; **12**: 447–51.

36. Nogueira MM, Neto JP, Sousa MF, Santos RL, Lacerda IB, Baptista MA, Dourado MC. Perception of change in sexual activity in Alzheimer's disease: Views of people with dementia and their spouse-caregivers. *Int Psychogeriatr* 2017; **29**(2): 185–93.

37. Tsatali M, Tsolaki M. Sexual function in normal elders, MCI and patients with mild dementia. *Sex Disabil* 2014; **32**(2): 205–19.

38. Abdo CH. Sexuality and couple intimacy in dementia. *Curr Opin Psychiatry* 2013; **26**(6): 593–8.

39. Roelofs TS, Luijkx KG, Embregts PJ. Intimacy and sexuality of nursing home residents with dementia: A systematic review. *Int Psychogeriatr* 2015; **27**(3): 367–84.

40. Simpson P, Wilson CB, Brown LJ, Dickinson T, Horne M. 'We've had our sex life way back': Older care home residents, sexuality and intimacy. *Ageing Soc* 2018; **38**: 1478–1501.

41. Tabak N, Shemesh-Kigli R. Sexuality and Alzheimer's disease: Can the two go together? *Nurs Forum* 2016; **41**(4): 158–66.

42. Simonelli C, Tripodi F, Rossi R, Fabrizi A, Lembo D, Cosmi V, Pierleoni L. The influence of caregiver burden on sexual intimacy and marital satisfaction in couples with an Alzheimer spouse. *Int J Clin Pract* 2008; **62**(1): 47–52.

43. Dourado M, Finamore C, Barroso MF, Santos R, Laks J. Sexual satisfaction in dementia: Perspectives of patients and spouses. *Sex Disabil* 2010; **28**: 195–203.

44. Hayes J, Boylstein C, Zimmerman MK. Living and loving with dementia: Negotiating spousal and caregiver identity through narrative. *J Aging Stud* 2009; **23**(1): 48–59.

45. Sanders S, Osterhaus J. Birth of a stranger: Intimacy, sexuality and dementia. In DeFord B, Gilbert R, eds. *Living, Loving, and Loss: The Interplay of Intimacy, Sexuality and Grief.* Amityville, NY, Baywood, 2013; 121–49.

46. Nilsson E. Facing dementia as a we: Investigating couples' challenges and communicative strategies for managing dementia (PhD dissertation). Linkoping University Press, Linkoping University, 2018.

47. Shavit O, Ben-Ze'ev AA, Doron I. Love between couples living with Alzheimer's disease: Narratives of spouse care-givers. *Ageing Soc* 2017; **39**(4): 488–517.

48. Donaldson C, Tarrier N, Burns A. Determinants of carer stress in Alzheimer's disease. *Int J Geriatr Psychiatry* 1998; **13**: 248–56.

49. Roelofs TS, Luijkx KG, Embregts PJ. Love, intimacy and sexuality in residential dementia care: A spousal perspective. *Dementia* 2019; **18**(3): 936–50.

50. Elias J, Ryan A. A review and commentary on the factors that influence expressions of sexuality by older people in care homes. *J Clin Nurs* 2011; **20**: 1668–76.

51. Tucker I. Management of inappropriate sexual behaviors in dementia: A literature review. *Int Psychogeriatr* 2010; **22**(5): 683–92.

52. Cipriani G, Ulivi M, Danti S, Lucetti C, Nuti A. Sexual disinhibition and dementia. *Psychogeriatr* 2016; **16**(2): 145–53.

53. Alagiakrishnan K, Lim D, Brahim A, Wong A, Wood A, Senthilselvan A, et al. Sexually inappropriate behaviour in demented elderly people. *Postgrad Med J* 2005; **81**(957): 463–6.

54. Wallace M, Safer M. Hypersexuality among cognitively impaired older adults. *Geriatr Nurs* 2009; **30**(4): 230–7.

55. De Medeiros K, Rosenberg PB, Baker AS, Onyike CU. Improper sexual behaviors in elders with dementia living in residential care. *Dement Geriatr Cogn Disord* 2008; **26**(4): 370–7.

56. Chapman KR, Spitznagel MB. Measurement of sexual disinhibition in dementia: A systematic review. *Int J Geriatr Psychiatry* 2019; **34**(12): 1747–57.

57. Nagaratnam N, Gayagay G Jr. Hypersexuality in nursing care facilities: A descriptive study. *Arch Gerontol Geriatr* 2002; **35**(3): 195–203.

58. Golander H, Raz A. The mask of dementia: Images of 'demented residents' in a nursing ward. *Ageing Soc* 1996; **16**(3): 269–85.

59. Mahieu L, Gastmans C. Sexuality in institutionalized elderly persons: A systematic review of argument-based ethics literature. *Int Psychogeriatr* 2012; **24**(3): 346–57.

60. Gott M, Galena E, Hinchliff S, Elford H. 'Opening a can of worms': GP and practice nurse barriers to talking about sexual health in primary care. *Fam Pract* 2004; **21**(5): 528–36.

61. Davies HD, Zeiss AM, Shea EA, Tinklenberg JR. Sexuality and intimacy in Alzheimer's patients and their partners. *Sex Disabil* 1998; **16**: 193–203.

62. Miller BL, Darby AL, Swartz JR, Yener GG, Mena I. Dietary changes, compulsions and sexual behavior in frontotemporal degeneration. *Dementia* 1995; **6**(4): 195–9.

63. Mendez MF, Shapira JS. Hypersexual behavior in frontotemporal dementia: A comparison with early-onset Alzheimer's disease. *Arch Sex Behav* 2013; **42**(3): 501–9.

64. Wilkins MJ. More than capacity: Alternatives for sexual decision making for individuals with dementia. *Gerontol* 2015; **55**(5): 716–23.

65. Kennedy CH, Niederbuhl J. Establishing criteria for sexual consent capacity. *Am J Ment Retard* 2001; **106**(6): 503–10.

66. American Bar Association/American Psychological Association. *Assessment of Older Adults with Diminished Capacity: A Handbook for Psychologists*. Washington, DC, American Bar Association/American Psychological Association, 2008.

67. Tarzia L, Fetherstonhaugh D, Bauer M. Dementia, sexuality and consent in residential aged care facilities. *J Med Ethics* 2012; **38**(10): 609–13.

68. Reynolds P. Seksuele toestemming ontrafeld (Sexual consent unravelled), *Ethiek & Maatschappij* 2010; **13**(1): 68–90.

69. Frederix N, Boerjan S, Verelst C. *Als Amor de draad kwijtraakt: Over seksualiteit en intimiteit bij personen met dementie (If Amor Is Lost: About Sexuality and Intimacy in Persons with Dementia)*. Leuven, Acco, 2017.

70. Kotter JP, Akhtar V, Gupta G. Change. How Organizations Achieve Hard-to-Imagine Results in Uncertain and Volatile Times. Hoboken, NJ, Wiley, 2021.

71. White MC. The eternal flame: Capacity to consent to sexual behavior among nursing home residents with dementia, *Elder Law J* 2010; **18**: 133–58.

72. International Planned Parenthood Federation. Sexual rights: An IPPD declaration (Internet). London (UK): International Planned Parenthood Federation, 2008. Consulted on 2 April 2021, available from www.ippf.org/sites/default/files/sexualrightsippfdeclaration_1.pdf.

73. Swinnen. *Seksualiteit van ouderen: Een multidisciplinaire benadering (Sexuality in Elderly: A Multidisciplinary Approach)*. Amsterdam, Amsterdam University Press, 2011.

74. Mahieu L, Anckaert L, Gastmans C. Intimacy and sexuality in institutionalized dementia care: Clinical-ethical considerations. *Health Care Anal* 2014; **25**: 52–71.

75. Bauer M, Fetherstonhaugh D, Tarzia L, Nay R, Beattie E. Supporting residents' expression of sexuality: The initial construction of a sexuality assessment tool for residential aged care facilities. *BMC Geriatr* 2014; **14**: 1–6.

76. Sensoa and Child Focus. Raamwerk seksualiteit en beleid (Sexuality and policy framework). Belgium: Sensoa and Child Focus, 2012. Consulted on 2 April 2021, available from www.sensoa.be/sites/default/files/digitaal_materiaal/2012j047raamwerkseksualiteitenbeleidprintable.pdf.

77. Makimoto K, Kang HS, Yamakawa M, Konno R. An integrated literature review on sexuality of elderly nursing home residents with dementia. *Int J Nurs Pract* 2015; **21**(2): 80–90.

Fathers and Sons

David Mason

Some things, they say,
one should not write about. I tried
to help my father comprehend
the toilet, how one needs
to undo one's belt, to slide
one's trousers down and sit,
but he stubbornly stood
and would not bend his knees.
I tried again
to bend him toward the seat,

and then I laughed
at the absurdity. Fathers and sons.
How he had wiped my bottom
half a century ago, and how
I would repay the favor
if he would only sit.

     Don't you –
he gripped me, trembling, searching for my eyes.
Don't you – but the word
was lost to him. Somewhere
a man of dignity would not be laughed at.
He could not see
it was the crazy dance
that made me laugh,
trying to make him sit
when he wanted to stand.

'Fathers and Sons', *reprinted from* The Sound: New and Selected Poems *(Red Hen Press, 2018) by David Mason. Reprinted by permission of the author.*

Informal Care for Persons with Dementia
Characteristics and Evidence-Based Support Interventions

Anja Declercq, Rose-Marie Dröes, Mary Mittelman
and Chantal Van Audenhove

1 Introduction

The proportion of people with dementia living at home is as high as 93–96% in lower- and middle-income countries and 69% in high-income countries [1]. The vast majority of people with dementia thus receive care at home, from either informal or formal carers or a combination of both. The annual global number of informal care hours provided to people with dementia living at home was estimated at about 82 billion hours in 2015. This equals 2,089 hours per year or 6 hours per day [1]. In the USA, friends and family provide 18.4 billion hours of care a year, an average of 21.9 hours of care per week per carer [2]. In the UK, 36% of informal carers of people with dementia care for more than 100 hours a week, and a similar percentage of dementia carers indicate they care day and night [3]. Unpaid care in the USA is valued at $244 billion, if the care were provided at the wage of a home care worker ($13.11/hour) [2]. Informal care thus is crucial for a vast majority of people with dementia. It allows them to stay at home and it has a huge impact on their quality of life.

Informal carers have multiple motivations for caring for a person with dementia. The care is seen as a natural part of family life based upon family relationships: love and wanting to reciprocate care received from the person with dementia in the past [4, 5]. A systematic review of motivations for caring for a person with dementia showed apparent similarity in carers' motivations, irrespective of their relationship with the care recipient, country of origin, ethnic or cultural background or gender [5]. Greenwood and Smith

[5] conclude: 'Caring for someone with dementia is a fluid, complex, often long-term role and it is likely that the motivations and the mixture or balance of motivations change as the health of the person with dementia, the carers' own health and their situations change.' The informal care process, in other words, is dynamic and as situations change, so does the support an informal carer may need [6].

In Section 1 of this chapter, the characteristics of informal care and care policies are discussed. Section 2 deals with the evolution of informal care in the different stages of the dementia process and the changing needs of the person with dementia and of the informal carer. Evidence-based interventions can support informal carers of people with dementia. In Section 3, such interventions are described. The chapter ends with the characteristics and effects of a successful multicomponent intervention, the New York University Carer Intervention (NYUCI).

2 The Provision of Care to People with Dementia

In general, about two-thirds of informal care hours are given by co-residing carers [7]. Women contribute 71% of the global hours of informal care, with the highest proportion in low-income countries [1]. Spouses who provide care are more likely to be female. Children who provide intensive informal care – defined as three hours or more daily – tend to be female, of working age, co-residing or living close to their parents, and they are less likely to hold a full-time job or be married and have fewer children than children who are not 'heavy helpers' [7].

2.1 Types of Support Carers Provide

Types of care given by informal carers differ with the stage of dementia (see further). Family carers usually start with instrumental activities of daily living, such as grocery shopping, administration or cleaning [8]. In the middle stages of dementia, carers have to cope with troublesome behaviours such as wandering and agitation. Later on, support is needed for activities of daily living such as toileting and personal hygiene. At this point, informal carers often seek formal help [9]. Typical for dementia is the need for supervision and safe-keeping [7, 9].

How much informal care is provided and by whom are also influenced by governmental choices and policy. In Europe, we see a north-south gradient with governments in Northern European countries and the Benelux spending the most on long-term care (at least 2% of gross domestic product (GDP)) and Southern European countries relying more on informal care (formal care is less than 1% of GDP). Twenty per cent of Belgian care-dependent people over 65 receive informal care, while this is the case for 62% in Italy [7]. However, we can assume that the chance of informal care increases when a person has dementia. In the Netherlands, for example, 70% of people with dementia live at home and receive informal care [10].

The growing number of older people causes concerns for public spending. In Western countries, governments attempt to promote informal caregiving. However, informal care is not without costs for the carers themselves (e.g. because they work fewer hours or leave the labour market either temporarily or permanently), and there is uncertainty about whether the availability of informal care will suffice in future years. Over the years, many studies have corroborated the societal and individual cost of dementia. From a financial perspective, it has been estimated that the worldwide costs of dementia exceeded 1% of global GDP in 2015, at US$818 billion [11]. The authors estimated that the direct medical costs were $159.2 billion (19.5%), the societal care costs were $327.9 billion (40.1%) and, most importantly from the perspective of the burden on families, the informal care costs were $330.8 billion (40.4%). Thus the medical costs of dementia are dwarfed by the societal and family costs (see Chapter 14).

2.2 The Availability of Informal Care Now and in the Future

With their 'Informal Care Model', Broese van Groenou and De Boer [6] describe a behavioural model for individual caregiving. The provision of informal care is a process in which individual, relational and contextual factors of both care recipient and carer are intertwined. Contextual factors include the availability of formal care and support services for informal carers.

While we rely heavily on the availability of informal care, societal changes in progress all over the world – shifting family structures, generational splits, migration and the increasing participation of women in the workforce – have an impact on the availability of informal carers now and in the future. Pickard [12] predicts a growing 'care gap' and states that the demand for informal care by older people will soon exceed the supply. For example, by 2060, there will be a deficit of approximately twenty thousand informal carers in the Netherlands, four hundred thousand in Germany and more than a million in Spain.

Demographic trends cause both a higher demand for informal care and a lower availability of informal carers. Population ageing – and age is the highest predictor of dementia – increases the number of people in need of informal care. At the same time, fertility declines and families become smaller, which diminishes the number of children who will be available for providing informal care in the future [13, 14].

Care for a person with dementia often requires being physically present, to be able to help the person if they feel disoriented, to answer questions and to keep the person safe. In our current society, a large proportion of people live alone. Between 2011 and 2020, the number of single adult households in Europe (EU-27) (i.e. households consisting of only one adult, living with or without children) increased by 16.2% from about 65,600 million to 76,250 million. When we look at age and gender, the increase is more pronounced for older people and for men in particular. The number of men between the ages of 55 and 64 living alone has increased 47.7% since 2010. Women in the same age category recorded an increase of 23.3%. The number of older men aged 65 or older and living alone grew by

34.7%. The corresponding increase for women was 11.3% [15].

Living alone in itself of course does not indicate an absence of informal care and support. Children or other family members living elsewhere also contribute and may have frequent contact with the older person with dementia. However, living alone is associated with having to move earlier to residential care for reasons of safety [16].

There is a gender informal care gap [17]. Women's greater involvement in informal care negatively impacts their participation in the labour market and increases their risk of economic dependency, poverty and social exclusion. In the European Union (EU), almost one third of women not participating in the labour market between the ages of 20 and 64, compared to just 5% of men in the same age group, are not in paid work because of family and care responsibilities [18]. However, the availability of unemployed women to provide this care is decreasing [12]. Women study longer and have professional careers. They have children later in life, which means they may have to take up many roles simultaneously: work, childcare and care for an older parent. This is often only possible with the help of formal care services and other types of support.

These changes in the timing of demographic events such as marriage and childbearing bring about changing family structures. Moreover, Western societies are experiencing rises in divorce and separation and declines in marriage and childbearing. The number of children who can share the care burden thus is lower and in families with stepparents, the number of parents needing help may be higher [13].

In many EU countries, the retirement age is increasing. German research shows that when women face an increase in their retirement age and prolong their working lives, they provide significantly less informal care. The probability of caregiving is reduced by almost 6%, mostly driven by a decrease in low-intensity care. The effects are larger for (full-time) employed or highly educated women [14].

Governments recognize the value of informal care. In some places, informal care is even formalized by rules and legislation. Informal carers are conceptualized as 'co-workers' and receive payment in the form of cash-for-care schemes or cash benefits. Many countries, regions and cities (e.g. UK, Ireland, Flanders (Belgium), Helsinki) have passed a type of 'Care Act' which intends to reinforce the concept that there is a need for recognition, support and valuing of informal care. The change of policy from 'de-familialization', with formal care services taking over caregiving responsibility from the family to 're-familialization', where the family 'takes back' caregiving responsibility from the state in a context of increasing need for care (as described before), has an impact on informal carers. In a context of cost containment, this policy change may also be perceived as reinforcing family obligations and responsibility to provide care [19]. These policies seem to be making efforts to strike a compromise between supporting and alleviating informal care and enforcement of informal care. Enforcement, however, may lead to overburdening and negative feelings towards informal care or the person in need of care. In the following sections of this chapter, we focus on the role of informal carers of people with dementia throughout the dementia process and on evidence-based interventions that may help them.

3 The Impact of the Stage of Dementia on Informal Caregiving Tasks and on Informal Carers

The process of dementia is accompanied by a decline in functioning and an increase in limitations in ability to carry out daily activities. As care needs increase, the role of the family carers becomes more and more important for allowing the person with dementia to keep living at home. In many cases, however, there comes a time when the burden of care exceeds the care capacity of the family, and a transition to a nursing home becomes inevitable.

Family carers and informal carers in general have knowledge and experience about the history, desires and needs and personality of the person with dementia, and they make the difference in quality of life and quality of care for that person when he is no longer able to easily express himself. However, their role is also often neglected or underestimated by government and the formal care system. In this section, we describe different aspects of family care throughout the stages of dementia. We focus on important contributions of family carers, as well as on risks of burden and abuse.

3.1 Different Caregiving Tasks at Different Stages

Depending upon the stage in the dementia process, the challenges have differing characteristics and the burden has a different face. We differentiate between the stage before the diagnosis, the phase of diagnosis, the phase of living with dementia and the end-of-life stage. Each stage is characterized by specific needs and problems for the person living with dementia and for the family members.

In the phase **before diagnosis,** most persons with dementia experience important changes in their functioning. These changes can reflect many physical or mental conditions such as physiological changes of the body, chronic diseases and effects of medication, loss of work or grief for beloved persons who passed away, loneliness, depressive feelings or depression and anxiety. Very often normal changes in memory related to emotional responses to these stressful situations can be very similar to symptoms of an early stage of dementia. Together with, among others, ignorance, embarrassment or the idea that nothing can be done anyway, this is one of the reasons why a correct diagnosis is not easy and often delayed. A comprehensive assessment of the characteristics of functional and cognitive decline and the sequence in worsening of mental conditions will bring clarity about the diagnosis.

Very often, memory problems are most prominent in this early stage: new information is very difficult to process and it becomes difficult to participate socially or to follow television programmes. Daily life becomes difficult and demanding. The experiences of persons with dementia in this stage are well known because persons with dementia themselves can testify. They start to doubt themselves and experience uncertainty, powerlessness, anxiety and despair. Their reactions to these experiences take different forms. Some people retreat from activities, while others express anger and blame someone else for what goes wrong. Still others behave as if everything is okay – for example, by filling in the gaps in their memory with fantasy or denying any problems. But overall, the phase of beginning dementia for many is a period of continuous grief. This grief is important in the process of saying goodbye to what one loses, but at the same time allows one to open up a new perspective [20].

The most nearby and trusted persons are strongly involved in this process, and they have an important role. Family carers share the uncertainties of their beloved partner or elder, their feelings of chaos and uncertainty, their anxiety and their grief. At the same time, they acquire responsibilities in caring for that person, whereas the person himself often is not (yet) able to face their care needs. Very often, well-intended offers of necessary support or care are met with refusal. This may lead to conflict and feelings of anger towards the person with dementia. Family carers in this stage need good access to information about what the stages of dementia are and about early signs of dementia, self-screening tools and decision aids to help them decide whether to seek help for a diagnostic assessment. They also need information about the availability of support services and of possibilities for connecting with peer groups.

A **timely diagnosis of dementia** is very important in order to exclude treatable causes of cognitive decline and also to make sure that the necessary support and care are planned and organized with shared decision-making that involves the person with dementia and their family. Unfortunately, very often a diagnostic assessment is not administered until very late in the dementia process, when cognitive decline no longer permits or hinders involvement in decision-making processes about future care. Particularly in persons with early-onset dementia [21], migrants from another cultural background [22] or patients who have a pre-existing chronic cognitive disability [23], the risk of non-diagnosis or very late diagnosis of cognitive decline is very high. Family carers have an important role in that diagnostic process. They are the first to detect alarming signs that may lead to early detection, assessment and diagnosis. A thorough assessment of their observations should therefore receive ample attention in the clinical discussion with a general practitioner (GP) or a geriatrician.

A timely diagnosis of dementia is important, but not sufficient. It should be accompanied by timely and professional communication about the meaning of dementia, prediction of the care needs and a process of advance care planning (ACP) to anticipate the period of high-intensive care needs and end of life. The European Association for Palliative Care defines ACP as a process which 'enables individuals to define goals and preferences for future medical treatment and care, to discuss these goals and preferences with family and healthcare providers, and to record and review these preferences if appropriate' [24].

De Vleminck and colleagues [25] identified barriers and facilitators in primary care relying to GP characteristics, perceived patient factors or healthcare system characteristics. Hindering factors include lack of skills to deal with patients' vague requests, difficulties with finding the right moment, the attitude that the patient should be the one initiating ACP and fear of depriving patients of hope. Factors facilitating initiation of ACP in general practice are accumulated skills, the ability to foresee health problems, skills to respond to a patient's initiation of ACP, personal convictions about who to involve in ACP and a long-standing patient–GP relationship. Since dementia gradually limits decision-making abilities [26], it is important to discuss goals and preferences for future care at an early stage with all stakeholders jointly. It is important to understand the preferences and wishes of the person with dementia in dialogue with family members, so that in later stages decisions can be taken on their behalf when they have become unable to decide for themselves (see further on).

Family members share the anxiety and fear that goes along with the symptoms of dementia. Various emotions evolve during the different stages of dementia: anger, frustration, sadness, grief etc. [27]. The process of dementia brings about important changes in their own lives as well. This may also impede them in searching an early diagnosis. When a diagnosis of dementia becomes real, many things must be organized to support the person with dementia in his daily activities and to prepare the care environment for the time to come. The involvement of informal and professional carers must be organized, as well as the coordination of home care. This entails different aspects such as safeguarding, for example, when the person with dementia drives or remains at home alone. Making financial decisions and using money are risky during that time. There also is a risk for abuse or mistreatment of persons with dementia, which can have different faces: it can be physical, mental or financial. In a situation where other people come into their home, persons with dementia with

continuing vulnerability cannot protect themselves against harm or exploitation. For family members, it is a real challenge to engage in activities that contribute to joint feelings of joy and well-being such as walking, singing or participating in social or cultural events. In all of this, family carers should be supported and informed in the early stages. At the same time, anxiety and grief can be very much present, which affects the mental well-being of family carers.

3.2 Supporting a Person with Dementia

Communication with a person with dementia changes with the progress of the cognitive decline. In the most advanced stage, contact will be more and more without words and language. Other senses such as tone of voice, music, eye and skin contact, smell and taste will become more important for making contact and creating positive feelings of connection. This requires a good understanding of the cognitive decline and of how to interact in a creative and innovative way. The so-called 'behavioural and psychological symptoms of dementia' (BPSD) such as shouting, (nightly) agitation or sleep problems are a huge challenge for family carers. Later on, the care needs include all activities of daily living such as bathing, eating and drinking and getting dressed. And of course this is very demanding for family carers, who themselves often are older or part of the 'sandwich generation' of working women with (grand)children.

With the progress of cognitive decline, the safety of the person with dementia becomes an issue for care at home. Persons with dementia cannot anticipate danger and are at risk for accidents that harm themselves or other people in their environment. Family carers are challenged to guarantee safety inside and outside the home environment. The risk factors are numerous: eating and drinking, medication, movement, falls, dangerous substances, participation in the community, banking and financial or administrative procedures, traffic, victimization and abuse. It is essential for carers to find an equilibrium between safety and overprotection. Quite often, well-intended and even necessary interventions are rejected by the person with dementia. A sophisticated communication style is needed when offering help and for securing safety in a way that is perceived as acceptable to the person with dementia. The quality of the previous interpersonal relation, as well as the understanding of dementia, communication skills and emotional and practical support, will contribute to the sustainability of a good, caring relationship in the home environment [28].

Nightly agitation and insomnia are frequently occurring problems in home care for persons with dementia. These affect the person with dementia, as well as family carers who have to wake up at night to address the needs of their family member suffering from insomnia. Insomnia and night-time agitation have many faces: difficulties falling asleep, getting up at night, walking around at night aimlessly, pacing or engaging in unusual activities or waking up others. Very often, these problems cause crises that can lead to a transition of the person with dementia to a nursing home. Besides causes related to dementia (such as disorientation), social factors (such as day-night rhythm in the household) and environmental factors (such as noise, light and temperature) are potential triggers of insomnia which should be addressed. Non-pharmacological solutions should be developed to better support and improve the quality of life of patients and carers, both during home care and in nursing homes [29].

As more problems arise and supervision becomes exceedingly necessary, in many cases the person with dementia fails to accept or forgets the need for support. This again requires inspiration for family members to acquire new styles of communication for which they need role models. The use of alarm systems and home automation such as telemonitoring is increasing. This supporting technology is in development, but the actual use in practice for persons with dementia has its limits: at a certain moment in time for many families, care at home will be less contributing to the quality of life of all involved than care in a well-organized and homely nursing home. Unfortunately, such a nursing home is not available everywhere.

Family care for a person with dementia is burdensome and at the same time rewarding in many aspects. In optimal conditions, family carers get sufficient access to necessary information concerning what dementia is about. In many countries and regions, 'expert by experience' groups of family carers have an important role in supporting these families. A lot of information and support is available in many ways: on the Internet, via memory clinics, general practice, social services etc. Besides the burden, caregiving can go along with feelings of resilience, belonging to a group and with receiving social support, respite care and feeling satisfied by giving support.

Caring for someone with dementia is generally not a choice. In most cases, there is no clear-cut decision to start giving informal care. In the later stages of dementia, caregiving often leads to high levels of burden. Emotional burden is about feelings of grief because of the loss of the partner, parent, family member or friend and other problems such as feeling overwhelmed. Feelings of guilt may arise when the caregiving burden becomes too high and transition to a nursing home becomes necessary. Sometimes the relationship becomes very difficult when the cognitive decline involves aggressive or socially unaccepted behaviour. Many factors determine the sustainability of dementia care such as the characteristics of the carer and the person with dementia, their (former) relationship, as well as the presence of peer support and professional support [28, 30]. It is important to help family carers in looking after themselves, and in anticipating what will happen later and how to deal with it.

When caring for a person with dementia becomes too demanding and emotionally and physically exhausting, it is important to get support in order to be able to cope with the situation. Friends and family can be helpful, and so can social and home care services or local support groups. Many countries have available helplines and assistive technology. In any case, the health and well-being of the family carer is a point of attention for the sustainability of care in the personal environment.

3.3 A Broad Vision of Care and Support

Good care for older people with dementia is focussed on quality of life or positive health rather than on cure. The concept of 'positive health' as defined by Huber [31] is 'the ability to adapt and self-manage in the light of life's physical, emotional and social challenges'. In the context of dementia, this implies much attention is needed to support mental well-being and social participation [32]. First and foremost, it helps the person to continue participating in society in the best possible way. Incorporating ordinary roles and activities and gaining appreciation for them are central. Initiatives such as dementia-friendly municipalities can contribute greatly to this by offering opportunities for inclusion in normative activities outside the home. Supporting the individual's autonomy in everyday choices and in dealing with the functional limitations they are confronted with is a second important aspect of good care. And thirdly, participation in social and meaningful activities, such as maintaining family ties, enjoying activities of interest and participating in cultural or religious activities is very important. It will be clear that the role of family members and other proxies is very important here [31]. In Section 4, effective interventions for psychosocial support of family carers are described.

3.4 Advance Care Planning in the Nursing Home

When the need for permanent supervision and support grows to a 24–7 challenge, for some home care is not possible anymore and the transition to a nursing home becomes an important topic of discussion between all stakeholders. Advance care planning for persons with dementia is a process that should start as soon as possible after diagnosis to make sure that the person is still able to express their preferences and wishes. Ideally this process will occur shortly after diagnosis if it hasn't occurred before then. Although ACP should have happened long before the transition to a nursing home, research shows it is still possible to initiate it there if necessary [33–37], although it will be much more difficult for the person with dementia to fully express his or her wishes.

End-of-life care decisions are rarely driven by the person with dementia [38]. In recent years, the concept of shared decision-making (SDM) has emerged to counter this trend [39, 40]. Shared decision-making (see Chapters 11 and 12) is an approach where clinicians and patients communicate using the best available evidence when faced with the task of making decisions [41, 42]. Involving persons with dementia and their family members in the decision-making process yields several benefits, including an increased sense of worth and an improved quality of life [43–45].

The intervention 'We Decide' (We Discuss End-of-Life Choices) has been developed to increase the level of SDM in ACP conversations in nursing homes [46]. It supports three steps to SDM [47]: creating insight into the availability of multiple options (Choice Talk), providing information on these options (Option Talk) and discussing preferences while working towards a decision (Decision Talk). The intervention consists of two workshops of four hours each, in which three modules are introduced, followed by implementation support. It provides theoretical information on ACP and SDM, role-play exercises and the internal ACP policy. A homework assignment between sessions allows the participants to practise the three-talk model during daily conversations with residents with dementia and their family members. First results showed that the context of the team, as well as the involvement of persons with dementia and their families, can be either facilitating or hindering factors in the implementation of the training [48].

In a second study [49], the 'We Decide' intervention was optimized by stimulating the discussion of SDM in teams and by involving families and persons with dementia more actively in the communication. At the organizational level, nursing home management needs to be committed to implement the intervention by participating themselves in training and by being prepared to review and update their internal ACP policies. Very important for a real implementation of SDM is an information campaign for residents and families about the openness and willingness for communication on ACP. Pocket cards, stipulating three possible questions to ask healthcare professionals, and posters, inviting all stakeholders to participate in SDM, appear to be important for sustainable approach in practice [50].

Professionals in nursing homes sometimes experience difficulties in providing residents and family members with detailed information on medical and care options, and instead rely on GPs to supply this knowledge. Research on GPs' attitudes and involvement in ACP [51–54], however, indicates resistance of GPs to attend ACP conversations. Consequently, when GPs are absent, nursing home staff feel left on their own and unable to provide sufficient insight to residents and family members. Since GPs are key figures in the healthcare trajectories of persons with dementia they could benefit from training in ACP and SDM [55].

3.5 Person-Centred as well as Relation-Centred Care in Nursing Homes

The interpersonal relationship between family carers and the person with dementia is a very important aspect of care in nursing homes. It not only contributes to opportunities for the maintenance of nurturing relationships in the wider community as opposed to the previous traditions of seclusion and total institutions [56], but also being involved in the long-term relationships with partners and family members may help to retain long-term habits and memories of the person with dementia. Partners, family members or friends also have knowledge and understanding of the person with dementia, which can help the professionals to better understand and value the person as an individual. Particularly at the stage in which the person with dementia cannot express himself with language, the people who knew him or her before dementia struck are well placed to help translate the 'silent voices'. The professionals also can model how to solve difficult relational situations or be available to family and friends to share their feelings of grief and mourning. By actively interacting with the informal carers as well as the person with dementia, professional carers can expand best practices to the broader community, which can lead to broader expertise and openness and acceptance for future persons with frailty.

4 Evidence-Based Interventions for Supporting Informal Carers

To support informal carers of the person with dementia, many supportive activities and programmes have been developed since the 1980s. Initially, the focus was on support groups, respite care and paid home care. Over the course of the 1990s and after 2000, the range became more varied with, among other things, the possibility of telephone support, specific training courses in, for example, coping with stress, dealing with behavioural and mood changes, communication skills training, online courses, case management and more comprehensive multicomponent interventions [57]. Also in the 1990s the first combined intervention programmes, focussing on both the person with dementia and family carers, were developed [58–61].

There were several reasons for setting up broader and more comprehensive support programmes, including the fact that respite care and support groups alone proved to have insufficient effect [62, 63]: informal carers indicated that in addition to practical support, they also needed help in learning to cope with their own emotions and stress [64, 65]. The need for emotional support and interventions tailored to the individual strengths, needs and wishes of informal carers also played an important role in the further development of composite, flexible programmes [60, 61, 66–68]. Carers differ in many ways and often have different needs and problems, which cannot all be solved with a 'one-size-fits-all' intervention or support programme [69].

Over the past decades, many carer support interventions and multicomponent programmes have been evaluated on their effectiveness on a range of carer outcomes, such as burden and stress, knowledge, caring skills, mood, mental health, physical health, self-efficacy, coping, sense of competence, resilience, well-being and quality of life. Here we provide a summary of the evidence for effectiveness of the most widely used interventions and programmes.

4.1 Respite Care

Regardless of the form in which it is provided (e.g. home care, day care or temporary admission of the person with dementia in a long-term care facility), the results of some studies suggest that respite care can offer temporary relief to the carer, decrease behavioural symptoms in the person with dementia and improve the mood of both. A meta-analysis by Knight et al. [70] showed that respite care has a significant influence on the feelings of burden of the carer. This was confirmed in five of the eight studies on respite care included in the review, which at the same time demonstrated that not all respite interventions were equally effective in reducing carers' feelings of burden. Conflicting evidence of effectiveness was also the result of a Cochrane review [71] on respite care which, based on (only) four studies, had to conclude that current evidence does not demonstrate significant benefits. However, the authors emphasize that these results should be treated with caution, as they may reflect the lack of high-quality research in this area rather than an actual lack of benefit.

A more recent review indeed showed that family carers experience day care as a respite service and to some extent as support service, improving their competence in caring for the person with dementia [72]. Not only the quality of the day care, but also the motivation of the family carers to care for the person with dementia influenced its use. The review suggested that to be effective, day care also had to provide carers with education, counselling and support and access to information; moreover, the professionals' expertise and the quality of their relationship with the persons with dementia affected the outcome for carers [73]. Compared to standard day cares, which focus only on the person with dementia, integrated support programmes for people with dementia *and* their family carers, such as the Meeting Centres Support Programme (MCSP) [74, 75], or a combination of day care and telephone support showed increased feelings of competence and confidence in carers [76] (see Section 4.4).

4.2 Alzheimer Cafés

The concept of Alzheimer cafés, also known as memory cafés, originated in the Netherlands in 1997 with the aim to provide people with dementia and their relatives the opportunity to openly discuss dementia and related problems, to receive information and have contact with peers and care and welfare professionals [77]. The cafés are organized monthly (2.5 hours) in community-based settings, starting with coffee or tea, followed by an interview with or presentation of an expert. Participants are again offered drinks and music and can exchange experiences and ask questions. The meeting ends in an informal atmosphere. The Alzheimer cafés have been widely replicated in Europe and elsewhere, and have taken on a variety of forms, including being organized by and for carers and people with dementia without including professionals.

While anecdotal evidence suggests the cafés are enjoyed by all participants, little systematic research has been done to evaluate their benefits for people with dementia and informal carers. Several qualitative studies suggest that the café prevents social isolation, provides the opportunity to exchange experiences with peers and to get information on available services, facilitates relationship building within care dyads as well as with other attendees, is perceived as a safe place where the experience of dementia can be reformulated

and brings back a sense of normalcy to the carers' lives [78–80], thus promoting attendees' social and emotional well-being [81]. The latter is confirmed in a recent pilot study of Merlo et al. [82], who demonstrated that carers who joined the Alzheimer café with their relative with dementia benefitted from learning strategies for daily care of the person with dementia, and in terms of overall well-being, vitality and emotional burden, compared to carers who did not participate in an Alzheimer café. This is in line with findings from a cross-sectional study which found significant differences between attendees at Alzheimer cafés and non-attendees in resilience and subjective well-being [83].

4.3 Support Groups

The most common form of support for carers of people living at home with dementia is the support group. The core of the support group is that informal carers share similar experiences with peers and thus experience support and gain information. Under the umbrella of the support group concept, a wide range of interventions is used – for example, groups focussed on education, groups focussed on mutual emotional support (peer groups), groups focussed on ventilating emotions and groups focussed on coping with the stress caused by the continuous pressure of care. Some support groups are led by skilled professionals and others are peer run. Of course there are also combinations of these forms (see Section 4.6).

Research into support groups shows that they have a small to medium effect on depression of informal carers, and they can reduce the burden and experienced stress to some extent. These effects persist after the support groups have ended [69, 84].

Studies into the effectiveness of the combined MCSP showed that informal carers who participated in the discussion groups with other carers, in addition to utilizing the social activity programme for the person with dementia, experienced a greater sense of competence after six months than informal carers who received respite care only by means of regular day care for their next of kin [74]. The carers who participated in the discussion groups also felt less burdened [74, 75]; 87% experienced emotional support from the support groups and 85% felt they received useful practical advice.

4.4 Telephone Support

Telephone support enables carers to receive customized information and support, tailored to their individual needs in their own homes, at a time of the day they prefer. This makes the intervention easily accessible for a large group of carers, including those who do not have services available nearby or who are not able to travel, for example, to support, counselling or education groups. It also gives them the opportunity to speak freely on the phone with an anonymous professional carer [76].

Telephone support and coaching has proven to be an intervention that on its own can reduce depressive symptoms and meet the support needs of carers [85], more specifically the need for information and education, emotional support, referral to other sources of support within the community and support that is easily accessible [86]. Van Mierlo et al. [76] showed that telephone coaching was more beneficial than respite care in reducing mental health problems in carers. However, burden telephone coaching in combination with respite care (day care for the person with dementia) proved more effective than telephone coaching alone in improving the carers' sense of competence and decreasing their feelings of burden. Also, a systematic review [87] showed that telephone support combined with internet delivery of multicomponent interventions proved more beneficial with regards to reducing depression and burden and increasing self-efficacy than telephone coaching or internet support alone.

4.5 Case Management

Case management in dementia is defined in the Dutch Standard of Dementia Care as:

> The systematic provision of coordinated guidance, care and support as part of the treatment, by a professional, preferably the same person from start to nursing home admission. This professional is part of a (multidisciplinary) partnership targeting home-dwelling people with dementia and their informal carers. The case management professional is involved from the start of the diagnostic process, as soon as the person with dementia wishes, without unnecessary waiting times or waiting lists. The aim is to involve case management on the basis of individual needs of the person with dementia and informal carer(s). These needs may vary over

time. Case management ends after admission in a residential care setting for people with dementia (such as a nursing home) by means of warm transfer, or if the person with dementia dies. The case manager offers after-care to the informal carers after the death of the person with dementia if desired. [88]

Although the implementation of case management may differ in practice and between regions and countries, the case manager is generally a specially trained nurse or social worker with knowledge and experience of dementia who acts as a personal coach and visits people at home as needed, thus gaining a good view of the situation. A familiar, easily accessible and ongoing point of contact is important because as the dementia process progresses the needs for care change and often become more complex.

Research into dementia case management is still very limited. The efficacy of case management among informal carers has been demonstrated in, amongst others, two systematic literature reviews [89, 90] and in a Dutch study among 13 regional networks of dementia care chains [91]. Reported positive effects include reduced feelings of strain, depression and loneliness [89, 90], being better able to deal with resistance, anxiety, anger and confusion of the person with dementia, and being better informed about dementia symptoms and care and support options [91]. Also effects on patients' time of institutionalization were found [90], as well as evidence of cost-effectiveness for intensive case management [92]. No effects were found on care burden or quality of life of the carer in the Dutch study. On the other hand, after starting with case management a significant change is seen in care use (i.e. fewer visits to the general practitioner, more use of home care and twice as much use of day care or meeting centre) [91].

4.6 Skills Training and Therapies

Skills training and therapy programmes aim to improve the skills of informal carers to the care for a relative or friend with dementia. A great variety of (psycho)educational programmes exist. Some are aimed at providing basic knowledge about dementia and its consequences in daily functioning in order to help carers better understand changes in behaviour of the person with dementia and their functional disabilities. Others are focussed on improving social and communication skills, providing cognitive stimulation, dealing with behavioural and mood changes of the person with dementia or coping with stress as a result of caring.

Research into programmes focussed on skills training shows that they have a medium effect on reducing the carer burden and a small effect on reducing depression in informal carers [93], and can improve their self-efficacy [94]. Only providing information about dementia proves not to be beneficial for the psychological health of carers. There is excellent evidence for the (long-term) efficacy in diminishing carer symptoms of individual behavioural management therapy (six or more sessions) focused on the person with dementia's behaviour [95]. Programmes specifically aimed at carer communication skills appear to increase these skills, as well as knowledge about dementia. In addition, there are some initial indications that these programmes can also lead to the reduction of depression in informal carers [96]. This also applies to coping-based psycho-educational interventions, individually or in a group, which teach informal carers to use adequate coping strategies [95, 97]. Both emotion-focussed strategies [98] and problem-focussed strategies [99] can, depending on the specific situation, have beneficial effects on the mental health of carers. Individual interventions appeared more effective than group interventions [95].

Cognitive behavioural therapy proved effective for increasing knowledge and caregiving-related self-efficacy and decreasing dysfunctional thoughts [97, 100], especially the 'cognitive reframing' which is an important element of this therapy and which aims to decrease carers' maladaptive, self-defeating or distressing cognitions about their relative's behaviour and their performance as a carer. A systematic review and meta-analysis on cognitive reframing showed beneficial effects over usual care for psychological morbidity (anxiety, depression) and subjective stress of carers [69, 101]. This was confirmed by a study of the 'Learning to Become a Family Carer' programme, in which carers were trained in cognitive reframing as a coping strategy, which resulted in less psychological distress and improved self-efficacy [102].

4.7 Internet-Based Support Interventions

Internet-based support interventions are promising to meet the educational and support needs of the increasing number of carers of people with dementia in the coming decades at relatively low costs. They vary from digital social charts, providing information on health and social services for people with dementia and carers, online courses and coaching, online or email support and information on a web portal, web-based multimedia interventions with educational videos, educational and peer-support website and chat forums, online stress management training programmes, online training workshops and videoconferencing [103, 104]. Recently a web-based dyadic supportive programme, FindMyApps, has been developed to train people with dementia and carers to use tablets and a selection tool to easily select apps for self-management and meaningful activities that match the person with dementia's needs, interests and abilities [105]. It is expected that this programme in addition to improving the self-management and social participation of people with dementia, will also positively impact the sense of competence, self-efficacy and experienced burden of their carers.

Regarding their aim, six categories of internet-based support interventions can be differentiated: interventions focussed on contact with healthcare or social care providers, peer interaction, provision of information, practical support, decision support and psychological support. Studies into their effectiveness have generally low quality, which makes it difficult to generalize their results. However, the studies suggest that multicomponent interventions tailored to the individual needs of carers can improve various aspects of carer well-being, such as confidence, depression, anxiety, self-efficacy and stress [103, 104]. Psychological support provided online proved especially beneficial in improving carers' mental health [104]. Provision of information online proved also beneficial when part of a multicomponent intervention and tailored for the individual [104]. Online contact with professionals is appreciated by carers because it provides easy access to personalized advice and emotional support [104]. The effectiveness of practical support for carers utilizing suitable dementia-friendly apps that may promote self-management and activities in people with dementia is yet unknown, but early pilot studies are promising and call for further research [106, 107].

4.8 Multicomponent Combined Interventions

Over the past three decades, a variety of multicomponent combined support programmes for people with dementia and carers have been developed and evaluated on their effectiveness [97, 108–112]. The components of such intervention programmes vary from, for instance, respite care at home, in a community centre or care setting, to cognitive rehabilitation therapy or occupational therapy for the person with dementia combined with different types of support activities for the carer such as psycho-education, individual assistance or counselling, informative group meetings, support groups aimed at education, skills training and/or emotional support, cognitive behavioural interventions, coping interventions, telephone coaching or internet-based support interventions. Some multicomponent programmes also include dyadic interventions such as case management, problem-solving classes, dyadic counselling and recreational or pleasant activities for people with dementia and their carers [111].

Several international systematic reviews have shown that especially interventions which are flexible and personalized, offer emotional and social support in addition to practical support, and provide support to both the person with dementia and the carer are more effective in supporting them both than interventions which do not meet these characteristics [108–112].

A widespread, successful and proven effective, multicomponent combined support programme in the Netherlands (which has also recently proved successful in Italy, Poland and England as part of a European study) is the Meeting Centres Support Programme (MCSP) [60, 74, 75, 113–115]. This programme, which aims to provide guidance in dealing with the consequences of dementia and is theoretically based on the adaptation-coping model [116], offers, in addition to day activities in the meeting centre for persons with dementia (one to three days a week), continuous discussion groups, a series of monthly information meetings and a weekly individual consultation hour for informal carers, and social activities such as outings for both. The support activities are offered by a small permanent staff and volunteers in an accessible, socially integrated place in the neighbourhood such as community or senior centres. Proven advantages of participating in MCSP compared to regular day care without an informal carer programme are reduced behavioural and mood problems, increased self-esteem and quality of life of the person with dementia and less experienced strain, emotional impact of behavioural problems of the person with dementia in carers, as well as fewer psychosomatic complaints in lonely carers. In addition, participation in MCSP increases the experienced support and sense of competence of informal carers [57], enabling them to maintain care for longer. This is shown, among other things, by the postponement of nursing home admissions (after six months, only 4% of the participants in the meeting centres were admitted compared to 30% of the participants in regular day treatment). Recently new elements were successfully added to the support programme (volunteer work for people with dementia outside the meeting centre), and an online course and telephone coaching for carers who are not willing or able to follow the group-oriented carer programme or of whom the relative is not interested or willing to participate in the meeting centre. This new individualized MCSP resulted in a decrease of neuropsychiatric symptoms and an increase of positive affect in the persons with dementia after six months of intervention, whereas carers experienced less emotional impact of neuropsychiatric symptoms [117].

Another successful example of a multicomponent intervention is the education and support group for carers (six months) in combination with case management and a professional support network in Hong Kong [118, 119]. A multidisciplinary group including a psychiatrist, social worker, case manager and researchers from the School of Nursing of the Faculty of Medicine listed intervention objectives based on dementia guidelines and designed an information and psychological support system linking case managers, care services, professionals and referrers. Each family was assigned one case manager who formulated a multidisciplinary education programme based on prioritized problem areas. The programme consisted of 12 sessions in six months with the following themes: orientation to dementia care, educational workshop about dementia care, family role and strength rebuilding, community support resources, review of the programme and evaluation. The case managers also conducted home visits (every other week) and monthly family health assessments. The programme improved quality of life of the carers and decreased carer burden and psychological and behavioural symptoms in people with dementia [110].

Several programmes offer integrated sessions focussed on people with dementia and their carers, such as occupational therapy at home, the Danish Alzheimer Intervention Study (DAISY) and problem-solving training classes. Occupational therapy at home provides carers with education, problem solving and technical skills and advice on simple home modifications (six monthly sessions) to support the functioning of the person with dementia, to reduce behavioural and mood disruptions and reduce carer burden [120]. Some occupational therapy programmes specifically guide persons with dementia and carers in performing prioritized meaningful activities they want to improve (10 sessions in five weeks [121]; six home visits in four months [120]). Several studies showed that these occupational therapy programmes resulted in less depression in carers [120, 121] and fewer behavioural and psychological symptoms in people with dementia [120].

The DAISY intervention [122] is a tailored programme which involves seven counselling sessions of which four or five families and carers attend, along with a group education course about dementia and its consequences with peer support, telephone support, written information and a journal. The intervention decreased depression in carers and improved their quality of life.

Problem-solving classes involved taking practical steps to manage day-to-day problems caused by the memory loss [123]. Dyads talked about troublesome situations, group leaders and other participants then made suggestions for managing these problems, taking into account the individual situation (severity of memory problems, living arrangements and personal resources). The classes met twice a week for one and half hours during three and a half weeks and resulted in a decrease of depression, burden and emotional impact in carers of behavioural and psychological symptoms of the person with dementia [110, 123].

To conclude, meta-analysis has shown that multicomponent interventions can reduce carer depressive symptoms, decrease experienced burden, reduce the emotional impact of symptoms of dementia on them and improve their quality of life [110], but can also reduce behavioural and psychological symptoms in the person with dementia. Although no significant differences

were found between combined/multicomponent interventions and multicomponent interventions focussed on carers only on most of the mentioned outcome variables, overall it appears that combined/dyadic multicomponent interventions are more effective in reducing carer burden [110]. This is of course plausible taking into account the interdependency of health and quality of life of people with dementia and their family members. However, studies in which the two types of multicomponent interventions are (directly) compared are required to provide a definite answer on this. A good example of a long-standing effective multicomponent intervention specifically for carers of people with dementia is the New York University Carer intervention, originally developed by Mittelman in the 1980s and evaluated on its short-term and long-term effects in several studies thereafter.

5 The New York University Carer Intervention As a Specific Example of a Successful, Evidence-Based Multicomponent Intervention

The goals of the New York University Carer Intervention (NYUCI) are twofold: (1) to improve the well-being of the family carer, and (2) to enable the carer to keep the person with dementia at home as long as he or she wants to do so. The NYUCI is a multicomponent intervention that includes counselling, support and education for both the primary carer and for other participating family members. The intervention is individualized to the needs of each family, includes the primary carer as well as other family members, is available when needed and as long as needed, and is geared to the stage of dementia and the strengths and limitations of the person with dementia and the family carers. The content of the sessions is based on the comprehensive intake assessment and the input of participating family members during counselling sessions, and emphasizes support for the primary family carer. It should be noted that, when the intervention was developed in the 1980s, there was no agreed-upon definition of the word 'counselling'. In 2010, however, a consensus conference agreed that 'Counselling is a professional relationship that empowers diverse individuals, families, and groups to accomplish mental health, wellness, education, and career goals' [124]. This definition is consistent with the NYUCI vision.

The NYUCI is made up of several components, each of which contributes to its success. There have been several randomized controlled trials of the intervention that have had clinically meaningful results. All of the components are necessary, and there is no evidence that removing one or more components would be equally successful. One can think of the totality of the components of the NYUCI like a recipe for a cake – if you leave out any of the ingredients, the cake is not likely to end up as good as if you follow the recipe exactly. Of course, after you've made the cake several times, you may think of ways to make it even better. This is the original recipe:

- A comprehensive assessment of the primary carer.
- Scheduled individual and family counselling sessions within a fixed period of time (four months from the intake assessment).
  - One individual counselling session.
  - Four family counselling sessions.
  - A second individual counselling session.
- Continuous participation in a support group that meets regularly (weekly in the original study).
- Ad hoc counselling – telephone consultation on request of carer or family member over the entire course of the disease.

The first individual session serves several purposes. Most importantly, the counsellor can tailor the intervention to the needs, strengths and limitations of the primary carer. Unlike a group intervention, individual counselling can occur in a time and place convenient for the carer. During the first counselling session, the carer can establish a relationship with the counsellor that makes it possible to seek further advice and support when needed, as he or she is not asking for help from a stranger. During the individual counselling session, emphasis is placed on the importance of involving other family members or close friends, and the carer is advised to think about who he or she would like to involve in the four family counselling sessions that follow.

The individual session is followed by four family counselling sessions that include family or close friends whom the carer has invited to participate. Family counselling is the linchpin of the NYUCI. While each family is different, and the counselling is guided by the expressed needs of its members, the general purpose of the sessions is to create a support system for the primary carer that can continue after the formal sessions are over. Many issues can be addressed in these sessions. Often, one or more family members do not understand that the person with dementia is ill. They may visit only occasionally or by phone, and the person with dementia can appear normal under those circumstances. One goal of the sessions is that all participating family members understand that the person with dementia is ill. This may also mean that he or she is no longer a sufficient source of social support for the spouse or partner who is now the carer. Family members learn about the needs of the primary carer, while the primary carer learns what kind of support other family members would like to and are able to give.

After the four family sessions have been completed, there is a second individual counselling session with the primary carer. This is a time for discussing what has changed since the person started with the NYUCI, whether the carer feels more supported by his or her family and friends, and what still could be improved. The intention is for the family to continue to have the kinds of conversations that occurred during the family session, and that issues can be resolved without the counsellor's guidance. During this second individual session, which is intended to occur within four months of the intake assessment, the counsellor advises the carer to join a support group that meets regularly.

Support groups are an important part of the NYUCI, as carers can provide each other with ongoing emotional support and practical information. Carers benefit from talking to others who have gone through similar experiences, and may be willing to discuss issues they are not comfortable discussing with their family members or friends. They can also get information about how to solve the problems they are currently facing from people who have had similar problems.

As the study of the NYUCI began, it became apparent that ad hoc counselling, or counselling on demand, was an essential aspect of the NYUCI, as it was another way to provide ongoing support. Carers know that the counsellor with whom they established a relationship through the individual and family counselling sessions is available for additional consultation when needed; the researchers found that this could be provided by phone or email. It meant that carers could receive help without leaving home. Since the effects of dementia change over course of illness; when a new problem arises, help is available. Family members who had participated in the family counselling were also able to use this service. And in a crisis, there is someone to call.

The first randomized controlled trial began in 1987. Between August 1987 and February 1997, 406 carers were enrolled. All carers in this study were spouses or partners of the person with dementia. These carers were followed and provided ad hoc counselling until they dropped out of the study, or until two years after the death of the person with dementia. There was a less than 5% dropout rate among carers whose relative with dementia was living at home, and some carers participated for as long as 18 years. This yielded a unique longitudinal database for analysis.

The intervention showed a long-lasting effect on carer depression. The first publication that reported on the first 200 participants described that in the first year after intake, the control group became increasingly more depressed while the treatment group remained stable, and that the differences between the two groups became significant at the 8-month follow-up and increased by the 12-month follow-up. Interestingly, although changes in depression were small for most carers, there were dramatic changes in a significant minority of carers by 12 months after intake. Among the 22 carers who became at least seven points less depressed by the 12-month follow-up, 15 (68%) were in the treatment group, while among the 22 carers who became at least seven points more depressed by the 12-month follow-up, 16 (73%) were in the control group, a statistically and clinically significant difference (Chi square = 7.4, $p < 0.05$) [124].

In a later paper, the results of analysis of outcomes for three years after intake with the larger sample of 406 carers were reported. After one year, 29.8% of carers in the enhanced treatment group had symptoms of clinical depression, compared with 45.1% of those in the usual care control group. Three years later, carers who received the NYUCI were found to still exhibit fewer symptoms of depression, on average, than those in the usual care control group [125]. An examination of the relationship between neuroticism, as measured by the NEO five-factor inventory, and the impact of the NYUCI on

depression showed that carers who were high in neuroticism showed a worse longitudinal course of depression compared to those low in neuroticism. However, the treatment had an impact on carer depression, regardless of neuroticism score. Those low in neuroticism responded to treatment with declining levels of depression, whereas those high in neuroticism maintained their baseline level of depression with treatment [126]. The intervention also reduced carer depressive symptoms and burden during the transition to a nursing home, even if this transition occurred many years after enrolment in the study [127], and persisted through bereavement as well [128].

In another evaluation that included the full sample of 406 carers over the first four years after intake, the NYUCI significantly reduced the severity of the carers' stress reaction to behaviour problems of the person with dementia, despite the fact that the intervention did not affect the frequency of these behaviour problems [129]. Carer physical health was another important outcome of interest. Carers who received the NYUCI had significantly better self-rated health and fewer illnesses than control group carers, and this significant difference was maintained for two years after enrolment [130].

Findings of a mediation analysis suggest that social support resources are at the core of the impact of the NYUCI. The outcomes observed were largely due to improvements in social support. Increased satisfaction with the social support network mediated a significant proportion of the intervention's impact on carer depression and changes in carer stress appraisals. The number of support persons, satisfaction with the support network and support persons' assistance with caregiving all increased significantly as a function of the intervention [131]. Further exploration of the impact of social support revealed that higher levels of emotional support, more visits and having more network members to whom carers felt close were all individually predictive of longitudinal changes in social support network satisfaction and that individuals in the intervention group reported higher levels of satisfaction with their social support network over the first five years of the intervention than those in the support group [132].

In 2006, sufficient data were available to examine the impact of the NYUCI on nursing home placement over a 12-year period. The intervention postponed nursing home placement of the person with dementia for a median time of 557 days compared to the usual care control group. Increased satisfaction with social support, reduced carer depression and a greater tolerance for patient behaviour accounted for 61% of the enhanced intervention's beneficial impact on delaying the placement of patients into nursing homes [133]. Thus delaying placement was not accomplished at the expense of the carer's well-being. Carers in the treatment group were not only able to keep their spouses at home with them longer, but as a result of the intervention they also had greater tolerance for patient memory and behaviour problems, improved satisfaction with the support provided by family and friends and fewer symptoms of depression.

One particular value of the long-term funding of the study of the NYUCI is that it made it possible to follow the progress of carers well beyond their intensive counselling period. Because the control group received ad hoc counselling and felt connected to the programme, they continued to participate in follow-up evaluations for many years, as did those who received the full intervention. Many of the effects of these therapeutic interventions are not felt immediately. For example, the two groups of carers began to show significant differences in their depression symptoms only after about 10 months had gone by since they enrolled in the study. The NYUCI has now been used in many locations in the United States. Findings have been replicated in randomized controlled trials in the USA, the UK, Australia and Israel. The results have also been replicated with adult child carers.

Many carers and their families requested help in locations where no NYUCI providers had been trained and certified. There also was a demand for family counselling for families who didn't all live in the same location. For example, sometimes adult children might live in the northern states of the USA, while their parents had retired to warmer climates in states like Florida or Arizona. Sometimes counsellors would include distant family members by telephone, although that was not in the original protocol. In response to these requests, training for online counselling using videoconferencing was developed. Reports from counsellors suggest that this modality can make family meetings much more accessible. In Virginia, a translation to online counselling, while not a randomized controlled trial, had positive results. The Virginia adaptation, FAMILIES, found similar results to those of the in-person study [134]. The online intervention had equal or greater benefits to caregivers than the in-person intervention, improving burden, depression and ability to manage reactions to the behavioural symptoms of dementia Moreover, the telehealth version overcame some of the common barriers to involvement in carer interventions (lack of time, distance to facility, transportation etc.).

6 Conclusion

While the value of informal care for persons with dementia is unquestionable, it is not self-evident that this type of care is sustainable in our current society. Governments stimulate informal care, often with a cost-containment motivation, but informal care will only remain feasible if support is available for the carers themselves. The tasks they perform change as the dementia process changes, and so does the burden they perceive. Evidence-based interventions, either singular or multicomponent, are available. They have proven positive effects. The costs associated with these interventions will easily be gained back as they diminish carer burnout and postpone nursing home admissions and avoid hospitalization of the person with dementia.

References

1. Wimo A, Gauthier S, Prince M. *Global Estimates of Informal Care*. London, Alzheimer's Disease International and Karolinska Institutet, 2018.

2. 2020 Alzheimer's disease facts and figures. *Alzheimers Dement* 2020 Mar 10. doi: 10.1002/alz.12068. Epub ahead of print.

3. Alzheimers Research UK. www.dementiastatistics.org/statistics/impact-on-carers.

4. Harris PB, Long S. Husbands and sons in the United States and Japan: Cultural expectations and caregiving experiences. *J Aging Stud.* 1999; 13(3): 241–67.

5. Greenwood N, Smith R. Motivations for being informal carers of people living with dementia: A systematic review of qualitative literature. *BMC Geriatrics* 2019; 19: 169.

6. Broese van Groenou MI, De Boer A. Providing informal care in a changing society. *Eur J Ageing* 2016; 13: 271–9.

7. Barczyk D, Kredler M. Long-term care across Europe and the U.S.: The role of informal and formal care. *Fiscal Studies* 2019; 40(3): 329–73.

8. Schneider J, Hallam A, Murray J, Foley B, Atkin L, Banerjee S, et al. Formal and informal care for people with dementia: Factors associated with service receipt. *Aging Ment Health* 2002; **6**(3): 255–65.

9. Ydstebø AE, Benth JS, Bergh S, Selbaek G, Vossius C. Informal and formal care among persons with dementia immediately before nursing home admission. *BMC Geriatrics* 2020; **20**: 296.

10. www.zorgvoorbeter.nl/dementie/cijfers

11. Prince MJ, Wimo A, Guerchet MM, Ali GC, Wu Y-T, Prina M. *World Alzheimer Report 2015. The Global Impact of Dementia: An Analysis of Prevalence, Incidence, Cost and Trends*. London, Alzheimer's Disease International, 2015.

12. Pickard L. A growing care gap? The supply of unpaid care for older people by their adult children in England to 2032. *Ageing Soc.* 2015; **35** (1): 96–123.

13. Agree EM, Glaser K. Demography of informal caregiving. In Uhlenberg P, ed. *International Handbook of Population Aging, vol. I*. New York, Springer, 2009; 647–68.

14. Fischer B, Müller K-U. Time to care? The effects of retirement on informal care provision. *J Health Econ.* 2020; **73**: 1–17.

15. Eurostat. https://ec.europa.eu/eurostat/statistics-explained/index.php/Household_composition_statistics#More_and_more_households_consisting_of_adults_living_alone

16. Lage DE, Jernigan MC, Chang Y, Grabowski DC, Hsu J, Metlay JP, Shah SJ. Living alone and discharge to skilled nursing facility care after hospitalization in older adults. *JAGS* 2017; **66**(1): 100–5.

17. Da Roit B, Hoogenboom M, Weicht B. The gender informal care gap. A fuzzy-set analysis of cross-country variations. *Eur Soc.* 2015; **17**(2): 199–218.

18. European Institute for Gender Equality. Gender Equality Index 2019. Work-life balance. https://eige.europa.eu/publications/gender-equality-index-2019-report/informal-care-older-people-people-disabilities-and-long-term-care-services

19. Zigante V. *Informal Care in Europe. Exploring Formalisation, Availability and Quality*. Brussels, European Commission, 2018.

20. Blendin K, Pepin R. Dementia grief: Theoretical model of a unique grief experience. *Dementia* 2017; **16**(1): 67–78.

21. Rosser MN, Fox NC, Mummery CJ, Schott JM, Warren JD. The diagnosis of early-onset dementia. *Lancet Neurol.* 2010; **9**(8): 793–806.

22. Tillman J, Just J, Schnakenberg R, Weckbecker K, Weltermann B, Münster E. Challenges in diagnosing dementia in patients with a migrant background: A cross-sectional study among German general practitioners. *BMC Family Practice* 2019; **20**(34): 1–10.

23. Krinsky-McHale SJ, Silverman W. Dementia and mild cognitive impairment in adults with intellectual disability: Issues of diagnosis. *Dev Disabil Res Rev.* 2013: **18**(1): 31–42.

24. Rietjens RL, Sudore M, Connolly JJ, Van Delden MA, Drickamer M, Droger M, et al. Definition and recommendations for advance care planning: An international consensus supported by the European Association for Palliative Care. *Lancet Oncol.* 2017; **18**(9): e543–e551.

25. De Vleminck A, Houttekier D, Pardon K, Deschepper R, Van Audenhove C, Vander Stichele R, Deliens L. Barriers and facilitators for general practitioners to engage in advance care planning: A systematic review. *Scand J Primary Health Care* 2013; **31**(4): 215–26.

26. Hugo J, Ganguli M. Dementia and cognitive impairment: Epidemiology, diagnosis, and treatment. *Clin Geriatr Med.* 2014; **30**(3): 421–42.

27. Sanders S, Adams KB. Grief reactions and depression in caregivers of individuals with Alzheimer's disease: Results from a pilot study in an urban setting. *Health Soc Work* 2005: **30**(4): 287–95.

28. Spruytte N, Van Audenhove C, Lammertyn F, Storms G. The quality of the caregiving relationship in informal care for older adults with dementia and chronic psychiatric patients. *Psychol Psychother.* 2002; **75**(3): 295–311.

29. Van Vracem M, Spruytte N, Declercq A, Van Audenhove C. Agitation in dementia and the role of spatial and sensory interventions: Experiences of professional and family carers. *Scan J Caring Sci.* 2016; **30**(2): 281–9.

30. Sutcliffe C, Giebel C, Bleijlevens M, Chester H, Challis D. Caring for a person with dementia on the margins of long-term care: A perspective on burden from 8 European countries. *J Am Med Dir.* 2018; **18**(11): 967–973.e1.

31. Huber M. *Towards a New, Dynamic Concept of Health. Its Operationalisation and Use in Public Health and Healthcare, and in Evaluating Health Effects of Food*. Maastricht, Maastricht University, 2014.

32. Dröes RM, Chattat R, Diaz A, Gove D, Graff M, Murphy K, et al. Social health and dementia: A European consensus on the operationalization of the concept and directions for research and practice. *Aging Ment Health* 2017; **21**(1): 4–17.

33. Hirschman KB, Kapo JM, Karlawish JHT. Identifying the factors that facilitate or hinder advance care planning by persons with dementia. *Alzheimer Dis Assoc Disord.* 2008; **22**(3): 293–8.

34. Tilburgs B, Vernooij-Dassen M, Koopmans R, Van Gennip H, Engels Y, Perry M. Barriers and facilitators for GPs in dementia advance care planning: A systematic integrative review. *PLoS One* 2018; **13**(6): e0198535.

35. Lund S, Richardson A, May C. Barriers to advance care planning at the end of life: An explanatory systematic review of implementation studies. *PLoS One* 2015; **10**(2): e0116629.

36. Ingravallo F, Mignani V, Mariani E, Ottoboni G, Melon MC, Chattat R. Discussing advance care planning: Insights from older people living in nursing homes and from family members. *Int Psychogeriatr.* 2018; **30**(4): 569–79.

37. Vandervoort A, Houttekier D, Van den Block L, Van der Steen JT, VanderStichele R, Deliens L. Advance care planning and physician orders in nursing home residents with dementia: A nationwide retrospective study among professional carers and relatives. *J Pain Symptom Manag.* 2014; **47**(2): 245–56.

38. Prince M, Comas-Herrera A, Knapp M. *World Alzheimer Report 2016: Improving Healthcare for People Living with Dementia Coverage, Quality and Costs Now and in the Future.* London, Alzheimer's Disease International, 2016.

39. Daly RL, Bunn F, Goodman C. Shared decision making for people living with dementia in extended care settings: A systematic review. *Brit Med J Open* 2018; **8**: e018977.

40. Miller LM, Whitlatch CJ, Lyons KS. Shared decision making in dementia: A review of patient and carer involvement. *Dementia* 2016; **15**(5): 1141–57.

41. Scholl I, Koelewijn-Van Loon M, Sepucha K, Elwyn G, Légaré F, Härter M, Dirmaier J. Measurement of shared decision making: A review of instruments. *Z Evid Fortbild Qual Gesundhwes.* 2011; **105**(4): 313–24.

42. Bae J. Shared decision making: Relevant concepts and facilitating strategies. *Epidemiol Health* 2017; **39**: e2017048.

43. Tyrrell JG, Genin N, Myslinski M. Freedom of choice and decision-making in health and social care: Views of older patients with early-stage dementia and their carers. *Dementia* 2006; **5**: 479–502.

44. Fetherstonhaugh D, Tarzia L, Nay R. Being central to decision making means I am still here! The essence of decision making for people with dementia. *J Aging Stud.* 2013; **27**(2): 143–50.

45. Hirschman KB, Joyce CM, James BD, Xie SX, Karlawish JH. Do Alzheimer's disease patients want to participate in a treatment decision, and would their carers let them? *Gerontologist* 2005; **45**(3): 381–8.

46. Ampe S, Sevenants A, Coppens E, Spruytte N, Smets T, Declercq A, Van Audenhove C. Study protocol for 'We DECide': Implementation of advance care planning for nursing home residents with dementia. *J Adv Nurs.* 2015; **71**(5): 1156–68.

47. Elwyn G, Frosch D, Thomson R, Joseph-Williams N, Lloyd A, Kinnersley P, et al. Shared decision making: A model for clinical practice. *J Gen Intern Med.* 2012; **27**(10): 1361–7.

48. Ampe S, Sevenants A, Declercq A, Van Audenhove C. Advance care planning for nursing home residents with dementia: Influence of 'We DECide' on policy and practice. *Patient Educ Couns.* 2017; **100**(1): 139–46.

49. Goossens B, Sevenants A, Declercq A, Van Audenhove C. 'We DECide optimised': Training nursing home staff in shared decision-making skills for advance care planning conversations in dementia care: Protocol of a pretest-posttest cluster randomized trial. *BMC Geriatr.* 2019; **19**(3): 33.

50. Goossens B, Sevenants A, Declercq A, Van Audenhove C. Improving shared decision-making in advance care planning: Implementation of a cluster randomized staff intervention in dementia care. *Patient Educ Couns.* 2019; **103**(4): 839–47.

51. Sinclair C, Gates K, Evans S, Auret KA. Factors influencing Australian general practitioners' clinical decisions regarding advance care planning: A factorial survey. *J Pain Symptom Manage.* 2016; **51**(4): 718–27.

52. Romøren M, Pedersen R, Førde R. How do nursing home doctors involve patients and next of kin in end-of-life decisions? A qualitative study from Norway. *BMC Med Ethics* 2016; **17**(5).

53. De Vleminck A, Pardon K, Beernaert K, Deschepper R, Houttekier D, Van Audenhove C, et al. Barriers to advance care planning in cancer, heart failure and dementia patients: A focus group study on general practitioners' views and experiences. *PLoS One* 2014; **9**(1): e84905.

54. Fosse A, Ruths S, Malterud K, Schaufel MA. Doctors' learning experiences in end-of-life care: A focus group study from nursing homes. *BMC Med Educ.* 2017; **17**(1): 27.

55. Corazzini K, Twersky J, White HK, Buhr GT, McConnell ES, Weiner M, Colón-Emeric CS. Implementing culture change in nursing homes:

An adaptive leadership framework. *Gerontologist* 2015; **55**(4): 616–27.

56. Goffman E. *Asylums: Essays on the Social Situation of Mental Patients and Other Inmates*. New York, Anchor Books, 1961.

57. Dröes RM, Goffin JJM, Breebaart E, De Rooij E, Vissers H, Bleeker JAC, Van Tilburg W. Support programmes for carers of people with dementia: A review of methods and effects. In Miesen B, Jones G, eds. *Care-Giving in Dementia III*. London, Routledge, 2004; 214–39.

58. Brodaty H, Gresham M, Luscombe G. The Prince Henry Hospital Dementia Carers' Training Programme. *Int J Geriatr Psychiatry* 1997; **12**(2): 183–92.

59. Moniz-Cook E, Agar S, Gibson G, Win T, Wang M. A preliminary study of the effects of early intervention with people with dementia and their families in a memory clinic. *Aging Ment Health* 1998; **2**(3): 199–211.

60. Dröes RM, Breebaart E. Amsterdamse Ontmoetingscentra; een nieuwe vorm van ondersteuning voor dementerende ouderen en hun verzorgers. Voorstudie. [Amsterdam meeting centres: A new form of support for older people with dementia and their carers. A preliminary study.] Amsterdam, Thesis Publishers, 1994.

61. Dröes RM, Breebaart E, Van Tilburg W, Mellenbergh GJ. The effect of integrated family support versus day care only on behavior and mood of patients with dementia. *Int Psychogeriatr.* 2000; **12**(1): 99–116.

62. Gendron CE, Poitras LR, Engels ML, Dastoor DP, Sirota SE, Barza SL, et al. Skills training with supporters of the demented. *J Am Geriatr Soc.* 1986; **34**(12): 875–80.

63. Hébert R, Leclerc G, Bravo G, Girouard D, Lefrançois R. Efficacy of a support group programme for carers of demented patients in the community: A randomized controlled trial. *Arch Gerontol Geriatr.* 1994; **18**(1): 1–14.

64. Zarit SH, Anthony CR, Boutselis M. Interventions with carers of dementia patients: Comparisons of two approaches. *Psychol Aging* 1987; **2**(3): 225–32.

65. Zarit SH, Stephens MA, Townsend A, Greene R. Stress reduction for family carers: Effects of adult day care use. *J Gerontol B Psychol Sci Soc Sci.* 1998; **53**(5): S267–S277.

66. Mohide EA, Pringle DM, Streiner DL, Gilbert, JR, Muir G, Tew M. A randomized trial of family carer support in the home management of dementia. *J Am Geriatr Soc.* 1990; **38**(4),446–54.

67. Vernooij-Dassen MJFJ, Persoon JMG. *Het thuismilieu van dementerende ouderen. Een interventie-onderzoek naar effecten van professionele ondersteuning van gezins- en familieleden van dementerende ouderen.* Nijmegen, Instituut voor Sociale Geneeskunde, Katholieke Universiteit Nijmegen, 1990.

68. Duijnstee M. *De belasting van familieleden van dementerenden.* Nijkerk, Intro, 1992.

69. Thomas S, Dalton J, Harden M, Eastwood A, Parker G. *Updated Meta-Review of Evidence on Support for Carers*. Southampton, NIHR Journals Library, 2017.

70. Knight BG, Lutzky SM, Macofsky-Urban F. A meta-analytic review of interventions for carer distress: Recommendations for future research. *Gerontologist* 1993; **33**(2): 240–8.

71. Maayan N, Soares-Weiser K, Lee H. Respite care for people with dementia and their carers. *Cochrane Database Syst Rev.* 2014; **1**: CD004396.

72. Tretteteig S, Vatne S, Rokstad AM. The influence of day care centres for people with dementia on family carers: An integrative review of the literature. *Aging Ment Health* 2016; **20**(5): 450–62.

73. Maffioletti VLR, Baptista MAT, Santos RL, Rodrigues VM, Dourado MCN. Effectiveness of day care in supporting family carers of people with dementia: A systematic review. *Dement Neuropsychol.* 2019; **13**(3): 268–83.

74. Dröes RM, Breebaart E, Meiland FJM, Van Tilburg W, Mellenbergh GJ. Effect of meeting centres support programme on feeling of competence of family carers and delay of institutionalization of people with dementia. *Aging Ment Health* 2004; **8**(3): 201–11.

75. Dröes RM, Meiland FJM, Schmitz MJ, Van Tilburg W. Effect of the meeting centres support program on informal carers of people with dementia: Results from a multi-centre study. *Aging Ment Health* 2006; **10**(2): 112–24.

76. Van Mierlo LD, Meiland FJM, Dröes RM. Dementelcoach: Effect of telephone coaching on carers of community dwelling people with dementia. *Int Psychogeriatr.* 2012; **24**(2): 212–22.

77. Miesen B, Jones G, eds. *Care-Giving in Dementia III*. London, Routledge, 2004.

78. Capus J. The Kingston dementia café: The benefits of establishing an Alzheimer café for carers and people with dementia. *Dementia* 2005; **4**(4): 588–91.

79. Greenwood N, Smith R, Akhtar F, Richardson A. A qualitative study of carers' experiences of dementia cafés: A place to feel supported and be yourself. *BMC Geriatrics* 2017; **17**: 164.

80. Teahan Á, Fitzgerald C, O'Shea E. Family carers' perspectives of the Alzheimer café in Ireland. *HRB Open Research* 2020; **3**: 18.

81. Dow B, Haralambous B, Hempton C, Hunt S, Calleja D. Evaluation of Alzheimer's Australian Vic Memory Lane Cafés. *Int Psychoger*. 2011; **23**(2): 246–55.

82. Merlo P, Devita M, Mandelli A, Rusconi ML, Taddeucci R, Terzi A, et al. Alzheimer café: An approach focused on Alzheimer's patients but with remarkable values on the quality of life of their carers. *Aging Clin Exp Res*. 2018; **30**(7): 767–74.

83. Jones SM, Killett A, Mioshi E. What factors predict family carers' attendance at dementia cafés? *J Alzheimers Dis*. 2018; **64**(4): 1337–45.

84. Chien LY, Chu H, Guo JL, Liao, YM, Chang LI, Chen CH, Chou KR. Carer support groups inpatients with dementia: A meta-analysis. *Int J Geriatr Psychiatry* 2011; **26**(10): 1089–98.

85. Lins S, Hayder-Beichel D, Rücker G, Motschall E, Antes G, Meyer G, Langer G. Efficacy and experiences of telephone counselling for informal carers of people with dementia. *Cochrane Database Syst Rev*. 2004; **9**: CD009126.

86. Salfi J, Ploeg J, Black ME. Seeking to understand telephone support for dementia carers. *West J Nurs Res*. 2005; **27**(6): 701–21.

87. Jackson D, Roberts G, Wu ML, Ford R, Doyle C. A systematic review of the effect of telephone, internet or combined support for carers of people living with Alzheimer's, vascular or mixed dementia in the community. *Arch Gerontol Geriatr*. 2016; **66**: 218–36.

88. Huijsman R, Boomstra R, Veerbeek M, Döpp C, eds. *Dutch Standard of Dementia Care [Zorgstandaard Dementie]: Samenwerken op maat voor personen met dementie en mantelzorgers*. Utrecht, Dementiezorg voor elkaar, 2020.

89. Mantovan F, Ausserhofer D, Huber M, Schulc E, Them C. Interventionen und deren Effekte auf pflegende Angehörige von Menschen mit Demenz – Eine systematische Literaturübersicht. *Pflege* 2010; **23**(4): 223–39.

90. Berthelsen CB, Kristensson J. The content, dissemination and effects of case management interventions for informal carers of older adults: A systematic review. *Int J Nurs Stud*. 2015; **52**(5): 988–1002.

91. Peeters JM, De Lange J, Van Asch I, Spreeuwenberg R, Veerbeek M, Pot AM, Francke AL. *Landelijke evaluatie van casemanagement dementie*. Utrecht, NIVEL, 2012.

92. MacNeil Vroomen J, Bosmans JE, Eekhout I, Joling KJ, Van Mierlo LD, Meiland FJM, et al.The cost-effectiveness of two forms of case management compared to a control group for persons with dementia and their informal carers from a societal perspective. *PLoS ONE* 2016; **11**(9): e0160908.

93. Jensen M, Agbata IN, Canavan M, McCarthy G. Effectiveness of educational interventions for informal carers of individuals with dementia residing in the community: Systematic review and meta-analysis of randomised controlled trials. *Int J Geriatr Psychiatry* 2015; **30**(2): 130–43.

94. Tang WK, Chan CY. Effects of psychosocial interventions on self-efficacy of dementia carers: A literature review. *Int J Geriatr Psychiatry* 2016; **31**(5): 475–93.

95. Selwood A, Johnston K, Katona C, Lyketsos C, Livingston G. Systematic review of the effect of psychological interventions on family carers of people with dementia. *J Affect Disord*. 2007; **101** (1–3): 75–89.

96. Eggenberger E, Heimerl K, Bennett MI. Communication skills training in dementia care: A systematic review of effectiveness, training content, and didactic methods in different care settings. *Int Psychogeriatr*. 2013; **25**(3): 345–58.

97. Vandepitte S, Van den Noortgate N, Putman K, Verhaeghe S, Faes K, Annemans L. Effectiveness of supporting informal carers of people with dementia: A systematic review of randomized and Non-randomized controlled trials. *J Alzheimer's Dis*. 2016; **52**(3): 929–65.

98. Li R, Cooper C, Barber J, Rapaport P, Griffin M, Livingston G. Coping strategies as mediators of the effect of the START (strategies for RelaTives) intervention on psychological morbidity for family carers of people with dementia in a randomised controlled trial. *J Affect Disord*. 2014; **168**: 298–305.

99. Gilhooly KJ, Gilhooly ML, Sullivan MP, McIntyre A, Wilson L, Harding E, et al. A meta-review of stress, coping and interventions in dementia and dementia caregiving. Review. *BMC Geriatrics* 2016; **16**(106): 1–8.

100. Pinquart M, Sörensen S. Helping carers of persons with dementia: Which interventions work and how large are their effects? *Int Psycogeriatr*. 2006; **18**(4): 577–95.

101. Vernooij-Dassen M, Draskovic I, McCleery J, Downs M. Cognitive reframing for carers of people with dementia. *Cochrane Database Syst Rev*. 2011; **11**: CD005318.

102. Ducharme F, Lachance L, Lévesque L, Zarit SH, Kergoat MJ. Maintaining the potential of a psycho-educational program: Efficacy of a booster session after an intervention offered family carers at disclosure of an relative's dementia diagnosis. *Aging Mental Health* 2015; **19** (3): 207–16.

103. Boots LM, De Vugt ME, Van Knippenberg RJ, Kempen GI, Verhey FR. A systematic review of internet-based supportive interventions for carers of patients with dementia. *Int J Geriatr Psychiatry* 2014; **29**(4): 331–44.

104. Hopwood J, Walker N, McDonagh L, Rait G, Walters K, Iliffe S, et al. Internet-based interventions aimed at supporting family carers of people with dementia: Systematic review. *J Med Internet Res.* 2018; **20**(6): e216.

105. Kerkhof Y, Pelgrum-Keurhorst M, Mangiaracina F, Bergsma A, Vrauwdeunt G, Graff M, Dröes RM. User-participatory development of FindMyApps: A tool to help people with mild dementia find supportive apps for self-management and meaningful activities. *Digital Health* 2019; **26**: 5.

106. Kerkhof Y, Kohl G, Veijer M, Mangiaracina F, Bergsma A, Graff M, Dröes ML. Randomized controlled feasibility study of FindMyApps: First evaluation of a tablet-based intervention to promote self-management and meaningful activities in people with mild dementia. *Disabil Rehabil Assist Technol.* 2020; **19**: 1–15.

107. Beentjes KM, Kerkhof YJF, Neal DP, Ettema TP, Koppelle MA, Meiland FJM, Graff M, Dröes RM. Process evaluation of the FindMyApps program trial among people with dementia or MCI and their caregivers based on the MRC guidance. *Gerontechnology* 2021; **20**(1): 1–15. https://doi.org./10.4017/gt.2020.20.1.406.11.

108. Smits CHM, De Lange J, Dröes RM, Meiland F, Vernooij-Dassen M, Pot AM. Effects of combined intervention programmes for people with dementia living at home and their carers: A systematic review. *Int J Geriatr Psychiatry.* 2007; **22**(12): 1181–93.

109. Olazaran J, Reisberg B, Clare L, Cruz I, Peña-Casanova J, et al. Nonpharmacological therapies in Alzheimer's disease: A systematic review of efficacy. *Dement Geriatr Cogn Disord.* 2010; **30**: 161–78.

110. Laver K, Milte R, Dyer S, Crotty M. A systematic review and meta-analysis comparing carer focused and dyadic multicomponent interventions for carers of people with dementia. *J Aging Health* 2017; **29**(8): 1308–49.

111. Van't Leven N, Prick A-EJ, Groenewoud JG, Roelofs PD, De Lange J, Pot AM. Dyadic interventions for community-dwelling people with dementia and their family carers: A systematic review. *Int Psychogeriatr.* 2013; **25**(10): 1581–1603.

112. Beentjes, KM, Neal, DP, Kerkhof Y, Broeder C, Moeridjan Z, Ettema TP, et al. Impact of the FindMyApps program on people with mild cognitive impairment or dementia and their caregivers: An exploratory pilot randomised controlled trial. *Disabil Rehabil: Assist Technol.* 2020; 1–13. Advance online publication. https://doi.org/10.1080/17483107.2020.1842918

113. Dröes RM, Meiland FJM, Schmitz M, Van Tilburg W. Effect of combined support for people with dementia and carers versus regular day care on behaviour and mood of persons with dementia: Results from a multi-centre implementation study. *Int J Geriatric Psychiatr.* 2004; **19**: 673–84.

114. Brooker D, Evans SC, Evans SB, Bray J, Saibene FL, Scorolli C, et al. Evaluation of the implementation of the meeting centres support program in Italy, Poland, and the UK: Exploration of the effects on people with dementia. *Int J Geriatric Psychiatry* 2018; **33**(7): 883–92.

115. Szcześniak D, Rymaszewska J, Saibene FL, Urbańska K, d'Arma A, Brooker D, et al. Meeting centres support programme highly appreciated by people with dementia and carers: A European cross-country evaluation. *Aging Ment Health* 2019; **5**: 1–11.

116. Dröes RM, Van Mierlo LD, Meiland FJM, Van der Roest HG. Memory problems in dementia: Adaptation and coping strategies, and psychosocial treatments. *Expert Rev Neurother.* 2011; **11**(12): 1769–82.

117. Dröes RM, Van Rijn A, Rus E, Dacier S, Meiland F. Utilization, effect, and benefit of the individualized meeting centers support program for people with dementia and carers. *Clin Interv Aging* 2019; **14**: 1527–53.

118. Chien WT, Lee YM. A disease management program for families of persons in Hong Kong with dementia. *Psychiatr Serv.* 2008; **59**: 433–6.

119. Chien WT, Lee YM. Randomized controlled trial of a dementia care programme for families of home-resided older people with dementia. *J Adv Nurs.* 2011; **67**: 774–87.

120. Gitlin LN, Hauck WW, Dennis MP, Winter L. Maintenance of effects of the home environmental skill-building program for family carers and individuals with Alzheimer's disease and related disorders. *J Gerontol A: Biol Sci Med Sci.* 2005; **60**: 368–74.

121. Graff MJL, Vernooij-Dassen MJM, Thijssen M, Dekker J, Hoefnagels WHL, Olderikkert MG. Effects of community occupational therapy on quality of life, mood, and health status in dementia patients and their carers:

A randomized controlled trial. *J Gerontol A: Biol Sci Med Sci.* 2007; **62**: 1002–9.

122. Waldorff F, Buss D, Eckermann A, Rasmussen M, Keiding N, Rishoj S, Waldemar G. Efficacy of psychosocial intervention in patients with mild Alzheimer's disease: The multicentre, rater blinded, randomised Danish Alzheimer Intervention Study (DAISY). *British Med J* 2012; **345**(7870): e4693.

123. Zarit SH, Zarit JM, Reever KE. Memory training for severe memory loss: Effects on senile dementia patients and their families. *Gerontologist* 1982; **22**: 373–7.

124. Mittelman M, Ferris S, Shulman E, Steinberg G, Ambinder A, Mackell J, Cohen J. A comprehensive support program: Effect on depression in spouse-carers of AD patients. *Gerontologist* 1995; **35**(6): 792–802.

125. Mittelman MS, Roth DL, Coon DW, Haley WE. Sustained benefit of supportive intervention for depressive symptoms in Alzheimer's carers. *Am J Psychiatry* 2004; **161**(5): 850–6.

126. Jang Y, Clay OJ, Roth DL, Haley WE, Mittelman MS. Neuroticism and longitudinal change in carer depression: Impact of a spouse-carer intervention program. *Gerontologist* 2004; **44**(3): 311–17.

127. Gaugler JG, Roth DL, Haley WE, Mittelman MS. Can counseling and support reduce Alzheimer's carers' burden and depressive symptoms during the transition to institutionalization? Results from the NYU Intervention Study. *J Am Geriatr Soc.* 2008; **56**(3): 421–8.

128. Haley WE, Bergman EJ, Roth DL, McVie T, Gaugler JE, Mittelman MS. Long-term effects of bereavement and carer intervention on dementia carer depressive symptoms. *Gerontologist* 2008; **48**(6): 732–40.

129. Mittelman MS, Roth DL, Haley WE, Zarit SH. Effects of a carer intervention on negative carer appraisals of behavior problems in patients with Alzheimer's disease: Results of a randomized trial. *J Gerontol B Psychol Sci Soc Sci.* 2004; **59**(1): 27–34.

130. Mittelman MS, Roth DL, Clay OJ, Haley WE. Preserving health of Alzheimer's carers: Impact of a spouse carer intervention. *Am J Geriatr Psychiatry* 2007; **150**(9): 780–9.

131. Roth DL, Mittelman MS, Clay OJ, Madan A, Haley WE. Changes in social support as mediators of the impact of a psychosocial intervention for spouse carers of persons with Alzheimer's disease. *Psychol Aging* 2005; **20**(4): 634–44.

132. Drentea P, Clay OJ, Roth DL, Mittelman MS. Predictors of improvement in social support: Five-year effects of a structured intervention for carers of spouses with Alzheimer's disease. *Soc Sci Med.* 2006 Aug; **63**(4): 957–67. PMID: 16616406

133. Mittelman MS, Haley WE, Clay O, Roth DL. Improving carer well-being delays nursing home placement of patients with Alzheimer disease. *Neurology* 2006; **67**(9): 1592–9.

134. Rice JD, Sperling SA, Brown DS, Mittelman MS, Manning CA. Evaluating the efficacy of TeleFAMILIES: A telehealth intervention for caregivers of community-dwelling people with dementia. *Aging Ment Health* 2021 Jun; **14**: 1–7. doi: 10.1080/13607863.2021.1935462. Epub ahead of print. PMID: 34125635

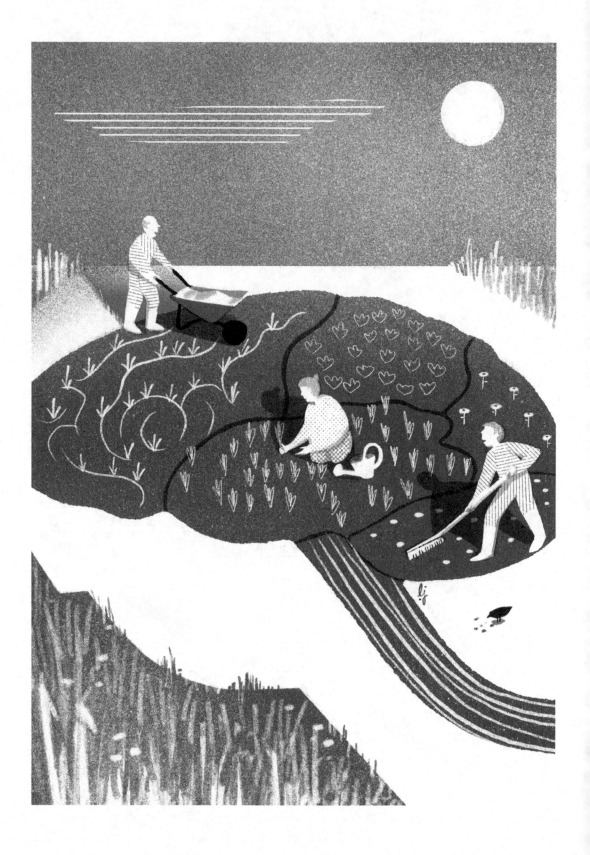

Risk Factors and Non-Pharmacological Prevention of Dementia

Rudi D'Hooge, Ann Van der Jeugd, Sebastiaan Engelborghs, Frans Boch Waldorff and Mathieu Vandenbulcke

1 Introduction

The quest to find a treatment for dementia is increasingly overshadowed by the search for risk factors and prevention. The World Health Organization (WHO) Ministerial Conference on Global Action against Dementia ranked prevention and reduction of risk highest among the top-ten research priorities to reduce the global burden of dementia by 2025 [1]. This shift towards prevention of dementia not only gains support amongst researchers, it also attracts the attention of policymakers and is becoming the focus of worldwide public health interventions. In the present chapter, we review the factors and measures that contribute to and promote healthy ageing. First, we want to distinguish between prevention and rejuvenation, and endorse the former strategy to mitigate the impact of dementia. We argue that prevention remains the most sensible course of action given the lack of effective treatment, and discuss the modifiable risk factors identified so far. We specifically address social isolation and loneliness given their importance from a psychological and societal perspective. Next, we describe prevention strategies followed by an overview of non-pharmacological interventions with increasing evidence of their effectiveness. We conclude that changing lifestyle might be an effective way to enhance tolerance to dementia and senescence in our ageing populations, but also represents one of the most formidable psychosocial and societal challenges.

2 Healthy Ageing without Rejuvenation

Even pop icons, who once hoped to die before they got old, now prefer to postpone death as long as possible. Indeed we find individuals and modern societies progressively unprepared to accept demise and *senescence* (i.e. the physical and mental decline that often attends ageing). Some people spend huge sums on unsupported remedies to reverse the effects of ageing. However, as we argue here, enhancing disease tolerance and prevention, in many different forms, is still the most sensible means to avert senescence and dementia. Compared to previous generations, many more elderly people nowadays maintain their quality of life, which indicates that healthy ageing can be achieved by prevention and lifestyle changes [2]. We are consequently convinced that the widespread implementation of these measures should feature prominently on our global public healthcare agenda.

Notably, the focus on prevention and healthy ageing is significantly different from the cause of rejuvenation activists, who want to 'cure' ageing. One of the most eloquent exponents of this anti-ageing movement, theoretical gerontologist Aubrey de Grey, tried to convince scientists as well as policymakers to reject the purportedly ageist opinion that accepts that we should get sick and die at a certain age [3]. Many people indeed feel that decline and dying are inevitable and essential aspects of our biology, and think that it would be disastrous to have people live much beyond their present lifespan (to which de Grey retorts that we have insufficient knowledge about our fertility and the planet's carrying capacity to know this for sure).

Even though de Grey found a lot of support among affluent baby boomers, many scientists regard his anti-ageing ideas as mere wishful thinking [4]. In a widely publicized debate at the 2012 meeting of the Oxford University Scientific Society, he discussed the possibility and desirability of using biomedical technology to have people live longer by repairing the molecular and cellular damage that attends increasing age. De Grey thinks much of this technology is already available, which he proposes to combine in a therapeutic programme (Strategies for Engineered Negligible Senescence (SENS)). His SENS Research Foundation wants to ensure public access to these SENS remedies. However, many neuroscientists doubt the potential of engineered treatment of senescence, and would call de Grey's programme a distraction. They consider the SENS programme utterly unrealistic, given the vast range of age-related diseases and the complexity of the ageing process. Defeating one cause of ageing would just have it replaced by another one, demonstrating that ageing is a multisystem and multifactorial process, an essential aspect of living.

Many experts agree that prevention and non-pharmacological interventions are still much more preferable than treatment, when it comes to ageing or age-related ailments such as dementia. We are still a long way from curing disorders of ageing or brain pathologies that cause dementia [5, 6]. In fact, no age-related neurological problem can be effectively treated for the moment. Even critical scientists, notably including board members of the SENS Research Foundation, have conceded that it remains impossible to reverse the damage of ageing. While arguing for further support to rejuvenation biotechnology, movements such as de Grey's might bolster complacency and misguided action of their own making. Rejuvenation ideas could distract from efforts to influence people change their lifestyle and habits in order to prevent senescence and dementia, rather than hope for some hypothetical cure.

3 Modifiable Risk Factors for Dementia

Dementia is one of the most important concerns in contemporary healthcare and social care. Some people are more at risk to suffer dementia in old age than others, which has been attributed to factors such as gender, genetics and ethnicity. Inheriting dementia directly is rare (e.g. through a single gene mutation), but genetic factors are thought to play some role in almost all cases of dementia. The most important risk factor is age, which can obviously be neither modified nor prevented. However, there is growing awareness among experts that a considerable proportion of risk factors for dementia could very well be modifiable. Such modifiable risk factors could be

important targets for preventive measures. However, dementia is a syndrome caused by various pathologies, from cerebrovascular through neurodegenerative (such as Alzheimer's disease, frontotemporal dementia, dementia with Lewy bodies) or mixed aetiology (as is often the case in elderly patients). About half of all dementia cases are supposed to be attributable to Alzheimer's disease that is presently often diagnosed in its prodromal stage of mild cognitive impairment. Preventive measures could thus delay further decline and conversion to dementia proper (i.e. secondary prevention, as interventions may only start after the occurrence of the first symptoms; see later in this chapter).

Prevention of dementia will have to take its etiological heterogeneity into account. For the time being, many dementias cannot, or can be only partially treated by available medication. There is some symptomatic treatment for Alzheimer's disease (that has positive effects in dementia with Lewy bodies as well), whereas no treatment is currently available for frontotemporal dementia. Despite formidable international research efforts, experts tend to be ambiguously optimistic about the possibility of disease-modifying therapeutics for Alzheimer's disease. Even if disease-modifying therapies eventually become available, they are unlikely to render prevention or tolerance enhancement obsolete. An extensive commission report in the journal *Lancet* reviewed the proven impact of modifiable risk factors for dementia [7, 8]. The authors found that about 40% of the identified risk factors could actually respond to prevention (see Figure 8.1). Risk factors that can be influenced by available medication include cardiovascular disease, diabetes and midlife hypertension. Although the evidence is still insufficient for firm conclusions and guidelines, it was shown that several of the modifiable risk factors could be or have the potential to be significantly influenced by non-pharmacological intervention.

It is a relatively recent concept to implement lifestyle as a modifiable risk factor for dementia. For example, a National Institutes of Health (NIH) expert panel concluded in 2010 that the association of lifestyle with dementia was not convincing, whereas merely three years later, the G8 World Dementia Council called for international focus on prevention by lifestyle modification. And again, two years later, the Alzheimer's Association

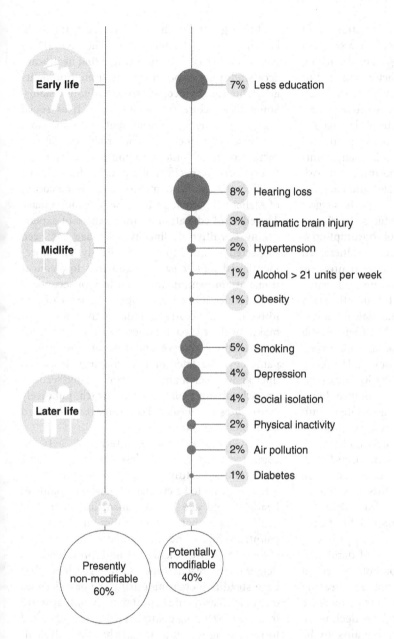

Figure 8.1 Different modifiable and non-modifiable risk factors for dementia. Modifiable risk factors at early life, midlife and late life could be important targets for interventions that do not aim to cure, but to attenuate or prevent the occurrence of risk factors and enhance tolerance to unavoidable risks. Adapted from [8].

concluded that there was compelling evidence to support the role of modifiable risk factors for dementia. In 2019, WHO launched a global action plan for the public health response to dementia. One of the targets was primary prevention, based on the popular adage that 'what's good for your heart is good for your brain'. Some of the risk factors for dementia are indeed also cardiovascular risks, such as current or midlife smoking, midlife obesity, hypertension and diabetes. Also notable is the relationship with emotional health, prompting healthcare organizations to promote projects that enhance psychological and emotional well-being in the elderly. It is clear from this that prevention and management of dementia should be multidisciplinary, implementing biomedical, psychosocial and societal strategies to address the wide scope of factors involved.

Not surprisingly, many modifiable risk factors for dementia are interconnected and eventually linked to impaired brain function. For example, diabetes mellitus increases inflammatory responses and causes high blood glucose concentrations, which are associated with vascular risk factors and neurodegeneration. Oxidative stress and inflammation impair cognition and are associated with Alzheimer brain pathology. Hypertension, a very significant systemic risk factor, can lead to vascular brain damage as well, which may ultimately lead to brain atrophy and neurodegeneration. Obesity is linked to prediabetes and metabolic defects, which can also enhance Alzheimer neuropathology. Smoking has decreased in many countries, but remains a prevalent and important risk factor classically linked with cardio- and cerebrovascular disease. Although some reports suggest that light drinking of alcohol reduces the risk of cognitive decline, excessive alcohol consumption is clearly associated with brain damage and increased risk for dementia. Besides the direct neurotoxic effect of alcohol, heavy drinking is often associated with nutritional deficiencies and traumatic brain injuries that impact brain health. Clinical depression could be a risk factor too, but there is still debate whether it is an actual risk for Alzheimer's disease or rather a prodromal symptom. However, there is some support for a pathophysiological connection, because depression does induce brain dysfunctions that have been associated with dementia, and some antidepressants decrease Alzheimer brain pathology in animal models.

Intriguingly, decreased sensorial input (e.g. caused by impaired hearing or vision) could be a risk factor as well. Hearing loss has indeed been recently recognized as a major risk factor for dementia. Whether it is a modifiable factor depends, among other things, on its presently equivocal role in the pathogenesis of dementia, since age-related vascular pathology could cause both dementia and peripheral hearing loss. Even mild hearing loss appears to increase progressively the risk of cognitive decline in later life and dementia, but it remains to be shown whether correction of hearing could actually prevent dementia. There is some evidence that traumatic brain injury or impaired sleep could be risk factors as well, but their pathophysiological mechanisms remain unclear. Environmental factors such as air pollution are thought to play a role too, and there is epidemiological evidence that people living near highways have a slightly higher risk to develop dementia. This association could be attributed to socio-economic factors, since houses near to highways might be cheaper.

More generally, the risk for dementia could be linked to social inequality. The COVID-19 pandemic has again demonstrated that healthcare accessibility and exposure to unsafe environments are influenced by people's socio-economic status. Some risk factors for dementia, such as social engagement, living environment and education, are closely entwined with the broad societal and socio-economic context. Living near busy roads or exposure to specific pollutants has been shown to affect the risk for dementia, or even the course of Alzheimer pathology, in vulnerable individuals. The effect of education on the chances of experiencing cognitive decline in older age has been suspected for quite some time already. The aforementioned *Lancet* panel found that low educational attainment, defined as a lack of secondary school education, makes people vulnerable to cognitive decline because it reduces their ability to maintain their capacities despite brain pathology (i.e. cognitive reserve and tolerance to neuropathology, see later in this chapter). It is still unclear whether higher education (after secondary school) and bilingualism, which putatively contributes specifically to cognitive reserve, afford additional protection.

Notably, the intricate interaction between cognitive reserve and disease tolerance on one hand, and a healthy and active lifestyle on the other, appears to be crucial to maintain cognitive health in old age [9]. A consortium of public health researchers from different European countries, Japan and the United States observed a decline in the incidence and prevalence of dementia in recent times [10]. Prevalence has been steadily increasing during the past decades due to increasing life expectancy. A similar trend in some developing countries has been attributed to increasing life standards. It has been difficult to determine exactly why this curve is now flattening. Possibly improved living conditions, education and healthcare influence physical, mental and cognitive health positively, thus reducing the risk of dementia in later life. Improved education and higher life standards indeed go hand in hand with a healthier lifestyle. In fact, some public health initiatives might have – rather inadvertently – contributed to primary prevention of dementia by this panoptic assumption that 'what's good for your heart is good for your brain'.

4 Pathophysiology of Social Isolation and Loneliness

There is increasing awareness about psychosocial factors and stress in emotional and cognitive health. The importance of a supportive and caring social circle at any stage of life has been well established. Also, the impact of physical factors such as hearing loss has been attributed to secondary psychosocial dysfunction and ensuing depression. Social isolation and loneliness appear to be associated with increased risk for dementia. Researchers at Harvard Medical School suggested that loneliness might actually be an early symptom of Alzheimer's disease. In a study using PET brain imaging in cognitively normal older individuals, they found an association between loneliness and cortical amyloid burden [11]. However, people's circle tends to decrease as they age, and older people regularly feel lonely. Social isolation often leads to stress and inactivity, which could aggravate depression and cognitive decline. Therefore, social isolation might actually be a prodrome of dementia as well as part of the set of interacting risk factors that increase the risk of depression, hypertension and coronary heart disease (all risk factors for dementia). The aforementioned *Lancet* panel concluded that the impact of social isolation as a dementia risk factor could be similar to that of physical inactivity and hypertension [7].

Social isolation and loneliness are fundamentally distinct [12, 13], but both could be linked to (a higher risk of) cognitive decline and a faster rate of decline. The conceptual and mechanistic difference between social isolation and loneliness and their impact has not been clearly made by all researchers. Social isolation indicates that an individual is physically alone, which can be quantitatively measured and defined as an objective lack of social contact and stimulation. Social isolation was found to raise the risk of morbidity and mortality with a similar or higher factor as high blood pressure, smoking, alcohol abuse, sedentary lifestyle and obesity [7]. Loneliness is a complex subjective feeling that depends on how a person evaluates communication with others or experiences isolation. Loneliness leads to hypervigilance to social threat and concerns about social rejection, and eventually, social avoidance and anxiety. Increased desire to connect with others and heightened sensitivity to social threats negatively impact cognitive ability [14, 15]. Research at the University of Leuven detailed the negative effects of loneliness on attributions, self-evaluations and self-efficacy [16]. Social cognition becomes impaired by isolation episodes that could further impoverish social interaction and hinder connection, which aggravates the condition and could render loneliness intractable to intervention.

The late social neuroscientist John Cacioppo (1951–2018) and his associates at the University of Chicago studied the effects of loneliness on general health and brain function most extensively [14, 15]. They confirmed that the experience of social connection, vital for human survival and welfare, is explained by subjective judgement and not the objective presence of others. Loneliness is often associated with unhealthy conditions such as sedentary lifestyle, hormonal changes, lower quality of sleep and impaired daytime functioning, and vascular defects. Cacioppo's prospective studies in elderly individuals without dementia demonstrate that loneliness, fewer close relationships and being unmarried all contributed to cognitive decline and/or risk of dementia. The harshness of social pain is illustrated by the observation that it shares brain and hormonal mechanisms with physical pain and stress [17]. Cacioppo and associates hypothesized that loneliness dysregulates the biological stress response, which includes activation of the hypothalamic–pituitary–adrenal (HPA) axis. Convergent with this putative pathophysiological mechanism, social isolation and/or loneliness were shown to increase cortisol levels, lower glucocorticoid receptor sensitivity and increase pro-inflammatory and lower anti-inflammatory processes.

Hypothalamic–pituitary–adrenal dysregulation has specifically been shown to affect the functions of the hippocampus, a region that plays a central role in cognitive processes. Hippocampal atrophy is a well-established characteristic of both non-pathological and pathological cognitive decline. Dysfunction of the hippocampus and related brain regions diminishes brain reserve, which could increase vulnerability to cognitive ageing. Recent research indicates that chronic social stressors also inhibit the generation of new neurons in the adult brain (i.e. adult neurogenesis). The functional role of adult neurogenesis remains a matter of debate, but it has been linked with cognitive and emotional functioning. Notably, the different steps in adult neurogenesis are known to be affected by stress, and specifically by HPA axis dysregulation. Fewer neurons can mature and integrate in stressful conditions. In fact, stressors experienced in adulthood are among the best-known suppressors of adult neurogenesis.

5 Models and Modes of Prevention

Canadian psychologist Stuart MacDonald and associates propose a multidisciplinary model for the management of dementia [18]. It largely relies on the integrated non-pharmacological approach of healthcare workers as well as social and community professionals. Given the complexity and the scope of the modifiable risk factors for dementia, the implementation of extensive preventive strategies is likely to benefit from such an approach. The team proposed by MacDonald provides integrated or parallel care from various healthcare workers and social service agencies as well as professionals from outside traditional healthcare. It consists of nurse practitioners, physical and occupational therapists, nutritionists and social workers, neuropsychologists and physicians from different medical specialties (e.g. neurology and geriatrics). Non-pharmacological prevention strategies that could be implemented

by such a team include cognitive, psychosocial and physical interventions in a variety of settings (e.g. domestic or institutional) and modalities (e.g. individual or collective).

Other models include disease-oriented approaches in specialized memory clinics. Notably, the importance of a strong primary healthcare approach by competent general practitioners (GPs) has been elaborated by one of the present authors [19–21] (see Figure 8.2). It is an essential component of dementia care, and one of the most prominent venues to achieve personalized prevention and health equity. For the majority of medical decisions, the GP tries to include patient preferences, which may be significantly different from a specialist approach. This particularly involves decisions about prevention, diagnosis and therapy for chronic conditions such as dementia. In hospitals, diseases stay and people come and go, whereas in general practice, people stay and diseases come and go. General practice often defines itself in terms of relationships, especially the GP–patient relationship. These relationships are instrumental to connect the generalizations of biomedical science to the unique individual experience of illness and disease. They could be essential to attain the lifestyle changes that decrease the risk of dementia.

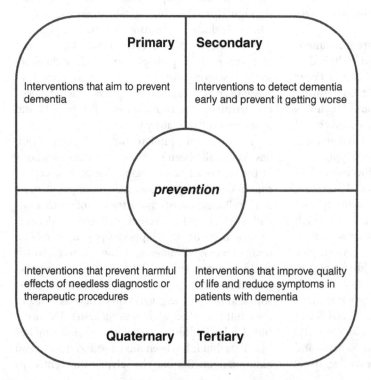

Figure 8.2 Different preventive interventions can help people maintain functional capacity in old age. The concept of quaternary prevention is relatively recent. It refers to the protection of patients against invasive healthcare interventions that may do more harm than good.

Primary — Interventions that aim to prevent dementia

Secondary — Interventions to detect dementia early and prevent it getting worse

prevention

Quaternary — Interventions that prevent harmful effects of needless diagnostic or therapeutic procedures

Tertiary — Interventions that improve quality of life and reduce symptoms in patients with dementia

Enhancement of disease tolerance and prevention of risk factors could both reduce the risk of dementia. Tolerance, a concept derived from infectiology, refers to an individual's ability to limit the impact of disease, whereas preventive interventions aim to prevent a disease from occurring or worsening. Primary prevention includes measures that aim to prevent people from getting a disease to start with, whereas secondary prevention includes interventions to detect a disease early and prevent it from getting worse. Tertiary prevention refers to interventions that improve quality of life and reduce the symptoms of a present disease. The concept of quaternary prevention was introduced by Belgian physician Marc Jamoulle, essentially to protect patients against over-medicalization and medical invasion. The concept could definitely be generalized to multidisciplinary therapeutic or preventive intervention in general. Jamoulle's model of four categories of prevention implements the distinction between disease (a pathophysiological construct) and illness (the subjective experience of poor health). Danish physician John Brodersen redefined quaternary prevention as actions to protect individuals from interventions that may do more harm than good [22].

The concept of quaternary prevention should be kept in mind by every healthcare professional, but it may be especially relevant in the prevention of dementia. A growing number of studies report a high prevalence of comorbidity in older people with dementia as well as the use of multiple prescription medication (i.e. polypharmacy). Healthcare services are typically organized around single conditions, leading to people with multiple conditions often receiving fragmented care that may lead to polypharmacy. Comorbidity and polypharmacy may affect cognition, physical function as well as survival in individuals with dementia. Both are more prevalent in the poor population than the affluent. Also, both are typically addressed in general practice, further confirming its crucial role in prevention as well as management of dementia.

6 Non-Pharmacological Interventions

Pharmacological interventions intended to cure neurodegeneration continue to fall short in clinical trials. It is often assumed that anti-amyloid therapies could halt or even prevent Alzheimer's disease, but the failure of potential anti-amyloid strategies, even in the earliest symptomatic stages, suggests that Alzheimer pathophysiology is more complex than previously thought [23]. A major issue in experimental therapeutics research may also be that patients enrolled in trials are already too far progressed and irreversibly damaged. Notwithstanding advances in symptomatic management, dementing diseases cannot be cured or significantly modified at present. The focus has therefore shifted to tolerance enhancement, or preventive efforts that target the asymptomatic stage, before the onset of significant decline. Prevention remains the preferred intervention strategy in treatable disorders such as heart disease or diabetes. It is almost certainly so that prevention and enhancement of disease tolerance will continue to be relevant and even preferable, even if modifying treatments for dementia become available. It has been noted that moderately delaying functional decline in brain function could already make a significant difference. In fact, a delay of just a single year in disease progression has been estimated to result in up to 9 million fewer cases by 2050 [24].

Few non-pharmacological interventions received such wide support as physical exercise [25]. Mayo Clinic neurologist Ronald Petersen said in a television interview that 'regular physical exercise is probably the best means we have of preventing Alzheimer's disease today, better than medications, better than intellectual activity, better than supplements and diet'. The famous Belgian nonagenarian and Nobel laureate Christian de Duve (1917–2013) explained his putative magic bullet to avert dementia in a 2004 interview: 'Most importantly, never stop ... just keep going ... Continue, both physically and mentally ... As long as you have the physical capabilities, it is possible.' Physical inactivity has been shown to be a major modifiable risk factor. People who exercise are more likely to remain in good health, both physically and mentally. Prospective studies do demonstrate that physical activity protects against cognitive decline at a more advanced age, but sceptics argue that there are still no controlled trials to support the preventive action of physical activity, and that exercise alone may not be sufficient.

Exercising in midlife is associated with a reduced risk for dementia, which suggests that it could enhance tolerance or have neuroprotective effects (e.g. by promoting release of neurotrophic factors and reducing vascular pathology). Animal studies do support a causal link between exercise and decreased risk of developing Alzheimer-like neuropathology as well as cognitive decline. Physical exercise has been shown to improve cognitive and behavioural performance in high-risk individuals. It also reduces falls and improves mood in elderly people, which has definite health benefits. Compared to other preventive interventions, physical exercise moreover has the advantage of being attainable and low cost, and does not have negative side effects of any real importance. Almost certainly, various mechanisms are involved in the putative beneficial effects of physical exercise, including effects on cardiovascular integrity and oxygen supply, and release of neurotrophic factors that enhance neuronal cell survival. Notably, exercise could benefit stress management and reduce the deleterious effects of stress.

The importance of social isolation and loneliness as risk factors for dementia emphasizes the importance of social engagement of older people, both for their physical and mental health. They may indeed be modifiable risk factors, but there is presently no evidence that improved or enhanced social functioning prevents, or protects against dementia. This might be attributed to largely the same factors playing a role in social isolation and cognitive decline alike. It is certain that social isolation is entwined with a large variety of health risks, as reflected by its association with mortality. However, once a state of isolation is reached, it may become an unfortunate downward spiral. It may be difficult for isolated individuals to reconnect, as poor social cognition hinders social integration. Consequently, the effectiveness of resocialization approaches is equivocal. According to some animal studies, isolation-induced behavioural, neurochemical and cardiovascular changes can be reversed by resocialization. Other studies found that resocialization reverses isolation-induced defects only partially at best, with especially persistent effects of isolation in early life.

Intellectual enrichment and education have been shown to be important to enhance tolerance or even act as primary prevention of cognitive decline. A research consortium at the Mayo Clinic examined the effect of a lifetime of intellectual enrichment, defined by educational and occupational attainment as well as late-life cognitive activity, in individuals with a genetic risk to develop Alzheimer's disease [26]. They found that cognitive impairment was delayed by more than eight years in their high-enrichment group, which indicates that being cognitively active could enhance the tolerance to or prevent the occurrence of decline. Whether cognitive activity could also be a therapeutic or secondary preventive procedure is still debated, but accumulating evidence steadily indicates that it might be cost-effective. A few randomized controlled trials indicate that cognitive intervention could enhance tolerance in elderly persons or prevent further cognitive decline in patients diagnosed with Alzheimer's disease [27]. A 2013 systematic review found some indication that global cognitive functioning improved after intervention, but no effects were observed in other functional domains. A later systematic review assessed 47 different trials and found indications that cognitive training using a reality orientation approach, moderately improved cognition [28]. Reality orientation helps patients reconnect and re-engage using conversational techniques that repeat environmental information to the patient. We refer to other chapters in this volume for examples of other psychosocial interventions with beneficial effects.

The benefits of a healthy diet have been widely endorsed by public health experts. The list of diets and (expensive) food supplements with putative effectiveness in averting age-related pathology is exceedingly long. Double Nobel laureate Linus Pauling (1901–94) spent a large part of his latter years to endorse the supplementation of large doses of antioxidants to prevent infections, cancer and old-age morbidity. Anecdotally, Pauling lived to a ripe old age in relatively good physical and mental health. Unfortunately, most of these regimes have not been evidence based; some have actually been demonstrated to be non-effective or harmful. Dale Bredesen, an Alzheimer researcher of the University of California at Los Angeles, proposes a more elaborate personalized programme that includes recommendations regarding diet, supplements (including antioxidants), exercise, sleep and cognitive activity [29, 30]. Bredesen's Metabolic Enhancement for Neurodegeneration (MEND) programme is certainly based on scientific insights and research about the factors that contribute to ageing and neural degeneration. His pilot study in a small group of patients with mild cognitive impairment suggested a sustained positive effect on functional performance, but a more extensive trial is needed before the programme can actually be scientifically and medically recommended.

7 Enhancing Tolerance and Influencing Lifestyles

Tolerance refers to an individual's ability to limit the impact of ageing and maintain functional capacity in old age. Several authors have written about the ways age-related functional decline can be compensated and proposed procedures to enhance tolerance. The scaffolding theory of ageing and cognition (STAC), expanded by psychologists Patricia Reuter-Lorenz and Denise Park, refers to compensatory processes that help the older brain counteract age-related neural and functional decline [31]. Cognitive training, education and an active lifestyle could engage or potentiate these processes to enhance the tolerance of the ageing brain to functional decline and morbidity. Obviously, this should be combined with other interventions that promote healthy ageing, prevent risk factors and disease, and increase well-being and life expectancy.

There is a vast literature about diets and lifestyle programmes with putative health benefits. Many of these recommendations are not based on scientific evidence. Some are ideologically or commercially inspired. In general, health experts propose to maintain a strong social network, refrain from smoking, exercise regularly and eat healthy, and consume moderate amounts of alcohol. It has been established that risk factors such as vascular disease, high blood glucose, oxidative stress markers and inflammation are positively influenced by low dietary intake of meat and dairy and high intake of fruit, vegetables and fish. The aforementioned *Lancet* panel decided not to examine dietary factors for dementia, but indicated that these factors could be important [7]. Consequently, no expert presently doubts that aspects of lifestyle represent important and potentially modifiable risk factors for dementia, but the way they could be sustainably influenced by intervention is still debated (see Figure 8.3).

Role models can present unrealistic goals to some, but help others to imitate healthy behaviours and demonstrate the sustainability and gratification of behavioural change. Luigi Cornaro (1464–1566) is one of the most famous

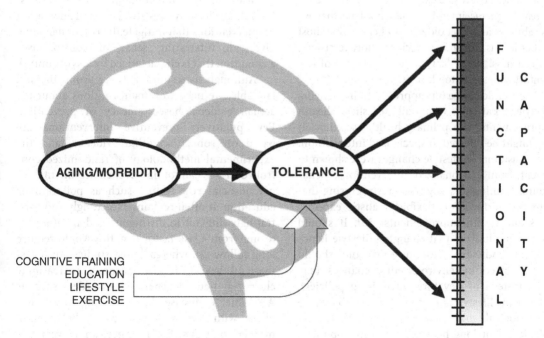

Figure 8.3 Various measures such as cognitive training, education, lifestyle changes and exercise could enhance tolerance to the possible morbidity that results from ageing. Tolerance thus refers to an individual's ability to limit the impact of ageing and maintain functional capacity in old age.

historical centenarians, who is still frequently cited to illustrate the health benefits of lifestyle changes [32]. For a Renaissance-era Venetian, living to an advanced age in good health was exceedingly rare. In several texts about lifestyle that he started writing from the age of 83, Cornaro promotes his decision to break with his professedly hedonistic lifestyle that left him increasingly exhausted and in poor health. Around the age of 40, he decided to devote himself to a 'sober and regular life', and switched to a strict and specific calorie-restriction diet. Cornaro also meaningfully testifies that he was able to maintain a cheerful and active state of mind, reporting enthusiastically that 'when [leaving] the table, [he] must sing, and after singing, [he] must write'. He clearly derived a lot of gratification and pleasure from his changed lifestyle.

Unfortunately, most of us find changing our habits and state of mind much more challenging. Convincing and supporting people to change their lifestyle has been notoriously difficult. For example, programmes for weight loss and physical activity typically lead to attrition and relapse to old habits [33]. Some primary caregivers and public health experts have been quite hard-lined and taxing, which may make patients feel guilty and does not promote sustainable behavioural change. Harvard neurologist Alvaro Pascual-Leone said in a 2017 *Wired Magazine* interview that 'It's true that we lose abilities as we get older, but I believe that most of that loss is driven by a lack of effort to sustain brain fitness. We're lazy, we don't get out of our comfort zones, we stop learning new things.'

We should revise our approach to influencing lifestyles. Patients who fail to show health improvements with primary healthcare counselling might be referred to specialized intervention. More sustainable lifestyle changes were shown to benefit from personalized interventions, behavioural training and cognitive restructuring that help people focus on flexible, realistic expectations and health improvements [33]. It should also be emphasized that changing lifestyle is not only an individual responsibility and should be supported by environmental changes (e.g. stairs instead of elevators, advertising policies). Influencing lifestyle and promoting health involve psychological, social and societal processes that help to adapt long-held attitudes and opinions to prevailing scientific insights. The gradual and beneficial alterations in lifestyle during recent times seem to be related to attitudes and opinions that view healthy lifestyle as socially acceptable and rewarding, rather than a punitive interruption of a more pleasurable way of life.

8 Conclusion and Disclaimer

Dementia has stopped being a late-life concern. In the present chapter, we endorse a life-course approach to enhance tolerance and prevent dementia, which is increasingly embraced by scientists, clinicians and policymakers alike. It is based on an actionable model of dementia and senescence prevention that would be cost-effective and converges with established public health programmes. It relates to central societal issues (such as social inequality and pollution), and translates to multidisciplinary professional interventions tailored to the individual. There is a central focus in these models on factors that contribute to healthy ageing. In many countries, private and governmental healthcare organizations are starting campaigns to raise public awareness about the relationship between lifestyle and dementia. For example, the Flanders Centre of Expertise on Dementia distributed a SaniMemorix medicine box to regional pharmacies (see Figure 8.4). It was styled as 'a vaccine against dementia', but contained a list of suggestions about healthy lifestyle. The implementation of interventions that mitigate the risk of dementia gives an interesting sense of control over a condition that is characterized by loss of control.

Although these initiatives are promising and laudable, we need to remain cautious about the actual, evidence-based efficacy of prevention. Few putatively preventive interventions are based on robust scientific evidence, and the experimental methodology of randomized controlled trials cannot involve environmental or psychosocial risk factors such as pollution or education. It often remains exceedingly and frustratingly difficult to distinguish a dementia prodrome from a risk factor (e.g. this would require long follow-up, whereas most studies cover less than 10 years). It also becomes increasingly clear that neurodegenerative disorders such as Alzheimer's disease have a long preclinical phase with largely undetermined behavioural markers or signs. For instance, an 18-year follow-up study failed to provide robust evidence for a protective association between leisure

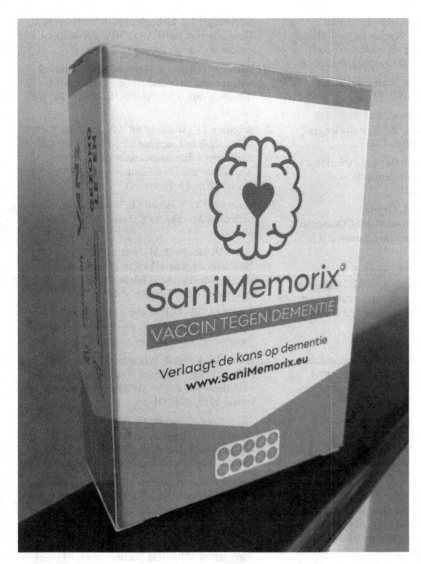

Figure 8.4 Example of a public campaign that aims to raise public awareness of the dementia risk factors. The box contains advice about a healthy lifestyle that could help reduce the risk for dementia. Translation of slogans: 'SaniMemorix. Vaccine against dementia. Lowers the risk for dementia'. www.SaniMemorix.eu (used with permission from the Flanders Centre of Expertise on Dementia)

activities and dementia, but pointed to declined participation in preclinical dementia [34]. Furthermore, there is considerable heterogeneity in terms of causes of dementia and their corresponding preventability. Early-onset dementia caused by frontotemporal degeneration has a significant genetic component, and is therefore unlikely to respond much to preventive intervention. As well, it becomes increasingly clear that the causative mechanisms underlying Alzheimer's disease differ considerably between subjects, with modifiable risk likely related to age of onset. This nuance is seldom mentioned in public campaigns, and could lead to false hope and frustration. Finally, we think that overestimating the efficacy of prevention could unjustly hold patients personally responsible for their condition. In many cultures, especially in sociocentric ones (see Chapter 1), dependency on others is often considered shameful, particularly so when deemed preventable.

References

1. Shah H, Albanese E, Duggan C, Rudan I, Langa KM, Carrillo MC, et al. Research priorities to reduce the global burden of dementia by 2025. *Lancet Neurol.* 2016; **15**: 1285–94.

2. Christensen K, Thinggaard M, Oksuzyan A, Steenstrup T, Andersen-Ranberg K, Jeune B, et al. Physical and cognitive functioning of people older than 90 years: A comparison of two Danish cohorts born 10 years apart. *Lancet* 2013; **382**: 1507–13.

3. Warner H, Anderson J, Austad S, Bergamini E, Bredesen D, Butler R, et al. Science fact and the SENS agenda. What can we reasonably expect from ageing research? *EMBO Rep.* 2005; **6**: 1006–8.

4. Vijg J, Campisi J. Puzzles, promises and a cure for ageing. *Nature* 2008; **454**: 1065–71.

5. Christensen K, Doblhammer G, Rau R, Vaupel JW. Ageing populations: The challenges ahead. *Lancet* 2009; **374**: 1196–1208.

6. Yaffe K, Hoang T. Nonpharmacologic treatment and prevention strategies for dementia. *Continuum* 2013; **19**: 372–81.

7. Livingston G, Sommerlad A, Orgeta V, Costafreda SG, Huntley J, Ames D, et al. Dementia prevention, intervention, and care. *Lancet* 2017; **390**: 2673–2734.

8. Livingston G, Huntley J, Sommerlad A, Ames D, Ballard C, Banerjee S, et al. Dementia prevention, intervention, and care: 2020 report of the Lancet Commission. *Lancet* 2020; **396**: 413–44.

9. Clare L, Wu Y-T, Teale JC, MacLeod C, Matthews F, Brayne C, et al. Potentially modifiable lifestyle factors, cognitive reserve, and cognitive function in later life: A cross-sectional study. *PLoS Med* 2017; **14**: e1002259.

10. Wu YT, Beiser AS, Breteler MMB, Fratiglioni L, Helmer C, Hendrie HC, et al. The changing prevalence and incidence of dementia over time: Current evidence. *Nat Rev Neurol.* 2017; **13**: 327–39.

11. Donovan NJ, Okereke OI, Vannini P, Amariglio RE, Rentz DM, Marshall GA, et al. Association of higher cortical amyloid burden with loneliness in cognitively normal older adults. *JAMA Psychiatry* 2016; **73**: 1230–7.

12. De Jong-Gierveld J. A review of loneliness: Concepts and definitions, determinants and consequences. *Rev Clin Gerontol.* 1998; **8**: 73–80.

13. Beller J, Wagner A. Loneliness, social isolation, their synergistic interaction, and mortality. *Health Psychol.* 2018; **37**: 808–13.

14. Cacioppo JT, Hawkley LC, Norman GJ, Berntson GG Social isolation. *Ann N Y Acad Sci.* 2011; **1231**(1): 17–22.

15. Cacioppo JT, Hawkley LC. Perceived social isolation and cognition. *Trends Cogn Sci.* 2009; **13**: 447–54.

16. Spithoven AWM, Bijttebier P, Goossens L. It is all in their mind: A review on information processing bias in lonely individuals. *Clin Psychol Rev.* 2017; **58**: 97–114.

17. Eisenberger NI, Lieberman MD, Williams KD. Does rejection hurt? An fMRI study of social exclusion. *Science* 2003; **302**: 290–2.

18. Grand JH, Caspar S, Macdonald SW. Clinical features and multidisciplinary approaches to dementia care. *J Multidiscip Healthcare* 2011; **4**: 125–47.

19. Sørensen LV, Waldorff FB, Waldemar G. Early counselling and support for patients with mild Alzheimer's disease and their caregivers: A qualitative study on outcome. *Aging Ment Health* 2008; **12**(4): 444–50.

20. Sørensen LV, Waldorff FB, Waldemar G. Coping with mild Alzheimer's disease. *Dementia* 2008; **7**: 187–99.

21. Due TD, Sandholdt H, Siersma VD, Waldorff FB. How well do general practitioners know their elderly patients' social relations and feelings of loneliness? *BMC Fam Pract.* 2018; **19**(1): art. 34.

22. Martins C, Godycki-Cwirko M, Heleno B, Brodersen J. Quaternary prevention: Reviewing the concept. *Eur J Gen Pract.* 2018; **24**: 106–11.

23. Honig LS, Vellas B, Woodward M, Boada M, Bullock R, Borrie M, et al. Trial of solanezumab for mild dementia due to Alzheimer's disease. *N Engl J Med.* 2018; **378**: 321–30.

24. Colantuoni E, Surplus G, Hackman A, Arrighi HM, Brookmeyer R. Web-based application to project the burden of Alzheimer's disease. *Alzheimers Dement.* 2010; **6**(5): 425–8.

25. Greene C, Lee H, Thuret S. In the long run: Physical activity in early life and cognitive aging. *Front Neurosci.* 2019; **13**: art. 884.

26. Vemuri P, Lesnick TG, Przybelski SA, Machulda M, Knopman DS, Mielke MM, et al. Association of lifetime intellectual enrichment with cognitive decline in the older population. *JAMA Neurol.* 2014; **71**: 1017–24.

27. Alves J, Magalhães R, Thomas RE, Gonçalves OF, Petrosyan A, Sampaio A. Is there evidence for cognitive intervention in Alzheimer disease? A systematic review of efficacy, feasibility, and cost-effectiveness. *Alzheimer Dis Assoc Disord.* 2013; **27**: 195–203.

28. Carrion C, Folkvord F, Anastasiadou D, Aymerich M. Cognitive therapy for dementia patients: A systematic review. *Dement Geriatr Cogn Disord.* 2018; **46**: 1–26.

29. Bredesen DE. Reversal of cognitive decline: A novel therapeutic program. *Aging* 2014; **6**: 707–17.

30. Bredesen DE, Amos EC, Canick J, Ackerley M, Raji C, Fiala M, Ahdidan J. Reversal of cognitive

decline in Alzheimer's disease. *Aging* 2016; **8**: 1250–8.

31. Reuter-Lorenz PA, Park DC. How does it STAC up? Revisiting the scaffolding theory of aging and cognition. *Neuropsychol Rev.* 2014; **24**: 355–70.

32. Cornaro L. *The Art of Living Long: A New and Improved English Version.* Milwaukee, WI, William F. Butler, 1915.

33. Hall KD, Khan S. Maintenance of lost weight and long-term management of obesity. *Med Clin North Am.* 2019; **102**: 183–97.

34. Sommerlad A, Sabia S, Livingston G, Kivimäki M, Lewis G, Singh-Manoux A. Leisure activity participation and risk of dementia: An 18-year follow-up of the Whitehall II Study. *Neurology* 2020; **95**: e2803–e2815.

From 'The Mother of the Muses'

Tony Harrison

And home? Where is it now? The olive grove
may well be levelled under folds of tar.
The wooden house made joyful with a stove
has gone the way of Tsar and samovar.
The small house with 8 people to a room
with no privacy for quiet thought or sex
bulldozed in the island's tourist boom
to make way for Big Macs and discotheques.

Beribboned hats and bold embroidered sashes
once helped another émigré forget
that Canada was going to get his ashes
and that Estonia's still Soviet.
But now the last of those old-timers
couldn't tell one folk-dance from another
and mistakes in the mists of his Alzheimer's
the nurse who wipes his bottom for his mother.

Some hoard memories as some hoard gold
against that rapidly approaching day
that's all they have to live on, being old,
but find their savings spirited away.
What's the point of having lived at all
in the much-snapped duplex in Etobicoke
if it gets swept away beyond recall,
in spite of all the snapshots, at one stroke?

If we are what we remember what are they
who don't have memories as we have ours,
who, when evening falls, have no recall of day,
or who those people were who'd brought them flowers.
The troubled conscience though's glad to forget.
Oblivion for some's an inner balm.
They've found some peace of mind, not total yet,
as only death itself brings that much calm.

Excerpt from 'The Mother of the Muses' by Tony Harrison
Published by Faber and Faber Ltd. Reprinted by permission of the publisher.

Chapter

9

An Empowering Dementia Environment

Jos Tournoy, John Keady, Mythily Subramaniam, Aline Sevenants, Chantal Van Audenhove, Iris Van Steenwinkel, Ann Heylighen and Maarten Van Den Bossche

1 Introduction

People with dementia flourish best in an environment adapted to their specific needs, the latter resulting from any impact of their condition. This environment contains different aspects and situates itself on different levels, discussed in this chapter by a multidisciplinary panel of authors. This diversity in authorship and specialism captures some of the opportunities and challenges in developing an optimal environment for people with dementia.

The chapter starts with a consideration of what makes an enriched environment of care for persons with dementia. This is tackled by reviewing the work of Mike Nolan and colleagues in the United Kingdom and the development of relationship-centred care and the Senses Framework which, we argue, provide the context for an enriched environment of care. This section includes a case study on care home practice.

Next, features of architectural design for people with dementia both in residential care homes and in community-dwelling settings are discussed, touching upon the importance of the physical environment in relation to dementia care and well-being. The chapter then moves to consider the importance of dementia-friendly communities and the societal aspects of dementia in relation to the person with dementia. This is demonstrated by an interesting case study of Singapore and introduces the role of technological innovation, an evolution taking up a fast-growing role in our society, specifically in the healthcare domain. Technology has a large potential influence on the environment in which we live and on our interaction with this environment, and we discuss this by elaborating on different aspects of healthcare technology for dementia.

Sleep disorders and night-time agitation, commonly occurring during the course of dementia, could also largely be influenced by environmental aspects. Because of the importance of sleep, we close this chapter by describing the interrelation between sleeping problems or night-time agitation and the environment, as an example on how the environment can impact this interrelation.

2 Enriched Environments of Care for People Living with Dementia

2.1 From Person-Centred Care to Relationship-Centred Care

The development of relationship-centred care [1] was a response to the person-centred care movement kick-started in the United Kingdom in the late 1980s by the social psychologist Tom Kitwood and his colleagues at the Bradford Dementia Group. Tom Kitwood's work culminated in 1997 with the publication of his seminal book *Dementia Reconsidered: The Person Comes First* [2] as the author died the following year at the still desperately young age of 61.

Enhancements to the vision and values of person-centred care have been taken forward since this time by other commentators. One of the most well-known was Dawn Brooker and her work on the 'VIPS' model [3]. As an acronym VIPS stands for: value of all human lives, individualized approach recognizing uniqueness, Seeing the world from the perspective of the service user and a social environment that promotes well-being. The acronym acts as an easy-to-remember mnemonic for front-line practitioners working with people living with dementia and showcases the essential elements of person-centred care. Brooker and Latham [3] have also extended the reach of the VIPs model to challenge the prevailing culture of care home attitudes and to highlight the importance of 'getting person-centred care into everyday practice' (p. 24).

Recently, in an editorial for *Aging & Mental Health* by Myrra Vernooij-Dassen and Esme Moniz-Cook [4], the authors suggested that person-centred care should 'not only be directed at compensating for what people with dementia cannot do, but also at facilitating their interests, pleasure and use of their capacities' (p. 667). This positive and affirmatory view of person-centred care has formed a foundation of policy and practice architecture in dementia care around the world.

As an illustration, in the United Kingdom, the most recent National Institute for Health and Care Excellence (NICE) dementia guideline published in 2018 (see www.nice.org.uk/guidance/ng97 (accessed 13 January 2021)) dedicated a section on the principles of 'person-centred care' which included 'respecting the individuality of people living with dementia' and 'acknowledging the importance of the person's perspective' (p. 10). Importantly, the shared principles were seen to underpin the whole of the dementia guideline and its communicated evidence base, thereby providing an accessible frame of reference for clinical practice.

On one hand it is indisputable that person-centred care has driven dementia care and studies forward over the past 30 years and has made a significant contribution to the betterment of people with lived experience. On the other there has been a growing concern that the lexicon and meta-narrative of person-centred care is too inward-looking and promotes a culture of individualism, self-reliance and personalization. This dichotomy was picked up in a comprehensive review of the literature on this topic area [5] which also concluded that person-centred care does not fully grasp the complexities of everyday life for people with dementia, especially when that life is situated within an embodied, relational and societal context. Moreover, the literature review also reported that person-centred care is presently conducted in a theoretical vacuum and that its evidence base is still to be fully tested.

An alternative model of care that embedded itself within a more relational, fluid and negotiated context was put forward by Mike Nolan and his colleagues working mainly from the University of Sheffield in the United Kingdom [1]. This approach drew on work conducted in the United States of America by the Tresolini and Pew Fetzer Task Force in the mid-1990s [6] where the Task Force were asked to consider how to create a healthcare system that could meet the future needs of the American population.

In sharing their findings, the Task Force suggested that instead of a focus on acute care – where most funding and services were targeted, a reality that is not confined to the United States of America – that designing services to meet the needs of people living with long-term conditions, which obviously includes people living with dementia, was the national priority. To do this, members of the Task Force argued that a completely new philosophy of care was needed, one they termed 'relationship-centred care'. To support this new direction, the Task Force [18] described the importance of relationships in the following way:

> [R]elationships are critical to the care provided by nearly all practitioners and a sense of satisfaction and positive outcomes for patients and practitioners. Although relationships are a prerequisite to effective care and teaching, there has been little formal acknowledgement of their importance and few formal efforts to help students and practitioners learn to develop effective relationships in health care. (p. 11)

In promoting this more holistic vision of healthcare, the Task Force focussed on several areas: the social, economic, environmental, cultural and political contexts of care; the subjective experience of illness; and the reality that relationships develop between practitioners, patients, families and the wider community. Moreover, the Task Force suggested that it was the interaction between these factors that should lie at the heart of a healthcare system based on relationship-centred care and that relationships form the 'foundation' of any therapeutic or curative activity. Refreshingly, the Task Force also recognized that the concept of relationship-centred care was still emerging and that further work was needed to put the concept into practice in ways that ensured an appropriate balance between the needs of everyone involved in healthcare relationships.

2.2 The Senses Framework as a Basis for an 'Enriched Environment of Care'

The Senses Framework [1] provides one way of achieving this balance whilst also acknowledging that, in the United Kingdom at least, the healthcare system extends to include services and support provided by social care (see www .scie.org.uk/dementia (accessed 13 January 2021)). This is important, as it is social care that offers the main post-diagnostic support for people living with dementia and their families, such as care in care homes and/or in the community through the provision of walking, art and singing groups.

That said, the early ideas that informed the Senses Framework were developed at around the same time as the Task Force report in the mid-1990s, especially the publication of the book *Understanding Family Care* [7] by Mike Nolan and his colleagues, one of whom was John Keady, one of the co-authors of this chapter. This work argued for a more multidimensional and longitudinal appreciation of caring relationships and that in paid care, it was essential to see care as both a positive choice and a rewarding experience.

This focus on staff well-being had previously been picked up by Tom Kitwood [2], who suggested that care was essentially about the maintenance of personhood for people living with dementia and that for 'good caring' to take place, it was vital for care staff to explore their own well-being and repair any past harmful events in their own lives. As Tom Kitwood went on to explain, failure to do this would result in care provision for people living with dementia not being person-centred and/or of good quality as care staff would be attempting to 'rescue' the person with dementia from being 'victims' of their diagnosis, rather than creating an authentic interaction based on equality, mutual respect and trust.

Towards the end of the 1990s, Mike Nolan picked up on the arguments about the importance for healthcare and social care providers to create a positive environment for all residents in long-term care (whatever their diagnosis or diagnoses) in order to ensure that the needs of frail older people were adequately met and that those providing care could experience feelings of job satisfaction and well-being. He suggested that in a positive long-term care environment older people should experience six 'Senses' [1]:

1. Achievement: to be able to achieve valued goals, to feel that your efforts are valued
2. Belonging: to maintain important relationships and to feel part of a valued group or community
3. Continuity: to be able to create links between the past, the present and the future, to experience consistent care delivered by known people
4. Purpose: to engage in valued activities, to have something to ensure the meaningful passage of time
5. Security: to feel safe physically, psychologically and existentially
6. Significance: to feel that you, who you are and what you do in some way 'matter' to others who are important to you.

However, Mike Nolan also argued that if staff were to create such an environment for older people then they too have to experience the 'Senses' for themselves [1]. So, for example, staff need to feel secure in their terms of employment and safe to raise any concerns they might have about standards of care. They have to feel they belong, not only to a staff team or group but also to a wider community of practitioners, something that is hard to achieve in many long-term care environments where staff turnover is often very high, compromising Senses of belonging and continuity.

During this and later studies an environment in which the Senses were met for all the major stakeholders, and not just one group such as older people or staff, was termed an 'enriched environment of care' [8] whose main elements are shown in Figure 9.1.

Senses \ Stakeholder	Person with long-term condition	Staff	Family carers	Students	Neighbourhood/ Community
Achievement					
Belonging					
Continuity					
Purpose					
Security					
Significance					

Figure 9.1 The components of an enriched environment of care. Adapted from Keady and Nolan [8]

The matrix on Figure 9.1 includes 'students' as it has been demonstrated that if students experience an enriched learning environment during their clinical placements, they are far more likely to choose to go and work with older people than if they experience an impoverished environment where the Senses are not created. Similarly, the matrix includes a column on the Neighbourhood/Community space as there is also much that could be done to 'enrich' the neighbourhood and community environment in which people with dementia and their families primarily live. This is because current strategies developed to account for the everyday lives of people with dementia that take place in public spaces such as streets, shops and civic amenities, and in care homes, are mainly positioned within a neighbourhood location but are rarely seen as part of that community.

We now share some pilot work that started to construct an enriched environment of care in a care home for people living with dementia. This brief case study is taken from a previously published report [9] where John Keady was a key contributor. It must be emphasized, however, that this case study is only intended to give an idea about how an enriched environment of care, underpinned by relationship-centred care and the Senses Framework, can begin to emerge.

2.3 Case Study

This case study is taken from a Bupa–funded study [8, 9] that involved two care homes in the north-west of England. One was a 'for profit' care home whilst the other was a 'not-for-profit' care home. The overall aim of the pilot practice development project was to develop a staff education programme that reflected the importance of relationships and provided participating staff with an opportunity to identify how they might produce an enriched environment of care using relationship-centred care and the Senses Framework. The project was called the Senses in Practice (SiPs) training programme and received all necessary ethical approval for its conduct and reporting (IRAS reference number 09/H1302/43).

The not-for-profit care home described in this case study had five 'houses' that allowed specialist care and attention, including to residents with dementia, with a total capacity of 150 residents. Four houses were registered for

nursing care and one house was registered for dementia nursing care. The care home had single-occupancy rooms and offered several different facilities on site, such as hairdressing. The day and timing of the session were negotiated with each care home in order to ensure maximum staff attendance and minimum disruption to the home. John Keady conducted each of the eight sessions of training in this care home along with a colleague from the University of Manchester, Dr Caroline Swarbrick.

Each training session focussed on a different Sense and was structured as follows:

Session 1: Knowing why we care. Focus: understanding the values and skills we bring to caring. Completion of an attitudes and values questionnaire.

Session 2: Creating a sense of achievement in everyday practice. Focus: understanding what makes people happy in their lives.

Session 3: Creating a sense of belonging in everyday practice. Focus: understanding the meaning of home.

Session 4: Creating a sense of continuity. Focus: the use of life story work.

Session 5: Creating a sense of purpose in everyday practice. Focus: understanding how we each define purpose in our everyday lives.

Session 6: Creating a sense of security in everyday practice. Focus: feeling safe with those around you.

Session 7: Creating a sense of significance in everyday practice. Focus: the use of memory chests.

Session 8: Putting it all together. Focus: highlighting and summarizing achievements.

Through this approach, staff attending the one-hour training sessions developed a 'Creating the Senses for . . . ' booklet which could be completed by residents, families and staff in order to enrich the environment of care and everyday life. The purpose of the booklet was to offer insight into a resident's current and past life, such as hobbies, holidays enjoyed and so on. The booklet was then located in the resident's room, giving the resident a sense of ownership and empowerment. Moreover, during the training sessions, the value of sensory and memory boxes was discussed and staff showed a keen interest in pursuing these ideas. Posters were displayed around the care home inviting staff, family members, members of the local neighbourhood and visitors to donate sensory items, particularly those with a reminiscence theme. Underpinned by the Sense Framework and the SIPs example in this case study, a focus on relationship-centred care started to build an enriched environment of care based on local custom, knowledge and practice.

2.4 Future Directions for Relationship-Centred Care

Nichola Hatton [10] has taken forward some of the ideas of relationship-centred care and has argued that wider social, environmental and cultural factors are also very important. Here, Hatton is developing ideas around the person with dementia's relationships with non-human artefacts, for example, through (i) familiar sounds and smells of the care home, and how a sense of belonging can start to be engendered through this sensory exposure, and (ii) the use of and access to familiar material possession(s) to help give the person a sense of security.

This addition helps to provide new directions for relationship-centred care and the Senses Framework and enables the work to continue to grow and evolve, much as Tresolini and Pew Fetzer Task Force [6] first envisaged in the mid-1990s. However, many new possibilities exist to develop an enriched environment of care informed by relationship-centred care and the Senses Framework and it is hoped that this contribution will help to inspire and enhance such future directions.

3 Insights into Living with Dementia: Five Implications for Architectural Design

3.1 Studying Architectural Design for People with Dementia

Researchers recognize the physical environment's potential in the context of persons with dementia. Multiple studies address architectural design for people with dementia (e.g. [11]). However, the fact that architects adopt the available scientific evidence only rarely [12] raises questions about its adequateness as design knowledge. Three possible limitations can be discerned:

1. Common discourses on quality requirements of housing and care for people with dementia address issues like personalization, privacy, hominess, scope for ordinary activities and small scale. To scientifically underpin the importance of such issues, the prevailing research on architectural design and dementia starts from a 'traditional' world view, which differs from the rich array of world views shaping environmental design [13]. Architectural features can be objectively correlated with behaviour disruptions and other outcomes in people with dementia [14], while the aforementioned environmental issues cannot be completely objectified as they reflect human values – the emancipation of people wanting to be valued as individuals, to continue their own life as much as possible and to participate in society [12]. By leaving little room for the voice of people with dementia and for individual human values to be taken into account, the prevailing research neglects clearly defining the phenomena studied. The resulting lack of robust theory development in environmental research [15] may hinder adoption of the findings by architects/designers, who prefer insight into why and how architectural features may affect people [16].

2. Prevailing studies may fail to uncover how and why people use spaces the way they do [17]. They provide little insight into experiences of living with dementia within the environments studied. Such insight, however, is indispensable to leverage the built environment's potential in supporting people in their daily lives.

3. Research outcomes specify insufficiently the physical environment studied [18]. Moreover, rather than addressing form and spatial organization [14], most studies deal with colour, signage and style of furniture. While affecting people's experiences, such features are secondary to architects' core business of organizing form and space [19, 20]: how spaces provide enclosure, interrelate and constitute a coherent whole.

These limitations highlight the importance of giving voice to people with dementia, offering insight into their experiences and daily life and bringing findings closer to architectural design. In this chapter, we explore how the built environment could support people with dementia in orientating in space, time and identity. Insight into living with dementia is provided, implications for architectural design are highlighted and potentials and limitations of the adopted approach are discussed [21]. This paragraph is based upon ethnographic case studies. Iris Van Steenwinkel collected and analysed data around three cases: two in private housing about Frances (77 years old) and Mary (47), and one in Woodside Residential Care Facility, with a focus on three residents, Irene (88), Miriam (74) and Gertrude (87).

Depending on each participant's competences, semi-structured interviews and participant observation (field notes and pictures) were used to collect data. Writing – from field notes, interview transcripts, labels, annotations and memos to the final written ethnographic account – was combined with analysing the architecture of each setting, guided by the work of Unwin [20] and Ching [19]. Assembling the textual and architectural analysis for each case study resulted in three ethnographic accounts [21], which provide insight into experiences of people with dementia in a format that allows architects to develop affinity with their perspective.

3.2 Beneficial Architectural Design Features Based on Ethnographic Case Studies

Dementia forces people to deal with symptoms changing their independence in daily life and to rely on others to take over where needed. It entails attempting to maintain, alter or discard activities and changing social roles and relations with other people (likely including loss of privacy and control), perspectives on life, priorities and appreciations. Moving to a residential care facility moreover entails losing home and related material things, living with unknown people and restructuring one's day according to the care organization.

People wish to remain involved in daily activities in a manageable and comfortable way. They make things easier for themselves (physically and cognitively), undertake alternative activities and maintain their routines. When distressed, they seek comfort in seclusion, the proximity of others or secure places.

Having dementia thus profoundly affects people's daily life. While their behaviour may seem peculiar, insight into their experiences suggests that their values, desires and expectations, and their interaction with others and the built environment, are often not that different and are understandable given the circumstances. Consequently, what they would like to change in their living environment may resemble what others would like in similar settings. Architectural features that benefit people in general also benefit people with dementia and might even be more important to them. Five implications for architectural design can be derived.

3.2.1 Create Strategic Places

When one's frailty increases, cognitively and physically, strategic places become increasingly important. These are places that allow a proper relation to the immediate surroundings by occupying this place and being occupied with an activity in a comfortable, more or less active way. Examples of strategic places derived from our case series include Mary's and Irene's strategic place.

Case Study 1

Mary needed to rest often, for which she created a comfortable and secure environment. Her armchair in the living room allowed her to take a nap with the chair reclined, look outside, read or watch TV. To this end, she had objects ready to hand: tissues, candy, a reading lamp, a magazine, the remote control and blankets and pillows she loved to wrap herself in and support her body with. Often her little dog sat on her lap.

Case Study 2

In Irene's private room, the sitting area offered a strategic place where she spent most of the day (Figure 9.2) watching TV, taking a nap, reading or, when the door was open, calling a caregiver passing by to help her. A side table provided the remote control, a phone, tissues, a magazine and a bottle and glass of water, while two chairs were available for when her sons visited.

A less fortunate position for Irene was in a circle in the living room, faced with co-residents she did not like and could hardly communicate with. From this position, she could not watch TV or look outside. Being seated in a wheelchair she could not move herself prevented her from going elsewhere. Irene withdrew: she closed her eyes and waited until someone would bring her to the table for dinner.

3.2.2 Articulate Proper Spatial Relations

While strategic places concern the smaller scale, articulating spatial relations is also important on the larger scale, especially for more complex programmes like residential care facilities. When several people and activities come together, it is important to define proper boundaries and connections, including boundaries between inside and outside, a dwelling unit, transitions between private, communal and public places, and connections with the neighbourhood.

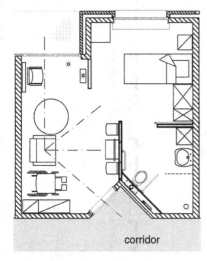

Figure 9.2 The armchair in Irene's private room offered her a strategic place.

corridor

Woodside, a small-scale residential care facility in Flanders, Belgium, has as its main organizational feature a U-shaped corridor running throughout the building, which leads along living rooms and service areas like storage rooms, bathrooms and the nurses' station. Secondary corridors that lead to private rooms branch from the long arms of the U (Figures 9.3 and 9.4).

The main corridor provides a convenient logistic thread, for example, for caregivers on night duty. However, by running through all dwelling units, it nullifies boundaries between them: it counters their articulation as separate spatial and social units and forms a rather public, interior passageway along private places (Figure 9.3b). While at one side the U allows connecting with the neighbourhood, its short segment turns its back on a residential area to the west of Woodside, where streets come to a dead end (Figure 9.3c) – a missed opportunity in terms of socio-spatial integration. Because corridors are frequently used to spatially organize residential care facilities, it is worth considering their desired and undesired roles of connecting and creating boundaries.

3.2.3 Include Everyday Places and Objects

People with dementia often want to and can be involved in daily activities provided that due places and objects are available. This is demonstrated in the case of Frances. The presence of everyday objects allowed her to continue to

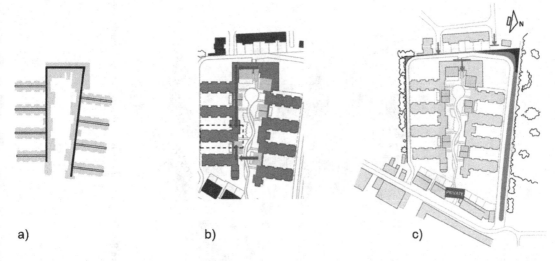

a)   b)   c)

Figure 9.3 (a) Woodside's spatial configuration. (b) The corridor offers a rather public passageway through the dwelling units. (c) Arrows indicate how Woodside turns its back on the neighbourhood; streets from that neighbourhood come to a dead end.

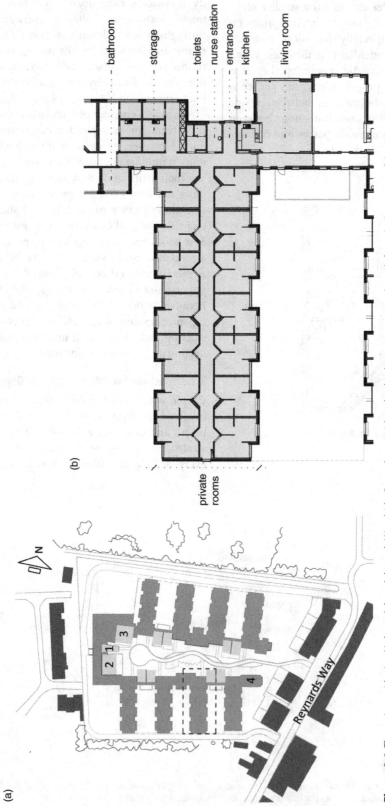

Figure 9.4 The main corridor is a U-shaped thread through Woodside. Secondary corridors that lead to private rooms branch from the long arms of the U.

participate in daily activities in ways that were manageable for her. When her husband asked her to fetch a bottle of water in the basement, she also found the clothesline and had the old tendency to check whether the clothes were dry, put them into a basket and bring them upstairs. She also helped preparing meals and could turn on music. Her husband had bought a CD player with an old-school turn button for the volume instead of a push button on a remote control. Besides a clothesline, kitchen and CD player, examples of everyday places and objects included a piano corner for playing music, a garden with a shed and an outdoor café in the neighbourhood for having a drink, enjoying being outdoors and social life.

The importance of meaningful occupation for social health has already been addressed (e.g. [22]). Considering everyday activities in their architectural context highlights the importance of everyday places and objects. This should be kept in mind when designing residential care facilities, which often have difficulties with transforming their hospital-like character into the everydayness of home environments.

3.2.4 Create Contemporary Architectural Qualities

A fourth implication for architectural design is to create architectural qualities found in contemporary housing – that is, light, roominess, relation with outdoors and an interior with few embellishments.

The importance of this is demonstrated by the case of Mary. When the living room felt too busy or oppressive, she could become angry or run outside in order to escape from it. Therefore she and her husband made the interior lighter, calmer and roomier by painting the walls white, replacing the dark-coloured antique cupboards with white and simpler ones, reducing the number of embellishments and keeping everything well ordered. There is more room 'to breathe', Mary said. When the weather was nice, she opened the windows, which gave her more energy, countered oppressive feelings and helped her to become more at ease.

While Mary's becoming angry or running outside may seem peculiar, the changes to their house are not. Many other people may make similar changes to this farm-style type of house (cf. an English cottage). Mary appreciated its secure

character, but also experienced its limitations – lack of light, roominess, strong relation to outdoors and the calmness of an interior with few embellishments. These are architectural qualities found more often in contemporary housing. The case study about Mary suggests that people with dementia can benefit from them.

3.2.5 Take into Account Social Dynamics

A fifth implication for architectural design concerns taking into account the social dynamics among people living together. When designing architecture, one should keep in mind that dementia likely affects social relations and the social environment.

The case of Frances highlights the importance of places for privacy and togetherness and how the house met changing needs. At first, Frances preferred to be alone from time to time and therefore retreated to her oldest daughter's former bedroom. Later, she preferred to have her husband nearby, while he also wanted to continue his daily activities. The living room's articulation into several 'corners' (a piano corner, sitting corner, a corner with a table and one with a desk) allowed them to be 'apart together'. Her husband could work at his desk while Frances watched TV in the sitting corner. He could pursue (some of) his own activities while his proximity offered her a feeling of security.

Where many people live together, like in residential care facilities, social dynamics are more complex. Moreover, wheelchair use requires more free circulation space and empty spaces in every seating configuration, which causes the configuration to partly fall apart when wheelchair users are absent. In addition, flexibility may be needed to accommodate different activities, change the configuration when more residents come to use a wheelchair or deal with changes in social dynamics among residents. Aspects like these make designing residential care facilities more challenging.

3.3 The Need for a Sociocultural Perspective in Architectural Design for People with Dementia

In general, experiences of people with dementia and associated architectural aspects can be comprehended better within a sociocultural context than in terms of objective (causal) relations. The study focussed on how daily life meshes with space rather than correlating architectural features with, for example, dementia symptoms. This resonates with the pursuit of people with dementia to continue their daily life as much as possible.

Moreover, it responds to architecture's potential to provide a proper framework for daily activities and social interaction, rather than countering the dementia process. Therefore, research on architectural design for people with dementia should look beyond dementia and take them into account as social beings within their cultural context. Broadening the scope in this way also offers the opportunity to draw from and develop knowledge from beyond the field of architectural design for people with dementia, which still largely lacks in theory development [15].

While it was possible to derive five implications for architectural design, the resulting ethnographies [21] are rather open-ended and descriptive. This may cause some frustration in those expecting design solutions or standards. However, it may also trigger interest from architects, who are often reluctant towards such standards [16]. Additionally, case studies, through their open and rich character, may inform readers from different backgrounds, like architects and caregivers, and facilitate a dialogue between them and with people with dementia. Such a dialogue is also facilitated by introducing architectural themes that allow linking experiences of living with dementia with architects' core business. In this way, case studies can broaden architects' and caregivers' insights into the possible roles of architecture in the daily life of people with dementia.

4 Dementia-Friendly Community

4.1 Empowerment, Support and Social Inclusion

Research suggests that there is significant public and family stigma towards persons with dementia emanating from fear and lack of awareness and understanding about the disease (see Chapter 2). Dementia-related stigma can cause significant negative effects such as avoidance of help-seeking behaviours, social isolation and reduced quality of life in persons with dementia and caregivers. The stigma associated with dementia has been highlighted as a significant concern for people living with the disease and their caregivers worldwide [23].

A raft of formal community services are available for a persons with dementia, including respite care, day care, home care and home help. However, research suggests that the uptake of services is not optimal as the informal carers of persons with dementia are either unaware of the services or the services are inaccessible, inadequate or prohibitively expensive [24]. Lack of a supportive environment leads to social alienation of the persons with dementia and their caregivers as many of them are forced to spend their time at home while caring prevents them from participating in social and community activities.

Alzheimer's Disease International (ADI) defines a dementia-friendly community (DFC) as 'a place or culture in which people with dementia and their carers are empowered, supported and included in society, understand their rights and recognise their full potential' [25]. However, the definitions of 'dementia-friendly community' vary quite widely. The concept of 'dementia-friendly' may focus either on persons with dementia or on both persons with dementia and their caregivers. On the other hand 'community' may represent a place, the social and physical environments, an organization, a society or a culture.

This diversity of definitions reflects the different sociocultural-political context of different communities and the shifts in the way these communities view and think about persons with dementia and their carers. A description by Crampton et al. [26] elaborates on the intent of a DFC as one that enables persons with dementia to navigate and feel safe in their community, which offers them easy access to amenities such as banks, shops, post offices, healthcare and social care agencies, and one that helps to foster and maintain their social networks. The concept of the community here is strength based – that is, leveraging the skills and abilities of persons with dementia rather than focussing on a 'deficit model' that tries to compensate for what they cannot do.

The origin of DFCs can be traced back to 2004 in Japan when the Japanese government launched a nationwide campaign, the '10-Year Plan to Understand Dementia and Build Community Networks', which led to the creation of DFCs. Notable activities and measures included renaming dementia from *chiho* (a pejorative word) to *ninch-isho* (which means cognitive disorder), initiation of the Ninchisho Supporters Programme which aimed to raise the public awareness of dementia and to train the populace to better support persons with dementia and their caregivers to live well in the community, as well as involving persons with dementia in various decision-making processes that affected their day-to-day life [25].

Dementia-friendly communities mark a paradigm shift in the understanding of dementia – that is, from a biomedical model to a more holistic approach of a biopsychosocial model so that persons with dementia can continue to have the best quality of life that is reasonably possible. Dementia-friendly communities can enable persons with dementia to live in the community for longer and delay if not obviate institutional care.

4.2 The Four Cornerstone Model

To establish and support a DFC, the Four Cornerstone Model posits that four elements are needed:

1. **Places**: This element is about how aspects of the physical environment such as housing, transport and information can support persons with dementia to move around independently with clear and legible signage and access to facilities. Persons with dementia must be involved so that those planning such services have a better understanding of their concerns and they are also included in the solution. Public transport must be designed with an ageing population in mind and to ensure their independence is maintained to the maximum extent possible.

2. **People**: This includes families, friends, communities and healthcare and social care professionals who need to understand and support persons with dementia. Initiatives launched as part of the community efforts to improve awareness of dementia and support must include involvement of persons with dementia and caregivers, who should guide and develop these activities. Healthcare and social care professionals should be adequately trained to understand the importance of timely diagnosis and support following a diagnosis of dementia, and training should also be provided to those in the community who are likely to provide services and support to persons with dementia.

3. **Networks**: This element refers to the broad network of organizations, businesses and individuals that come together to ensure cross-sectoral support and coordinated action to support persons with dementia. Such networks can be top-down, such as those led by leaders in the community or funded by an agency, or a bottom-up effort where small groups or even a single organization leads the formation of the network within a community.

4. **Resources**: The European Union Joint Action on Dementia identified time, energy and leadership as the three main resources needed to support a DFC. The need for a committed budget has been debated, with proponents arguing that funding is needed to ensure the sustainability of these initiatives, while others suggest that a committed community can provide support with little budget. Resources needed range from logo-branded material to guides and templates for projects, toolkits and a database of good practices [27].

The impact of DFCs has been measured using various outcomes, such as improvements in the community's knowledge and skills, persons with dementia's ability to access community resources, their sense of being valued and their ability to advocate for themselves. Improvement in networks between organizations and agencies working with persons with dementia has also been evaluated. While there is good evidence for the implementation and impact of DFCs in North America and Europe, the evidence from Asia is limited. Japan and Taiwan have made significant strides in this area but there is little literature from other countries. Singapore is a multi-ethnic, multireligious, multilingual city state which serves as a microcosm of East, South and Southeast Asia ethnic groups. The rapid development of DFCs in this country, with its cultural diversity and focus on innovative technology-based solutions for dementia care, make it an interesting case study.

4.3 Case Study: Dementia-Friendly Communities in Singapore

Singapore is a developed Southeast Asian country with a multi-ethnic resident population of 3.8 million comprising Chinese, Malay, Indian and other ethnicities. The population demographics are similar to the global trend seen in developed economies, which is a rapidly ageing population and declining birth rates. According to the Department of Statistics, Singapore, the proportion of residents aged 65 years and over increased from 8.5% in 2007 to 13% in 2017. By 2030, one in four Singaporeans will be aged 65 years and older.

A national study identified the prevalence of dementia as 10% among those aged 60 years and older [28]. This prevalence is expected to increase with the ageing population – a development that imposes several challenges for the medical and social care arrangements needed for persons with dementia. Local data have also found that recognition of dementia is reasonable in the adult population of Singapore and it is less stigmatized as compared to other mental disorders [29].

As the understanding of dementia grew in Singapore, the need to provide person-centred care to persons with dementia was recognized. The dementia-friendly Singapore (DFSG) initiative was initiated and led by the Ministry of Health of Singapore, the Agency of Integrated Care and key stakeholders to create awareness of dementia and empower people and communities to better support persons with dementia and their caregivers. The Senior Minister of State of Health of Singapore described a DFC as:

> a neighborhood where residents, businesses and services, and the community at large, are aware of dementia and understand how to better support persons with dementia and their caregivers. It is a place where resident persons with dementia feel respected [and] valued, and where help is within easy reach so that they can continue to lead independent lives. It is also an environment which persons with dementia will be able to move around safely and with ease. A Dementia Friendly Community can also better support caregivers of persons with dementia by helping to look out for their loved ones and thus reduce the stress and fatigue they may face.

Since its inception in 2015, eight DFCs have been created across Singapore.

The DFCs in Singapore comprise four components that are somewhat different from the Four Cornerstone Model. These components are outlined next.

Dementia Awareness

Community-wide talks, workshops, posters at common areas and door-to-door outreach have been used to create awareness. A network of Dementia Friends comprising volunteers are trained to recognize the key signs and symptoms of dementia. They are also trained to communicate with persons with dementia, serve as community lookouts and lend a helping hand when needed to assist disoriented or lost persons with dementia. Dementia Friends are encouraged to download the mobile application described in what follow. This app alerts the volunteers to look out for missing persons with dementia and report the missing person's sightings through the app. These trained volunteers also support persons with dementia by befriending or engaging them in activities.

Technology

The key component is the Dementia Friends mobile application, which serves as a resource portal that provides access to useful information on dementia and events for caregivers. It also provides information about support in the community and, finally, it serves as an avenue for caregivers to post cases of lost persons with dementia that is broadcasted to Dementia Friends who are asked to keep a lookout for the persons with dementia.

Go-To Points (GTPs)

Go-To Points located in community centres and senior activity centres serve to provide information and resources on dementia. These also serve as 'safe return' points where one can bring persons with dementia who may appear lost or are unable to identify themselves. The staff at the GTPs assist in reuniting them with their caregivers.

Infrastructure

The design of the built environment is widely recognized as a major aid for persons with dementia. This component focusses on making the physical environment accessible and safe for persons with dementia. This includes installation of ramps and railings to facilitate mobility, clear colour contrast signage with larger text, appropriate lighting to prevent disorientation etc.

4.4 Evaluating the Success of Dementia-Friendly Communities

While the development of DFCs across multiple countries is a positive one, concerns remain about the impact of such communities. The evaluation of such communities requires the development of appropriate indicators and reliable and valid measures. Since DFCs vary considerably in terms of structure, key activities and priorities, it would be naïve to imagine a universal assessment tool that can work across different settings.

The DEMCOM study was funded to carry out a national evaluation of DFCs in England. The case studies used a refined evaluation framework originally meant to evaluate age-friendly communities. An example of this approach was the evaluation of Sheffield's overall dementia friendly city initiative [30]. Data gathered from documentary evidence as well as conversations and interviews with key informants were used to assess the performance in 10 key areas – political support, leadership and governance, financial and human resources, the involvement of people affected by dementia, priorities based on needs assessment, application of existing frameworks for assessing dementia friendliness, provision, interventions rooted in evidence, coordination, collaboration and linkages, and monitoring and evaluation.

Applying this tool to assess Sheffield's dementia friendliness, the authors identified strengths in several key areas. These included coordination, collaboration and linkages, as well as the involvement of people affected by dementia. On the other hand, performance in applying existing frameworks to assess dementia friendliness was not systematic and the financial and human resources area was also identified as one that needed further strengthening.

These outcomes resulted in targeted recommendations that further improved the dementia friendliness of the city. Other communities have adopted simpler outcome measures such as the number of participants involved in initiatives, the number of talks/workshops held on dementia awareness, dementia knowledge and dementia attitudes evaluation questionnaire results, media coverage, and quality of life of persons with dementia.

The DFCs in Asia are unique and culturally rooted. For example, Singapore, a small country with high mobile penetration, leveraged social media and a custom-designed app to promote dementia friendliness. Community centres that are easily identified and well connected were identified as GTPs. Political support for DFCs was clear and consistent. Japan too has built DFCs by focussing on areas where connections can be created between persons with dementia and communities. The innovative use of cafes, libraries and schools has made the community inclusive and services accessible. Public-private partnerships are another key feature of Japan's DFCs. The private enterprises support awareness initiatives, ensure access to services such as banks and convenience stores and employ people with dementia in suitable jobs.

However, there remains a paucity of research on the evaluation of DFCs in Asian countries. A recent study from Taiwan used a qualitative approach to identify indicators of a DFC from the perspective of persons with dementia and their caregivers. The indicators included dementia-friendly hospitals, dementia-friendly community environment, dementia-friendly transportation, dementia-friendly stores and shops, dementia-friendly community members and opportunities for people with dementia to contribute to and be involved in the community [31].

Most of these indicators were similar to and overlapped with those identified in Western countries, suggesting that persons with dementia and their caregivers have similar expectations of the essential components and indicators of DFC. However, these indicators must be used across DFCs to evaluate their effectiveness and identify the gaps that need to be met.

4.5 The Road Ahead

While DFCs are emerging globally, several challenges have also been identified, and these need to be addressed. Adequate and appropriate resources are vital for the establishment of DFCs, which involves long-term commitment from local governments, healthcare organizations and charities. However, there is little information on the nature and amount of resources needed by DFCs to ensure improved awareness and meaningful participation of persons with dementia in their communities.

Evaluation of outcomes and especially cost-effectiveness analysis could help in the appropriate allocation of scarce resources to DFCs. However, monitoring and evaluation are often not given the attention they deserve. An evidence-based evaluation tool would support systematic reporting and lead to better planning and focus on the critical needs of persons with dementia and their caregivers.

Dementia-friendly communities must remain open to breakthrough innovations, and especially adopt technological innovations (see Section 5 of this chapter) and other novelties such as the accident relief system adopted by Kobe, Japan – an insurance scheme covering persons with dementia and other Kobe citizens when they suffer accidental damages or losses from dementia. As DFCs mature, it is hoped that persons with dementia remain not just the passive recipient of services, but active contributors to the community with the agency to seek and support the change needed to ensure that their rights are respected, and they are truly and meaningfully involved and in decisions that involve them – that nothing about persons with dementia should be without persons with dementia.

5 Technology and Dementia

In this paragraph we discuss recent developments and the current status of new technologies for dementia, as well as privacy, societal and ethical aspects of this matter. In the current flow of negative clinical trials for new disease-modifying drugs for (Alzheimer's) dementia, we have to broaden our focus. A wider, better dementia approach should also take into account the actual wishes and needs of people with dementia and their family/friends/caregivers to optimize daily living and quality of life. We briefly discuss how technology can play a role in offering support for the individual in interaction with their environment, and more specifically discuss technologies for assessment and monitoring, followed by assistive and therapeutic devices.

In general, the widespread use of technologies for persons with dementia is currently relatively limited and fragmented, but the potential is there and should be further explored. In addition, the evolution from smartphones to smart homes and environments includes technologies that may not primarily be intended for persons with dementia, but they could be a specific end-user group of interest.

Several aspects in current and future development of these technologies deserve adequate attention. First, as the concept often first grows within knowledge institutions, commercial settings or the healthcare field, there should be an early and continuing interaction in the development process of all involved players. Involving all stakeholders in the development process from idea to market-ready technology should be pursued when appropriate. This to ensure that the technology is developed to cover the right needs, is fit for purpose and is adapted to the end user. The technology should demonstrate a sufficient level of market readiness and be welcomed by users or caregivers.

Secondly, as evidence-based practice is an important concept in healthcare, creating the necessary evidence that the new technology has added value and real impact should be incorporated early in the research and development plan. Defining the role in the existing diagnostic, support or care environment should be anticipated, as should its place in the existing healthcare financing framework. Lastly, we stress the importance of types of care we want to offer to persons with dementia, as due to country or culture differences the need for supportive technologies might well vary and therefore be pushed further forward in some countries compared to others. In addition, technologies should be adaptive to fulfil individual needs – which might evolve over time – be capable of multiple tasks and must be sustainable over the course of different levels of cognitive impairment. In this chapter, we discuss aspects of two broad categories of technologies – assessment and monitoring, and assistive and therapeutic devices – and their related ethical and privacy aspects.

5.1 Assessment and Monitoring

5.1.1 (Mobile) Technologies for Diagnosis and Monitoring

Technology and the 'virtual' environment is taking up more and more space in our existence and expanding our natural environment. This provides us with a whole new range of possibilities for assessment and early diagnosis of mild cognitive impairment (MCI) and dementia [32]. In fact, one of the earliest uses of technology in dementia was in the domain of assessment. This started with digital modifications or expansions of the traditional neuropsychological evaluation.

Touchscreen-based cognitive assessment batteries like the Cambridge Neuropsychological Test Automated Battery and the Examen Cognitif par Ordinateur were developed in Europe already in the 1980s and 1990s [33].

Since then digitized versions of pen-and-paper tasks have been developed. For example, a digital clock-drawing task and clock-drawing pen became available. The much-used pen-and-paper test for cognitive evaluation, the Alzheimer's Disease Assessment Scale – Cognitive Subscale (ADAS-Cog), formed the basis for the Touch Panel-Type Dementia Assessment Scale (TDAS) [34]. Validity was shown and the TDAS can serve as a substitute for the ADAS-Cog while having several advantages. The TDAS can be administered in 30 minutes instead of the 45 minutes required for the ADAS-Cog, and it doesn't require the supervision of a qualified clinical psychologist. Over the years, several computerized neuropsychological batteries have been developed, like the Cogstate Brief Battery, Mindstreams (NeuroTrax Corp., NY, USA) and the Computerized Self-Test (CST). Several tests are now also available in web-based or app-based versions.

Cognitive assessment could also be built into specially designed so-called serious games that test a number of cognitive functions [35]. The same games can also be used for cognitive training. Similarly a SmartWalk system has been designed to assess and train sustained auditory attention while the patient walks [35]. A SmartTapestry system can assess episodic verbal memory and as the task involves auditory, visual-spatial and kinaesthetic information the consolidation-retrieval process is stimulated [35].

However, with the explosion of mobile technology and the increasing 'digitalization' of everyday life, assessment and early diagnosis by technology can be taken a few steps further. Indeed, one possible explanation for the relative failure of finding disease-modifying drugs for dementia is that currently the disease is detected only late in the neurodegenerative process. Existing neuropsychological tests are sometimes less effective in detecting a neurodegenerative process in the early stages of disease and have other possible flaws like being rater dependent, being labour-intensive and providing only snapshot evaluations [32].

On the other hand, current technological investigations like scans, profiling of cerebrospinal fluid

biomarkers or genetic tests are often expensive and/or invasive, which makes repetitive use of these techniques as a way of screening vulnerable individuals less feasible [32]. However, new and mobile technologies now offer enormous possibilities for early diagnosis. Subtle cognitive, sensory and motor changes may precede clinical manifestation of (Alzheimer's) dementia by as many as 10–15 years. At the same time, people, also elderly people, nowadays constantly tend to carry with them mobile electronic devices equipped with a whole array of sensitive sensors that can potentially detect data on behaviour, mobility and cognition, which can show subtle changes years before clinical manifestations of a dementia [32].

They also use personal computers and are surrounded by all kinds of electronic appliances that can be connected to the Internet. Mobile technology could be used for both active (prompted) or passive (unnoticed) data collection [32]. In active data collection, the patient is prompted to enter a value or to perform a measurement of a feature previously linked to a disease. In passive data collection, metric values are gathered without the patient noticing and without the need for actions by the patient. Passive data collection has several major advantages: the possibility to gather high-frequency or even continuous data sets, objectivity and lower patient or caregiver burden (hopefully leading to higher adherence) [32].

Several studies already show promising results of how data gathered from the use of personal electronic devices could help in early diagnosis. Fine motor control, speech and executive functioning can be measured frequently or even continuously from smartphone or personal computer use. Slower typing, more pauses and more mouse clicks, for example, can help to differentiate between those with and without cognitive impairment.

Automatic speech analysis is another tool that could be used to detect cognitive decline. Features such as pause and vocal reaction time can be used to distinguish between healthy controls, MCI patients and patients with Alzheimer's disease [32]. Web search data could be used to create digital phenotypes for detecting neurodegenerative disorders. Features on queries (e.g. how much time there is between repeat queries), combined with other features like click and scrolling behaviour, can be taken into account to create such digital phenotypes [32].

The technology built into cars or cell phone data on location could provide another tool for early diagnosis as this technology can detect subtle changes in driving behaviour that could point to early cognitive impairment. For example, driving speed relative to the rest of traffic, mileage close to home or habitual location patterns can all provide clues for early stage dementia [32].

The possibility to integrate technology in the daily life at home offers even more ways for assessment and diagnosis but also for follow-up of patients, and eventually also for interventions. Technology also offers the possibility for naturalistic assessment of everyday activities. At the same time, technology can detect when assistance is needed for successful completion of such tasks and deliver reminders or prompts to the patient when needed [33]. In this way, technology can be used for both continuous monitoring and for personalized assistance. To this end, the daily home environment of the patients with dementia can be equipped with technology capable of assessing and monitoring them. Again, the possibilities are numerous: motion detection can be installed in the house of patients, toilets and faucets can be equipped with sensors, carpets or other floor coverings could be used to detect falls or measure gait speed etc. [36].

5.1.2 Smart Home Technologies

The advancements in the so-called Internet of Things (IoT) make it possible to create smart systems in which physical objects, people and electronic devices are connected [37]. Passive sensors embedded in a patient's home, combined with electronic or medical devices measuring specific parameters, record real-time data that can be sent over Wi-Fi and Bluetooth and through gateways to the backend systems [37]. At the backend systems, the integrated data are processed by an advanced analytical tool that uses machine learning and data analytics algorithms to generate alerts and notifications on the patient living in the smart environment [37]. Clinical knowledge and experience can be used to set the parameters for these notifications and alerts. The information can be monitored around the clock by healthcare professionals.

This kind of advanced IoT platform was used in the United Kingdom to create a technology-integrated health management (TIHM) system [37]. This system allows for real-time insights into the health status of a person with dementia. Instead of having to rely on anecdotal accounts at clinic visits, immediate intervention with the right level of support is possible at the earliest point of need, which could also prevent escalating crisis. What's more, such systems could prolong the time people with dementia can live at home, while at the same time increasing quality of life and decreasing caregiver burden. It could eventually also lead to a reduction in healthcare costs (by reducing hospital admissions and delay institutionalization in nursing homes) and provide one of the solutions for staff shortage [37].

One of the first projects to use smart home technology for dementia was the Gloucester Smart Home. At the university of Surrey, IoT technologies are used in a TIHM home monitoring system. The TIHM uses machine learning and data analytics algorithms that combine physiological and environmental data [38]. Higher-level activity patterns can be detected and can then be used to detect changes in a patient's routine. This system could be used, for example, to detect early manifestations of a urinary tract infection in order to avoid hospital admission or delirium [38]. A network using different sensors could also be used to monitor behavioural problems in dementia like agitation or apathy.

Depending upon the level of cognitive and functional impairment, increasing levels of directive assistance can be given. Progressive levels of assistance starting with a low level of assistance may be important to maintain a better sense of autonomy and independence in the person with dementia. Technological assessment of tasks like making coffee or tea and toast or instrumental activities of daily living have been designed. An important prototype example of prompting is the Cognitive Orthosis for Assisting aCtivities at Home (COACH), which prompts people with dementia to take them through hand-washing procedures by combining computer vision (for tracking the current stage of activity) with artificial intelligence (AI) (for deciding what prompt is required) [33]. However, so far, these technologies are not yet in widespread use in the general population. There is no golden standard on which kind of sensors to use, how to integrate data, which algorithms to use etc. We believe there is a need for international collaboration to create widely applicable systems, however still being able to take into account personal and cultural preferences.

5.1.3 General Data Protection Regulation and Ethical Aspects of Assessment and Monitoring Technology

The use of technology for assessment and monitoring also brings several possible risks. It is important to stress that computerized neuropsychological tests need their own validation studies; it cannot be just assumed that they will have the same validity and psychometric properties as pen-and-paper tests [39]. The interface must be useable for elderly with varying degrees of cognitive impairment and computer skills. Adequate supervision by healthcare professionals is necessary. These tools can be used in a clinical context, but we should be wary of commercial exploitation without appropriate clinical supervision as this can lead to inaccurate self-diagnosis and adverse health consequences [39].

The processing of personal data generated by smart technology in a big data context has to be done in compliance with data protection rules, in particular given the sensitive nature of personal health data [40]. It has to be clearly defined for which purposes the data can – and cannot – be used. Data should be processed in an efficient but nevertheless completely secure way, avoiding all leakage to unauthorized third parties [40]. The use of big data for data mining should also be done in full compliance with legal requirements. It is very important that adequate informed consent is acquired before personal health data are used.

Liability is another concern. In the use of technology, an adverse outcome could result from different sources: a device not working properly, a wrong diagnosis based on inaccurate data gathering, a technical error by an information technology (IT) specialist, inappropriate use of a device by the patient etc. The tele-monitoring of patients by smart home technologies raises its own concerns, as who will be ultimately responsible for the monitoring and timely detection of changes in the health situation of the patient? [40]

Safety of a certain technology, application or monitoring system could be demonstrated by using specific standards and corresponding quality labels. Certification could be reliable indicators towards both professionals and patients. Reimbursement of these technologies is needed but also often warranted, and certification procedures could help in determining which technologies could be eligible for reimbursement by health insurances [40].

Finally, it is pivotal to guarantee equal access to new technology for all patients. Patients with certain disabilities, cultural backgrounds or socio-economic status may have poorer access to technological possibilities or healthcare systems. However, technological innovation can also contribute to a more equitable access to healthcare as it could be specifically geared towards the care of people who have otherwise more difficult access to the healthcare system [40].

It is advisable that the various stakeholders – patients, caregivers and healthcare professionals – are involved in the design and application of new technologies from the beginning. What's more, the principle of 'ethical adoption' – that is, the deep integration of ethical principles into the design, development, deployment and usage of technology – will be crucial [41].

5.2 Assistive and Therapeutic Devices

5.2.1 Technologies to Assist in Living with Dementia

An assistive technology for persons with dementia could be defined as an item, piece, product or system driven by electronics and used to help persons with dementia in dealing with the consequences of the condition [42]. The technology can but should not necessarily be purposefully designed for dementia, as also more widely used technologies could be of value here. Technologies can offer support on several not mutually exclusive domains, including cognitive or functional support or engagement in psychosocial support and interaction [43].

In brief, all of these technologies include devices supporting activities of daily living or domestic services, including electronic calendars or reminders (e.g. for medication) for activities, robotics and navigation systems and technologies that stimulate to engage in meaningful and pleasurable activities such as cognitive stimulation, exercise or any physical activity. Technologies can also support social participation, emotional or behaviour management and contact with others or combine one or more of all of these.

The general purpose of these technologies would be to empower persons with dementia, to improve quality of life and to support the identity, independence and social engagement of persons with dementia within their own environment. In this process, often the caregiver is of crucial importance, and these technologies could also support caregivers in largely identical domains. In addition, a caregiver is often required for initiating, training and using the technology, and often the early introduction in the process of dementia is beneficial in order to get the user acquainted with the technology.

In general, technical solutions should be considered where indicated and possible provide holistic and multilevel support and assistance due to the nature of the disabilities that come along with a diagnosis of dementia. They should also be adaptive, as the needs of persons with dementia are likely to change over the course of time. An interesting emerging concept here is the rise of 'zero-effort technologies', where due to the use of advanced techniques (computer vision, artificial intelligence, machine learning etc.) the device can offer support with little or no effort from the end user. This is obviously particularly interesting in the framework of dementia.

5.2.2 User-Centred Design and Creation of Evidence

In the development phase and where applicable, one must make sure that the technology is a good match for the person with dementia as often a top-down approach may result in a mismatch as the approach was, for example, too general and not individualized or even stigmatizing. Here, co-creation or participatory approaches open the possibility to incorporate needs, wishes and user-friendliness but also to detect potential shortcomings or limitations early in the development. Currently, less than 50% of technologies use this user-centred design, and the low prevalence of such joint approaches is seen as a co-determinant for low adaptation rates of certain technologies.

A different aspect is the creation of evidence regarding the outcome of these technologies. Where the approval of new drugs is strictly regulated by controlling authorities such as the US Food and Drug Administration (FDA) and the European Medicines Agency (EMA), this is often not the case for assistive technologies, and only applies to the commercialization of medical devices. Where the authorities demand evidence for safety and efficacy of drugs and medical devices, this is often not so with most assistive technologies. Clinical trials that demonstrate safety and/or effectiveness are, if they are available at all, often of low methodological quality and demonstrate methodological flaws such as inadequate design, low power, short duration and high dropout rates. Currently, clinical validation of technologies is poor and 50% of all cases have not been validated in clinical trials with persons with dementia. Here, evaluation of cost-effectiveness should also be incorporated, as this would be a crucial aspect to take into account in the implementation and possible reimbursement discussions, at least in countries where (partial) reimbursement for these technologies would be an option.

Due to the diversity of available technologies or technologies in development, it is difficult to gain and maintain a good overview for both end users and caregivers. Some items may be sold by a specific (medical or care) industry, while others are more widely available in do-it-yourself (DIY) or electronics stores, or sold by software providers (e.g. apps). A point of attention would be to increase transfer of information about new technologies. Clinical staff, even when working in specialized dementia settings such as memory clinics, are often unaware of all the technologies or devices available to support persons with dementia, in contrast to drug treatments, for example, where the information is more readily available and their use actively promoted. Here, a comprehensive and regularly updated index of technologies that are available or in development would be a large step forward.

As comprehensive and up-to-date websites already exist providing a complete overview of, for example, drug compounds in development, biomarkers or risk factors (e.g. www.alzforum.org/databases), these formats could be used for that purpose and locally translated and adapted where needed. Fortunately, national and local examples of technology and aids databases already exist (see www.alzproducts.co.uk and https://hulpmiddelen wijzer.nl/informatie/hulpmiddelen-bij-dementie), but these do not represent the full available spectrum.

5.2.3 Examples of Technologies

As hundreds of assistive and therapeutic technologies are available or in development that would be of value for persons with dementia [44, 45], a complete overview of the current state of the industry is beyond the scope of this chapter. Most technologies focus on systems composed of sensing and processing technologies including the ambient assisted living systems, and second most are robotics that assist in personal care, domestic services or social interaction. Striking is the fact that often marketed technologies are only available in one country. For example, care technology solutions such as VITAL or VALERE (https://senso2.me) were manufactured in Belgium and are not (yet) commercialized in other countries.

This reflects a dispersed, non-globalized introduction, contrary to, for example, drugs or specific medical devices, that are widely available. One of the few technologies that is available within different countries is PARO. PARO is a socio-emotional robotic seal developed in Japan and one of the robots with the longest history and most widespread use for persons with dementia. Evidence on its effects and acceptance of use is mixed. What's more, the device is relatively expensive and the studies on cost-effectiveness are not convincing.

Another concern is hygiene and infection prevention, especially when the device is to be used in residential care by different residents. Also lacking is data on how older adults themselves experience the use of robots in their care and what their attitudes are towards these sophisticated machines. Another example would be the Robotic Assistant for Mild Cognitive Impairment (RAMCIP), a service-oriented robot developed through the pan-European Horizon 2020 Project (https://ramcip-project.eu). RAMCIP can detect falls, support medication use, bring water and assist with video calls. However, as several of these research projects are investigator driven, it is unclear how further development and marketing will be continued once the temporary financing is halted.

Numerous apps have also been developed for cognitive stimulation, cognitive training, reminiscence, art, music, games etc., but most of these are only available in the English language. During recent years, it became clear that technologies and robotics involve several legal, privacy and ethical aspects that are discussed next.

5.2.4 Ethical Aspects of Technologies

Several of the (advanced) technologies automatically lead to ethical issues and questions among all stakeholders of aged and dementia care, from managerial personnel to older adults, from caregivers to older adults' family. In general, respect for autonomy, beneficence and non-maleficence should define the ethical standards, and several levels require ethical consideration [46].

First, at the *individual level*, how does the use of technology fit into the user's views on care? The technology should support a person's autonomy and if the technology is not wanted, alternatives should be explored. Within the same line, the privacy of the users and others should be sufficiently guaranteed, and this is often a delicate balance between privacy/autonomy on one hand and safety/minimizing risks on the other.

Older persons with dementia show an important dynamic of their disease over time, a fact that should be taken into consideration. Where one technology (e.g. a certain app) might be very stimulating and beneficial in early stages, this same app might become frustrating and disadvantageous once the dementia evolves. Here, the potential and supposed effects of any technology on behavioural and psychological symptoms of dementia require specific attention (e.g. irritability and agitation arising from a technology that is too cognitively demanding so it cannot be used properly), as we should be sure of the beneficial effects. In the case of humanized robots, additional aspects come into play. People can get attached to these robots, but this type of relation should not threaten other (established or new) relations, and even potential deceit deserves attention.

On the *organizational level* (e.g. nursing homes, home care), technology should be embedded in the vision and mission and fully be in agreement with local practices of good care. For the latter, the role of the technology in the care process should be defined and delineated within an (integrated) care process. This should also be a dynamic process where the (changing) voice of the older person with dementia is heard.

On a *societal level*, we should consider which technologies contribute to the flourishing of persons with dementia and cannot be any threat in the long term (e.g. with a dehumanizing effect). Here, a reflection on whether the technology is motivated out of a care imperative or a technological-economic imperative is desirable.

Several countries have local or national dementia policy plans and reflection is warranted on how the use of technologies could optimally be incorporated into existing and future policy plans for dementia. Here, an ethical and legal framework should exist concerning safety and privacy (e.g. data access and storage).

Lastly, the financial /economical impact should be known and (knowledge on) cost-effective technologies should be accessible independent of socio-economic status. Future work in this matter should include a framework for better and integrated private–public collaboration, and focus on a multinational plan for technology development, policy and accessibility.

6 Night-Time Agitation in Dementia and the Influence of the Environment

Approximately one person with dementia in three will experience sleep problems (e.g. sleep fragmentation, difficulty falling asleep, reduced deep sleep, increased daytime sleep and early awakening) and night-time agitation (e.g. general restlessness, wandering or verbal agitation) [47]. This night-time restlessness is often problematic for persons with dementia and their family caregivers. The characteristics of the physical environment are important determinants for the orientation in time and space of people with dementia [48], and could contribute in different ways to agitation during the night.

In people with dementia, sleeping problems can lead to dangerous situations such as falls at night, feelings of depression and anxiety and reduction in the overall quality of life. Accumulating evidence demonstrates that insomnia is a significant risk factor contributing to the progression of dementia [49]. Good sleep hygiene can help to prevent progression of dementia. Family caregivers are affected as they are worried about the situation, have to wake up at night to intervene and sleep less well themselves, causing fatigue and feelings of depression [50].

When these problems persist for a long time, the situation eventually becomes unbearable and care at home will be no longer tenable. Exhaustion in family caregivers is often a reason for moving the person with dementia to a nursing home. After transferring to a residential care facility, the sleeping problems generally persist, leading frequently to the overuse of sleep medications [51].

Current treatment options for insomnia in people with dementia are unsatisfactory, leaving patients, carers and doctors with few tools to manage this issue. Pharmacological solutions have limited effect and are accompanied by side effects whereas non-pharmacological solutions are often overlooked. In this section, a brief overview is given of possible causes of night-time restlessness and non-pharmacological solutions that may contribute to a good night's sleep of people with dementia at home as well as in nursing homes [52].

6.1 Causes of Night-Time Agitation and Sleeplessness

Night-time agitation in people with dementia may have different causes. It sometimes seems pointless behaviour but it can equally well be the expression of a certain perception or need. Based on our research, three groups of triggers of night-time agitation are distinguished: triggering factors in (1) the person, (2) the social environment and (3) the spatial and sensory environment [53, 54].

6.1.1 Triggering Factors in the Person with Dementia

Changes in the brain cause various problems in the functioning of persons with dementia which may, in interaction with the environment, trigger night-time agitation. Memory problems disturb the ability to remember or recognize places, objects, people or events and consequently lead to a loss of control over the world and difficulty in orienting in time and space. Significant changes in the course of the day (such as a visit or a trip outside the nursing home) may overstimulate or bring the person out of balance. This can lead to a changed day-night rhythm and subsequently to reduced sleep at night and more sleep during the day.

Lack of activity during daytime may also lead to being awake and active during the night. Some people suffer from 'sundowning', a condition in which people with dementia become restless when the sun goes down as it triggers people in their need to go to a safe place where they feel at home. Dementia in some cases is also accompanied by hallucinations. When during the night the person sees or hears things that are not there which induce anxiety, this may cause night-time agitation.

Furthermore, pain or other physical needs can cause sleeping problems or restless behaviour. For example, hunger or thirst are reasons for people with dementia to get out of bed at night. Due to their orientation problems, they may get lost along the way. On the contrary, eating too much or too heavily and drinking caffeine or alcohol in the evening can cause night-time agitation as well. The feeling of having to go to the toilet at night can also be a cause. Understanding previous sleep and wake habits and routines is helpful to identify possible causes of sleep problems in a person with dementia and to find solutions to restore the sleeping rhythm. For example, when someone used to read a book or drink a glass of milk before going to bed, these actions may calm the person and reduce night-time agitation.

6.1.2 Triggering Factors in the Social Environment

Persons with dementia often have difficulty to interact with others, which may lead to anxiety or distress and contribute to night-time restlessness. It may be difficult for them to understand long or complex sentences. Speaking clearly and slowly to persons with dementia during the night may help to reduce stress. When spoken language can no longer be processed, body language and non-verbal communication (e.g. speaking softly, whispering and giving a hug) can help to calm the person with dementia down.

Bringing structure in daily routine and the organization of care can also reduce the night-time restlessness and sleep problems. People with dementia benefit from a fixed evening ritual which reminds them that sleep time is coming. Unexpected events such as a surprise visit in the evening break the routine and cause confusion. Moreover, routine care provided during the night (e.g. checking safety or incontinence materials) is best tailored to the individual needs of the person with dementia and accompanied by telling the person what will happen in order to increase predictability [55].

6.1.3 Triggering Factors in the Spatial and Sensory Environment

People with dementia are more sensitive to elements in the spatial and sensory environment than others. Absence of light and noise are important contributing factors for a good sleep. Clear light during the night may contribute to the confusion between day and night. Disrupting the normal rhythm or experiencing too little daylight can disturb the sleep-wake cycle. Getting outside during the day, seeing enough daylight and having indications for the course of the day such as the smell of coffee or soup, closing the curtains and dimming the light gives people with dementia markers of time and supports a good sleep-wake rhythm.

Placing a night light in the room can be important when the person with dementia needs to go to the toilet at night. It could prevent falling or getting lost. Music and sounds have potential to connect with persons with dementia. Singing songs, listening to music and reminiscing can have a calming effect. Environmental noise during sleep time (e.g. loud televisions, noisy trolleys or loud conversations) should be avoided. Furthermore, both body and room temperature can cause disturbed sleep. When a person with dementia is too hot at night, he or she may start sweating and perhaps even undressing to cool down, disturbing a good night's sleep. The 'ideal' room temperature depends very much on individual preferences. Finally, it is important to let the person sleep in a comfortable position and to prevent strange tactile sensations in bed such as itchy blankets.

6.2 A Stepwise Non-pharmacological Approach to Improve Sleep

Every person is unique. Sleeping problems in persons with dementia may have different causes and not everyone will react in the same way to solutions. Therefore, it is important to analyse what triggers night-time agitation so adjustments can be made accordingly. Family or professional caregivers in nursing homes can rely on the 'ABC' model to distinguish and investigate causes of night-time restlessness and to search for solutions.

The acronym ABC refers to antecedents behaviour, and consequences of sleeping problems. Antecedents refer to what happened prior to the sleeping disturbance, including what happened earlier in the day (e.g. a visit from the grandchildren). Behaviour is defined as how the night-time restlessness manifested itself and what behaviour the person displayed (e.g. difficulty going to bed or getting up frequently at night). Consequences refer to how the night-time restlessness was solved (e.g. the person relaxed again after drinking a cup of tea or after turning on a night light).

A first step is to observe the sleeping pattern of the person with dementia for a certain period of time followed by looking for triggers. The three groups of triggering factors just described can be used as a source of inspiration to decide what triggering factors cause the night-time restlessness and provide starting points for tackling the sleeping problems. Often the sleeping problems are provoked by a combination of factors. However, it is recommended to focus on only one factor at a time and to investigate whether it can be tackled by a certain solution (e.g. a small action or change in the sleeping routine).

To investigate whether a solution works, it is best applied for a few days to see whether it generates change. When the solution seems to work, it can become a daily routine. Accordingly, new solutions tackling the same or different factors can be tried out and added to the daily routine. An important point here is to keep sufficient time between the try-out of different solutions and to avoid too drastic solutions or actions to prevent the patient with dementia from being overwhelmed.

According to the scientific literature, the following solutions are evidence based and generally applicable to improve sleep [56]:

- Reduce naps or time in bed during the day.
- Be physically and socially active during the day.
- Get outside or sit in daylight during the day.
- Sit in bright daylight in the morning.
- Work with more or less fixed time blocks to go to bed and get up.
- Pay attention to food and beverage.
- Reduce light and noise during the night.

In addition to these evidence-based solutions, inspiration to improve the sleeping and living pattern of a person with dementia can be found in his or her past. Questioning family members about earlier habits and preferences may result in new insights and effective solutions. Finally, it is important to keep evaluating the chosen solutions as a person with dementia evolves over time. Hence, solutions that are currently effective may become ineffective later on and need to be replaced.

When nursing homes want to rely on this step-wise non-pharmacological approach to improve the sleep quality of residents with dementia, it is important that employees from different disciplines work together. Everyone has his or her own responsibility and observes other things. When developing a daily routine or a treatment plan, it is therefore crucial to integrate the observations of different staff members, including those of the cleaning personnel or the logistics assistant, as they are equally well placed to notice crucial triggers or changes. In particular, sharing relevant information observed during day and night shifts is critical. Setting up a working group for discussing night-time restlessness of habitants may encourage a good exchange of information. Finally, as staff often alternates in nursing homes, it is important to communicate regularly about the agreements that are made.

It is self-evident that night-time agitation has enormous impact on the health and well-being of carers. This applies to family carers as well as to professional carers. In both care at home and in nursing homes, the support of carers should be a point of attention. General tips and methods are described in Chapter 7.

6.3 Getting a Better Grip on the Situation

The environmental aspects contribute strongly to the feelings of safety and well-being of the persons with dementia. We reviewed aspects concerning the person centredness and the relation centredness of the social environment such as the DFCs that make persons with dementia feel respected and recognized as full citizens. Aspects of the spatial and sensory environment may still be underestimated in their contribution to the feelings of belonging and well-being of persons with dementia. Often they are even the cause for (night-time) agitation. Here, assessment and monitoring technologies as discussed in Section 5 of this chapter might be helpful to provide a safe and pleasant environment facilitating better sleep and reducing night-time agitation.

7 Concluding Remarks

Due to new scientific insights and the growing global attention on dementia, the landscape for persons with dementia is gradually changing. Here, the environment plays an important role in encouraging persons with dementia to live a qualitative and independent life in connection with their closest ones and broader social network. This chapter dealt with several important aspects of this environment, starting off with enriched environments of care. As an example, the Senses Framework could provide new directions to individualize and create the optimal environment for each individual on different levels, including the community level.

Subsequent to that, insights for the physical environment and architectural design were discussed, where the road is still largely open for further research and implementation of good practices. Next, the role of the community can now be better identified as the cornerstones for DFCs were laid out and good examples were discussed in this chapter. It is to note that no generic models exist, as these need to be adapted to local communities. However, more research is definitely needed, especially implementation (research) and evaluation of outcomes and cost-effectiveness.

We debated the growing role technologies play for persons with dementia and affiliated ethical and privacy aspects. It became clear that the number of universally implemented and accepted technologies is still relatively small, due to several aspects discussed here, but a bright future awaits and technology will definitely play an important role as an environmental factor to improve the life of persons with dementia and their carers. Lastly, we discussed the importance of the social and physical environment for night-time agitation and sleep, where aspects of the other parts of this chapter (architecture, aspects of care, technology) all need to be integrated, but may not always be able to solve this often difficult problem.

References

1. Nolan MR, Brown J, Davies S, Nolan J, Keady J. *The Senses Framework: Improving Care for Older People through a Relationship-Centred Approach*. Getting Research into Practice (GRIP) Series No. 2. Sheffield, University of Sheffield, 2006.

2. Kitwood T. *Dementia Reconsidered: The Person Comes First*. Buckingham, Open University Press, 1997.

3. Brooker D, Latham I. *Person-Centred Dementia Care: Making Services Better with the VIPS Framework*. Second edition. London, Jessica Kingsley, 2015.

4. Vernooij-Dassen M, Moniz-Cook E. Person-centred dementia care: Moving beyond caregiving. *Aging & Mental Health* 2016; **20**: 667–8.

5. Harding E, Wait S, Scrutton J. *The State of Play in Person-Centred Care: A Pragmatic Review about Person-Centred Care Is Defined, Applied and Measured. Featuring Selected Key Contributors and Case Studies across the Field*. London, Health Foundation, 2015.

6. Tresolini CP, Pew-Fetzer Task Force. *Health Professions Education and Relationship-Centred Care: A Report of the Pew-Fetzer Task Force on Advancing Psychosocial Education*. San Francisco, Pew Health Professions Commission, 1994.

7. Nolan MR, Grant G, Keady J. *Understanding Family Care: A Multidimensional Model of Caring and Coping*. Buckingham, Open University Press, 1996.

8. Keady J, Nolan MR. Person and Relationship centred dementia care: Past, present and future. In Dening T, Thomas A, Stewart R, Taylor JP, et al., eds. *Oxford Textbook on Old Age Psychiatry*. Third edition. Oxford, Oxford University Press, 2021; 233–48.

9. Keady J, Brown Wilson C, Swarbrick C. Developing the senses in practice: A pilot practice development project involving two care homes in the north west of England. Final report to BUPA Giving. Leeds, BUPA, 2011.

10. Hatton N. Re-imagining the care home: A spatially responsive approach to arts practice with older people in residential care. *Research in Drama Education: Journal of Applied Theatre and Performance* 2014; **19**(4): 355–65.

11. Day K, Carreon D, Stump C. The therapeutic design of environments for people with dementia. *Gerontologist* 2000; **40**(4): 397–416.

12. Mens N, Wagenaar C. *De architectuur van de ouderenhuisvesting*. Rotterdam, NAi Uitgevers, 2009.

13. Diaz Moore K, Geboy L. The question of evidence. *Architectural Research Quarterly* 2010; **14**(2): 105–14.

14. Marquardt G, Bueter K, Motzek T. Impact of the design of the built environment on people with dementia. *Health Environments Research and Design Journal* 2014; **8**(1): 127–57.

15. Diaz Moore K. The role of theory in furthering evidence-based practice. *Health Environments Research and Design Journal* 2011; **4**(2): 4–6.

16. Gray DB, Gould M, Bickenbach JE. Environmental barriers and disability. *Journal of Architectural and Planning Research* 2003; **20**(1): 29–37.

17. Chalfont GE. Building edge. *Alzheimer's Care Quarterly* 2005; **6**(4): 341–8.

18. Van Hoof J, Aarts MPJ, Rense CG, Schoutens AMC. Ambient bright light in dementia. *Building and Environment* 2009; **44**(1): 146–55.

19. Ching FDK. *Architecture: Form, Space, and Order.* Second edition. New York, Van Nostrand Reinhold, 1996.

20. Unwin S. *Analysing Architecture.* London, Routledge, 2009.

21. Van Steenwinkel I. Offering architects insights into living with dementia. Unpublished PhD thesis, KU Leuven, 2015.

22. Zingmark K. Experiences related to home in people with Alzheimer's disease. Unpublished PhD thesis, Umea University, 2000.

23. Herrmann LK, Welter E, Leverenz J, Lerner AJ, Udelson N, Kanetsky, et al. A systematic review of dementia-related stigma research: Can we move the stigma dial? *American Journal of Geriatric Psychiatry* 2018; **26**: 316–31.

24. Forbes D, Markle-Reid M, Hawranik P, Peacock S, Kingston D, Morgan D, et al. Availability and acceptability of Canadian home and community-based services: Perspectives of family caregivers of persons with dementia. *Home Health Care Services Quarterly* 2008; **27**: 75–99.

25. Alzheimer's Disease International. *Dementia Friendly Communities: Key Principles.* London: Alzheimer's Disease International, 2016. Available from www.alz.co.uk/adi/pdf/dfc-principles.pdf

26. Crampton J, Dean J, Eley R. Creating a dementia friendly York. Report for the Joseph Rowntree Foundation, 2012.

27. European Union Joint Action on Dementia. Evidence review of dementia friendly communities, 2017.

28. Subramaniam M, Chong SA, Vaingankar JA, Abdin E, Chua BY, Chua HC, et al. Prevalence of dementia in people aged 60 years and above: Results from the WiSE Study. *Journal of Alzheimer's Disease* 2015; **45**: 1127–38.

29. Subramaniam M, Abdin E, Picco L, Pang S, Shafie S, Vaingankar JA, et al. Stigma towards people with mental disorders and its components: A perspective from multi-ethnic Singapore. *Epidemiology and Psychiatric Sciences* 2017; **26**: 371–82.

30. Buckner S, Mattocks C, Rimmer M, Lafortune L. An evaluation tool for age-friendly and dementia friendly communities. *Work Older People* 2018; **22**: 48–58.

31. Wu SM, Huang HL, Chiu YC, Tang LY, Yang PS, Hsu JL, et al. Dementia-friendly community indicators from the perspectives of people living with dementia and dementia-family caregivers. *Journal of Advanced Nursing* 2019; **75**: 2878–89.

32. Kourtis LC, Regele OB, Wright JM, Jones GB. Digital biomarkers for Alzheimer's disease: The mobile/wearable devices opportunity. *Npj Digital Medicine* 2019; 2.

33. Astell AJ, Bouranis N, Hoey J, Lindauer A, Mihailidis A, Nugent C, et al. Technology and dementia: The future is now. *Dementia and Geriatric Cognitive Disorders* 2019; **47**(3): 131–9.

34. Brando E, Olmedo R, Solares Canal C. The application of technologies in dementia diagnosis and intervention: A literature review. *Gerontechnology* 2017; **16**(1): 1–11.

35. Mancioppi G, Fiorini L, Timpano Sportiello M, Cavallo F. Novel technological solutions for assessment, treatment, and assistance in mild cognitive impairment. *Frontiers in Neuroinformatics* 2019; **13**: 58.

36. Carrillo MC, Dishman E, Plowman T. Everyday technologies for Alzheimer's disease care: Research findings, directions, and challenges. *Alzheimer's and Dementia* 2009; **5**(6): 479–88.

37. Enshaeifar S, Barnaghi P, Skillman S, Markides A, Elsaleh T, Acton ST, et al. The internet of things for dementia care. *IEEE Internet Computing* 2018; **22**(1): 8–17.

38. Enshaeifar S, Zoha A, Skillman S, Markides A, Acton ST, Elsaleh T, et al. Machine learning methods for detecting urinary tract infection and analysing daily living activities in people with dementia. *PLoS One.* 2019; **14**(1): e0209909.

39. Robillard JM, Illes J, Arcand M, Beattie BL, Hayden S, Lawrence P, et al. Scientific and ethical features of English-language online tests for Alzheimer's disease. *Alzheimer's & Dementia (Amsterdam, Netherlands)*. 2015; **1**(3): 281–8.

40. Commission E. Green paper on mobile health. 2014.

41. Robillard JM, Cleland I, Hoey J, Nugent C. Ethical adoption: A new imperative in the development of technology for dementia. *Alzheimers Dement.* 2018; **14**(9): 1104–13.

42. Meiland F, Innes A, Mountain G, Robinson L, van der Roest H, Garcia-Casal JA, et al. Technologies to support community-dwelling persons with dementia: A position paper on issues regarding development, usability, effectiveness and cost-effectiveness, deployment, and ethics. *JMIR Rehabilitation and Assistive Technologies* 2017; **4**(1): e1.

43. Kenigsberg PA, Aquino JP, Bérard A, Brémond F, Charras K, Dening T, et al. Assistive technologies to address capabilities of people with dementia: From research to practice. *Dementia.* 2019; **18**(4): 1568–95.

44. Ienca M, Fabrice J, Elger B, Caon M, Scoccia Pappagallo A, Kressig RW, et al. Intelligent assistive technology for Alzheimer's disease and other dementias: A systematic review. *The Journal of Alzheimer's Disease.* 2017; **56**(4): 1301–40.

45. Moyle W. The promise of technology in the future of dementia care. *Nature Reviews Neurology* 2019; **15**(6): 353–9.

46. Vandemeulebroucke T. *The Use of Socially Assistive Robots in the Care for Older Adults: A Socio-historical Ethical Analysis.* Leuven, University of Leuven, 2019.

47. Cipriani G, Lucetti C, Danti S, Nuti A. Sleep disturbances and dementia. *Psychogeriatrics* 2015; **15**: 65–74.

48. Van Steenwinkel I, Van Audenhove C, Heylighen A. Spatial clues for orientation: Architectural design meets people with dementia. In Langdon P, Clarkson PJ, Robinson P, Lazar J, Heylighen A, eds. *Designing Inclusive Systems: Designing Inclusion for Real-World Applications.* London, Springer, 2012; 227–36.

49. Wunderlin M, Züsta M, Fehér D, Klöppel S, Nissen C. The role of slow wave sleep in the development of dementia and its potential for preventive interventions. *Psychiatry Research Neuro-imaging* 2020. https://doi.org/10.1016/j.pscychresns.2020.111178

50. McCurry SM, Song Y, Martin JL. Sleep in caregivers: What we know and what we need to learn. *Current Opinion in Psychiatry* 2015; **28**: 497–503.

51. Hope T, Keene J, Gedling K, Fairburn CG, Jacoby R. Predictors of institutionalization for people with dementia living at home with a carer. *International Journal of Geriatric Psychiatry* 1998; **13**: 682–90.

52. Spruytte N, Van Vracem M, Van Audenhove C. *Naar een omgevingsaanpak van nachtelijke onrust bij dementie in woonzorgcentra.* Leuven, LUCAS, 2017.

53. Van Vracem M, Spruytte N, Declercq A, Van Audenhove C. Agitation in dementia and the role of spatial and sensory interventions: Experiences of professional and family caregivers. *Scandinavian Journal of Caring Sciences* 2015; **30**(2): 281–9.

54. Van Vracem M, Spruytte N, Declercq A, Van Audenhove C. Nachtelijke onrust bij personen met dementie in woonzorgcentra: een verkennende veldstudie. *Tijdschrift voor Gerontologie en Geriatrie* 2016; **47**(2): 78–85.

55. Ellmers T, Arber S, Luff R, Eyers I, Young E. Factors affecting residents' sleep in care homes. *Nursing Older People* 2013; **25**(8): 29–32.

56. Brown CA, Berry R, Tan MC, Khoshia A, Turlapati L, Swedlove F. A critique of the evidence-base for non-pharmacological sleep interventions for persons with dementia. *Dementia* 2011; **12**(2): 210–37.

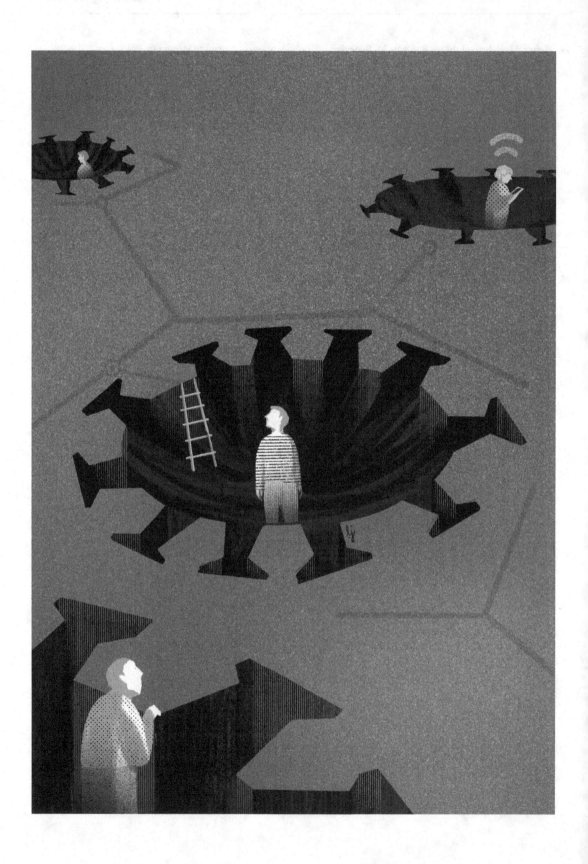

The Impact of the COVID-19 Pandemic on the Well-Being of People Living with Dementia

Debby Gerritsen, Henriëtte van der Roest, Shirley Evans, Ruslan Leontjevas, Marleen Prins, Dawn Brooker and Rose-Marie Dröes

1 Introduction

At the time of the writing of this book, the world was in the grip of the COVID-19 pandemic. As we write this chapter, many people living with dementia have just received their vaccinations and many countries have experienced two lengthy 'lockdowns' where contact with others was significantly curtailed. This had a great impact on all citizens but especially on older and vulnerable people, such as many people living with dementia, and those who provide care and support. The long-term impact is still unknown but the short-term effects have been significant. In some European countries, 20–30% of COVID-19 deaths have been in people living with dementia [1]. The social distancing measures introduced to prevent further spread of the virus (e.g. keeping a distance of 1.5 meters from others, shielding, less accessibility to healthcare and social care and lockdown measures) may have resulted in loneliness and confusion as well as a deterioration of symptoms in people living with dementia.

In addition, the negative impact of losing daily routines and contact with family and friends placed people living with dementia at greater risk for self-neglect and social isolation, especially where healthcare and social care interventions were curtailed due to the pandemic [1]. Social isolation can be defined in terms of the size of the social network and the frequency of social contacts [2], which generally tend to decrease in people living with dementia due to changing abilities over time. Further restrictions of social contacts may therefore more likely induce loneliness and evoke anxiety, especially among those living alone [3], which will negatively impact their quality of life and well-being [4]. Many care and welfare organizations as well as national Alzheimer's associations made great efforts to continue providing support to people living with dementia and their carers by means of alternative services, particularly where in-person support was not possible.

In this chapter, based on studies done inside and outside Europe, and more specifically in the United Kingdom and the Netherlands, we reflect more in depth on the consequences of the COVID-19 pandemic for people living with dementia, their families and professional caregivers in different care settings. We first consider what impact the lockdown and the continuing social distancing measures have had on the social and mental health of home-dwelling people living with dementia and their carers. As a substantial number normally participates in group-oriented support activities, we also describe how care providers of such activities have delivered support in alternative ways – that is, mostly at a distance – and how this was experienced by the participants. Secondly, we consider the impact of the lockdown and social distancing measures on the well-being of people living with dementia in nursing homes.

2 The Impact of COVID-19 on Home-Dwelling People Living with Dementia and Their Carers

2.1 The Impact on Social and Mental Health

The COVID-19 pandemic has put the social health of community-dwelling people living with dementia and their family carers highly at risk. During the lockdowns people were/are advised to stay home, especially when they were/are vulnerable, and only to go out for necessary shopping or some fresh air. Many people living with dementia depend on support from home-care teams coming into the home, sometimes on a daily basis, to provide help with daily living activities and personal care. Together with their families, they had to make a choice between doing without this support or running the risk of infection from daily visits.

Early in the pandemic, confusion and short supply of personal protective equipment (PPE) made this a particularly difficult decision for many families. Relatives not cohabiting with the person living with dementia, neighbours and friends were urged not to visit them or to stay outside when visiting them. A study of Thyrian et al. [5] conducted during the first lockdown showed that in a convenience sample of community-dwelling people with cognitive impairment, on average seven activities decreased in frequency. Social activities related to meeting people, dancing or celebrating birthdays decreased significantly. Talking with friends by phone and activities like gardening increased. Utilization of healthcare services decreased, as did visits to general practitioners.

All group support activities for people living with dementia and carers, which are, for example, in the Netherlands used by about 40% of the people with dementia living at home [6], were stopped under governmental rules to prevent further spread of the virus. This included Alzheimer's cafes, Meeting Centres and other day care services which normally are used one to four days a week. Consequently, the carefully constructed social structure with daily physical encounters, opportunities to participate in meaningful activities with peers and respite care for family carers suddenly disappeared.

The positive outcomes of person-centred care and national initiatives like dementia-friendly neighbourhoods, supported by ministries of health, local governments and national Alzheimer's associations over the past decade, were at risk of being negated. When the centres were allowed to open again after the first lockdown, due to the social distancing rule of staying 1.5 metres away from others, the majority could welcome only half of the visitors at the same time due to limited space. They therefore had to decrease the hours participants could visit the centres in order to provide all participants at least some hours of support and their carers some respite.

As social contact and meaningful activities are crucial to maintain the social health [7, 8] and quality of life of people living with dementia [9, 10], social isolation and under-stimulation are likely to result in an increase of behaviour and mood disruptions such as agitation, depression, anxiety and apathy. A review study of Simonetti et al. [3] into alterations in behaviour and mood during COVID-19 – which included 20 studies carried out during the lockdown between March and June 2020 – showed this was indeed the case. Apathy, anxiety and agitation were the most frequently reported neuropsychiatric symptoms. They were mainly triggered by the protracted isolation. Cohen et al. [11] reported a deterioration of behavioural symptoms in older people living with dementia in the community in Argentina and suggested this was related to a combination of social isolation, lack of outpatient rehabilitation services and increased stress of family carers.

The health of family carers came under pressure without respite or support. Research before the pandemic in the Netherlands showed more than half of family carers feel burdened, of which 13% feel heavily burdened and 4% overburdened [12]. During the pandemic these numbers inevitably grew even higher: 61% of the carers felt more burdened [6]. This clearly resulted from receiving less support: 45% reported receiving less support from day care services, 42% received less support from volunteers and 'buddies' and 20% received less support from their case manager. On the other hand, 27% received more support from neighbours [6]. The increased carer burden and decreased formal support has been confirmed by the study of Van Maurik et al. [13], which showed carers experienced more psychological symptoms. Increased carer burden, anxiety and depression were associated with increased behavioural and psychological symptoms in the person with dementia [14].

A study of Roach et al. [4] in Canada showed many carers experienced feelings of burnout and stress around coping with daily living activities, which was partly due to no longer receiving formal home care service and having only limited support from their own network of family and friends because of the social distancing measures. Carers were understanding of the changes in healthcare services, but it was clear some degree of ongoing contact and support was crucial. They did not feel well informed or supported regarding protective equipment such as masks, and this resulted in feelings of anxiety about the pandemic and about leaving the house.

Furthermore, some carers expressed concerns about the person living with dementia experiencing more cognitive decline since the start of the lockdown because of the decrease in social interaction. The remote support offered had some advantages for carers such as not feeling rushed, having options presented such as the telephone or Zoom and the ability to be more candid with the care provider or doctor if the person living with dementia did not participate in the call.

2.2 Impact on Support Services That Rely on Bringing People Together in Groups

Supporting people living with dementia and their carers to live as well as possible in their communities, with timely psychosocial support, is a global public health goal. Even prior to COVID-19, there were significant gaps in social care for people affected by dementia in many countries [15], with an associated reliance on informal carers (e.g. family members) to provide support [16] and a growing recognition that informal carers' own health and well-being is often negatively impacted by their caring activities [17].

The detrimental health impact of social isolation and loneliness is also increasingly being recognized [18–20]. Regular social activity, where people can leave their homes and gather in a communal setting on a frequent and ongoing basis, is seen as beneficial to social and mental health for people living with dementia and the people who care for them [8, 21]. For those with more significant care needs, many countries provide day care with a focus on providing a break for family carers and activity and companionship for those with dementia. For people who are earlier in their journey with dementia, there has been a proliferation of groups and activities that provide social connection and support for people and families.

To maintain the social health of people living with dementia and carers during the COVID-19 pandemic, many support services for community-dwelling persons with dementia, Meeting Centres and Alzheimer's cafes have been urgently looking for remote support alternatives, such as telephone/ video calling, online support and WhatsApp and Facebook groups, to compensate for the lack of face-to-face meetings. Also, the use of tablets and apps which can support people in finding meaningful and pleasant activities has increased. This necessitated teaching and support for persons with dementia and their carers, and sometimes also for professional caregivers, who had no experience in the use of tablets and apps.

The rapid move towards virtual care provision may have influenced the quality of care provided. It is therefore important to evaluate the changes in care provision from different perspectives – that is, from the perspective of the care providers, but also from the experience of persons with dementia and their carers. Some of the authors of this chapter have been particularly engaged in the spread of the combined Meeting Centre Support Programme (MCSP) for people living with dementia and carers in different countries in Europe and beyond. They have particular knowledge of the alternative support provided by the meeting centres and how these were experienced by their participants. This is shared in what follows.

2.3 Impact on Meeting Centres for People Affected by Dementia and Their Carers

In normal times, meeting centres provide a comprehensive support programme consisting of person-centred recreative, creative and therapeutic activities for people with dementia in a social club (three days a week) – based in an ordinary community building in order to stimulate social integration -, informative meetings and support groups for their carers, as well as individual consultation and social activities for both (monthly meetings, outings etc.). The meeting centres provide an opportunity for participants to socialize with peers, build friendships, discuss problems, get practical help and emotional support and prepare for the future.

We were impressed by how the meeting centres continued to support people in their communities during the first lockdown, even when it was not possible to meet physically. A survey of meeting centres connected to the MeetingDem Network in different parts of the world (www.meetingdem.eu), conducted during 2020, showed a wide variety of alternative activities were undertaken so as to fulfil the meeting centre aims of supporting people living with dementia in the process of practical, emotional and social adjustments [22] (see Section 2.4).

In the Netherlands, meeting centres continued to support participants at a distance through telephone and video calling, WhatsApp groups, postcards and visiting people at their homes to provide food and treats, activity materials and music making. There were also examples of facilitating people getting out of the house by going on a walk or cycle ride. The strong relationships the meeting centres have built with their participants appeared very important to continue the support at a distance during the lockdown.

Nevertheless, it was clear the more limited support sometimes had a negative impact on the person with dementia (more apathy, agitation, lack of understanding as to why they could not go to the meeting centre) and led to a greater burden on their carers. Many centres also started using tablets and apps for meaningful activities, thus stimulating people to stay active and enjoy themselves at home. Several care organizations and local governments provided funding for this, which helped to stimulate the usage of tablets and apps, while a 'train-the-trainer' course for tablet use for the meeting centres' staff, offered by researchers of the VU University medical centre in Amsterdam (which is specialized in assistive technology for people living with dementia), helped them to effectively assist their participants.

In Spain, the meeting centres provided the carers of people living with dementia with a weekly programme activities guide. They provided all families with a computer and gave those inexperienced with computers instructions on how to use it. They made video calls with the person living with dementia several times a week, during which they talked with them, engaged them in cognitive exercises and had reminiscence therapy sessions.

In addition, they organized video sessions with the caregiver in order to provide guidance with activities and advice on solutions for specific behaviour difficulties and to provide emotional support. They composed different types of infographics to facilitate care, such as: tips for quarantine with a person living with dementia, protection of the carer of a person living with dementia in confinement, an activity routine for the person with cognitive impairment, and behavioural treatments of dementia. Moreover, they

offered participants an activity notebook based on reminiscence that provided continuity to the programme in the video calls but with the participation of the whole family, which was much appreciated.

In Italy, the participants of the meeting centres received information on how to stay active during the lockdown period and a tutorial for music therapy, dance and cognitive stimulation was sent to the participants. In some cases, interventions at home to support carers or the person living with dementia were undertaken. In this way the interaction between participants and staff was maintained and highly appreciated by all.

In Sydney, Australia, the two meeting centres had to close altogether, which affected more than 40 families. As the staff understood the consequences of social isolation and the anticipated additional pressure on family carers they decided to restructure from a group-based level to an individual, one-to-one support for their members and online and telephone support for the carers. This resulted in the new integrated, tailor-made Individual Dementia Support Programme for people with mild to moderate dementia and carers, which was delivered at the home of the person living with dementia and included two weekly visits (one and a half to two hours).

The programme is based on the principles of the MCSP and Individual Cognitive Stimulation Therapy (iCST). Although members of the meeting centres and the staff experienced anxiety in the first couple of weeks, this eased within a short period of time as they all knew each other very well and the clients were very happy to receive a visit and to see a familiar face.

In Singapore, with the required safety measures in place, meeting centres still managed to organize several activities, such as music and movement, discussing photos along with families, current affairs discussion, scrapbooking and workshop and interest groups for carers. They also organized outings, such as a photo contest with a group of members with young-onset dementia. Furthermore, groups of student volunteers engaged the members through activities such as Bingo and exercise over Zoom on a regular basis.

A qualitative study carried out among meeting centres in the UK investigated the extent to which these centres were still able to operate when physical meetings were not possible and how they succeeded in achieving their goals. In the next paragraph we describe the results of this study in more detail from the perspective of support aims and how the adjusted support was experienced by people living with dementia and their family carers.

2.4 Adaptations in the Support Provided to People Living with Dementia by Meeting Centres in the United Kingdom and Their Experiences

In the UK, funding from the National Lottery is currently being utilized to accelerate the number of meeting centres. All meeting centres were prohibited from providing face-to-face support from 23 March to 30 June 2020. Four well-established meeting centres gathered data and provided interviews so as to enable deeper understanding of the challenges faced and how they overcame some of them for the three-month period at the beginning of the pandemic [23].

This study focussed on whether it was possible to provide opportunities that would help people and families adapt to and cope with the challenges dementia brings. All of the features of a meeting centre are geared up to help people make the best emotional, social and practical adjustments to living with dementia. Dröes [24–27] developed the adaptation-coping model as a framework for understanding mood and behaviour difficulties in people with mild to moderate dementia and as a theoretical foundation for psychosocial interventions (see also Chapter 1). Meeting centres have been shown to support this with their usual face-to-face delivery [28]. It is of interest to learn how much this differed when people could no longer meet face to face.

During the first three months of total lockdown, the four meeting centres supported 76 people living with dementia and 72 family carers. The most common contact was via email, telephone and newsletters. There was less dependence on Zoom, WhatsApp and FaceTime initially. Certainly at the beginning of lockdown people either did not have the relevant technology and/or skills to participate virtually. However, all of the meeting centres ran Zoom meetings with more than 100 of these involving both the person living with dementia and the family carer. Around 60 of these Zoom sessions delivered an online activity

of the type usually delivered at the meeting centre. Groups tended to be small, comprising one to five people living with dementia. Seventy Zoom sessions were provided specifically for carers.

2.4.1 Support for Practical Adjustment

Many of the activities at the meeting centre help people to adjust to the cognitive symptoms of dementia and the practicalities of living with dementia. A lot of the activities in newsletters and in Zoom sessions therefore focussed on providing cognitive stimulation. People were encouraged to do activities outside of sessions and/or take photographs for a particular theme such as watching nature in the garden or baking and share them during group sessions. Many group sessions also included short quizzes or singing for people to join in with, much as would be done in a usual face-to-face session.

Keeping physically active was also encouraged through seated exercise in Zoom group sessions alongside items and challenges in newsletters. Outside activities, meeting in gardens for dancing and going for walks were permitted during the summer months, all of which encouraged physical activity. Meeting centre staff were more available on the phone and through email for families to be in contact. Regular contact via telephone calls providing tailored practical information and discussion of problems was particularly appreciated. The calls and newsletters were used to keep people up to date on COVID guidance/rules and plans for reopening, enabling clear, effective and timely communication. The clarity of the information around reopening was particularly appreciated by both carers and members.

2.4.2 Support for Emotional Adjustment

One of the key areas meeting centres work on is helping people to make good emotional adjustment in living with dementia. The newsletters and email contacts often contain ideas for different activities for people to try at home, providing opportunities for people living with dementia and family carers to do something different from their everyday lives and be engaging and fun. The garden visits also provided carers a chance to come out of caring mode for a while. The carer Zoom sessions were also a chance to relax and have fun, as the atmosphere was very relaxed with carers feeling comfortable enough to laugh and joke with each other.

People living with dementia and family carers both had fun with the activities and games during the Zoom group sessions. Singing proved a particular draw with some people living with dementia. An approach that worked well over Zoom was 2–2–1 support with two members of staff engaging the person living with dementia for a chat or a creative activities, with the family caregiver in the background. This facilitated a different type of relationship with this three-way interaction in terms of building confidence and relaxing and having fun as well as the opportunity for the family caregiver to have some time to themselves.

Some people living with dementia and family carers felt isolated and worried about leaving the house. Meeting centre staff were able to provide some reassurance during telephone calls and garden visits to reduce anxiety about the pandemic itself and the specific concerns affecting particular families. Use of Zoom also helped to maintain continuity with familiar faces for when meeting centres would reopen. Three of the meeting centres ran regular online carers meetings, which were highly supportive for family carers. Some carers were not getting a break from caring or support during lockdown and were missing the reassurance that they were not alone in their situation and that they were not the only ones feeling guilty. One caregiver commented:

> You might laugh at this but after we came off of the iPhone, I felt honestly as if I've been out. And I thought, well, I haven't been anywhere, why should I feel like that? But I suppose relaxation and that sort of thing, just talking, listening to other people.

2.4.3 Support for Social Adjustment

Meeting centres in usual times provide lots of social contact. The degree of social contact was undoubtedly more limited through lockdown. Some people living with dementia and family carers had been used to up to four days of contact per week and this was reduced for some to two or three Zoom sessions a week (if they had access to the technology) and a weekly phone call, a newsletter and an email. People had differing levels of contact with family, friends, neighbours, the local community and professionals during

lockdown. For some, the meeting centres staff were a more significant part of the social circle than in normal times. Being able to visit people in their gardens was very useful in terms of providing social interaction and of being able to physically see the people living with dementia and carers. Some people reported high levels of isolation and loneliness. This contact, although limited, provided a real lifeline.

One meeting centre ran hour-long Zoom sessions four days a week and this helped some people living with dementia to recognize each other and stay in touch. Carers also enjoyed seeing everyone during the online sessions and some reported their relationships with other carers had actually grown stronger during carer Zoom sessions. Two of the meeting centres took on much more of a wider community role during lockdown, supporting other organizations working with people with other conditions. Meeting centres were still receiving new referrals during lockdown and the remote support enabled new people living with dementia and family carers to become part of the meeting centre even though they had not actually 'met' anyone or visited the physical premises.

2.5 Lessons Learned

Overall, the worldwide survey among meeting centres and the study among meeting centres conducted in the UK demonstrated the centres could continue to support people affected by dementia to adjust to change during a period when no or limited face-to-face contact was possible. The meeting centres were able to adapt much of what they do in usual circumstances by introducing remote support with continuity and consistency having been maintained to some extent.

However, the study in the UK showed key aspects such as group activities were only open to a minority of attendees and as such the majority were digitally excluded. In some cases, support was enhanced in terms of availability and flexibility as were relationships between family carers and between people living with dementia, family carers and staff, but this was again largely only to the benefit of the minority. Non-technological approaches such as newsletters and garden visits were vital in terms of bridging that gap.

All of this could not prevent the fact that for some people with dementia, the sudden decrease in social activities and contacts with peers they had in the meeting centres had a negative impact on their mental and social health and on the burden on their carers. Also, this level of engagement was only possible because people with dementia and their families had already established strong and trusting relationships with meeting centre staff over a considerable length of time in regular face-to-face activity.

Moving forward, a blended approach using remote and regular meeting centres face-to-face methods means person-centred support could be optimized, reaching those who cannot attend meeting centres, and it could be used in rural areas to address social isolation. This would enable flexibility and consistency should there be future lockdowns. Digital upskilling of meeting centres' staff, people living with dementia, family carers and volunteers is essential not only to mitigate against the impact of a similar lockdown situation in the future but also to help address both social inclusion and digital exclusion in usual times.

3 The Impact of COVID-19 on People Living with Dementia in Nursing Homes

People who live or work in nursing homes are particularly vulnerable to COVID-19 and its consequences [29–31]. The risk of spreading COVID-19 infections is particularly high in long-term care settings [32, 33]. The disease may, for instance, be spread by sharing physical space and bathroom facilities, having physical contact during care provision or caring for those using catheters or who have continence issues. Residents with cognitive impairments may be unable to uphold preventive measures such as social distancing [34]. Moreover, residents are vulnerable to infection due to their overall frailty and immunosuppressive medications [30]. To prevent the spread of COVID-19 and to protect not only residents and their visitors but also staff in nursing homes, during the first lockdown, the Dutch government and other European governments put nursing homes under quarantine from 20 March to 15 June 2020 [35]. This necessitated a visitor ban and restrictions on going outside and participating with others in activities [36]. Also, after the first lockdown, many nursing homes kept restrictive measures in visiting arrangements for residents and their family and friends.

Several studies in Europe and beyond investigated the impact of the measures during the first lockdown on people living with dementia and found negative effects for their psychosocial well-being [3, 37–41]. In this chapter we discuss the results of two of these studies in more detail. Both studies, carried out in the Netherlands, were large-scale surveys focussing on well-being from the perspectives of professionals, care staff, families and residents. Leontjevas et al. [37] studied the views of practitioners (n = 323), including psychologists, elderly care physicians, nurse practitioners, occupational therapists and physiotherapists who are multidisciplinary team members working in Dutch nursing homes. Van der Roest et al. [39, 40] focussed on the perspectives of care staff (n = 811) and family (n = 1,609) and residents without dementia (not included here) in nursing homes and residential care facilities.

Leontjevas et al. [37] contacted professionals through digital networks such as LinkedIn, the Netherlands Institute for Psychologists, Amsterdam University Medical Centre (Department of Medicine for Older People) and the Psychogeriatric Service (a network on expertise in elderly care: www.pgdexpertise.nl). A subsample of practitioners who participated in the survey was subsequently approached by email and interviewed via a video platform. Participants were drawn from all Dutch provinces.

Van der Roest et al. [39, 40] invited 357 long-term care organizations to participate via email. Respondents came from all but one of the Dutch provinces. In this study target group-specific surveys were developed in order to gain insight into the impact of the COVID-19 measures in Dutch nursing homes among several stakeholders, with a focus on social contact with family and friends and on changes in affect (mood and emotions) and behaviour. Respondents were questioned about the current situation and, where relevant, to make comparisons to before the implementation of the visitor ban.

3.1 Changes in Social Contact and Experienced Loneliness

Due to the COVID-19 measures, the social well-being of people living with dementia may have

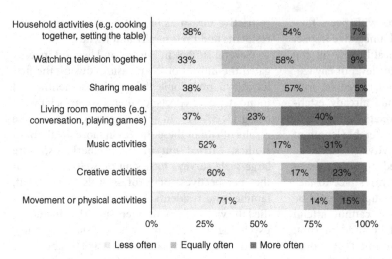

Figure 10.1 Changes in organized activities during the visitor ban as compared with before the visitor ban based on staff reports [39, 40].[1]

been compromised. The absence of face-to-face contact with relatives and the prohibition of meeting others may have resulted in social isolation and loneliness, which may in turn have induced distress behaviour. There was also a considerable decrease in regular group activities such as physical or movement activities, creative activities and music activities for many residents. These types of activities normally stimulate social contacts amongst residents. Because of the difficulty in maintaining social distancing measures among people living with dementia, regular homelike activities such as enjoying a meal together or watching television occurred less frequently.

On the other hand, activities that could be done easily in social areas with sufficient social distancing, such as conversations and playing, were undertaken more frequently during the lockdown as compared to the period before COVID-19 started (see Figure 10.1). Also, alternative music activities were offered more often, such as garden concerts, which were organized outside many facilities for residents to enjoy from inside the facility or from a balcony.

The most common ways to maintain contact with family and friends were via telephone (80%), video calls (62%) or window contact (often with an audio connection) (46%). Despite great efforts by nursing homes to facilitate such contact, not all residents were able to stay in touch with their relatives and friends. For about 20% of the residents, digital communication was not suitable. The reasons for this included the severe level of cognitive impairment, heightened sadness or restlessness provoked by the contact, the inability to understand digital communication or audio-sensory impairment of residents. Staff reported around one in five residents did not have any contact with relatives in the previous four weeks during the lockdown. In addition, 25% of staff reported the new ways of maintaining contact was a barrier for especially spouses, since they also experienced difficulties in utilizing digital means of communication.

In general, the social contacts of residents changed because of the visitor ban. According to relatives of the residents who received visits from grandchildren, siblings, and friends and acquaintances before the visitor ban, one out of three residents had not had any contact with their grandchildren in the four weeks before the survey. Additionally, about 20% of the residents had no contact with siblings, and half had no contact with friends or acquaintances. Residents' social contacts became less varied. Although the average contact frequency of residents via alternative means was comparable with the frequency of visits before the visitor ban, those who had daily visits before the visitor ban had significantly less frequent contact during the visitor ban.

Importantly, there were reports of an increase in cohesion and social connectedness among residents and between care providers and family as this quote illustrates:

[1] Reprinted from J Am Med Dir Assoc., 21(11), Van der Roest HG, Prins M, van der Velden C, Steinmetz S, Stolte E, van Tilburg TG, et al., The impact of COVID-19 measures on well-being of older long-term care facility residents in the Netherlands [Research Letter], p. 1570, Copyright (2020), with permission from Elsevier.

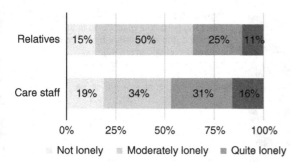

Figure 10.2 Relatives and care staff reports on categories of loneliness of residents during the visitor ban [39, 40].

Solidarity. Residents and the care staff make compliments to each other. They thank each other in words or with a gesture. In some situations, there is now a better relationship [between caregivers and residents] because of mutual understanding.

(Psychologist)

During the lockdown and visitor ban, the majority of residents – more than 80% – were perceived to be lonely by care staff and relatives. However there were differences. Residents with cognitive impairment were less often perceived to be lonely (71%) than residents without cognitive impairment (89%). Nevertheless, when this happened it could have great impact both on the person living with dementia and on the relative. These percentages are much higher and seem contrary to what has been reported in previous research that showed people with dementia in residential care homes generally have less unmet needs for company and people with dementia more often have unmet needs for company than people without dementia (see Figure 10.2) [42].

They say we have to protect the vulnerable elderly. When she does not die from corona, then she will die from grief and loneliness. It is unbearable for me as a daughter. I want to have nice, cosy moments with her as long as she still lives.

(Relative)

It is difficult to make contact with people living with dementia to whom it is not possible to explain that we can't have physical contact. They get emotional because they don't understand it.

(Care staff member)

3.2 Impact on Affect

In general, quarantine is an unpleasant experience that may result in confusion, fear, anger, grief, depressive symptoms and anxiety-induced insomnia [43]. This is also likely for people living with dementia. Research shows social isolation can also increase apathy [3, 44]. Public media information about high numbers of deaths in nursing homes caused by COVID-19 (e.g. [45]) and deaths of fellow residents can amplify sadness, fear and panic reactions [46]. Evidence on mood alterations in people living with dementia during the lockdown is still scarce and mixed, and some anecdotally described, varying from depressed mood, hopelessness and increased suicidal ideation [3].

In the Dutch studies, changes in residents' affect (mood and emotions) were reported by care staff and practitioners as well as the majority of relatives who could remain in contact with the residents. At least half of the staff reported increased severity levels for depression (68%), anxiety (66%) and irritability (65%) in residents within their facility. Furthermore, increases were mentioned in boredom, sleeping problems, apathy, withdrawal and negativity. On the other hand, staff also reported elevated mood and a decrease in sleeping problems in residents.

During the lockdown, many of the relatives also saw negative affect in residents more often than before. This accounted especially for sadness and anger. Positive affect was seen less often: more than half of the relatives noticed the residents were less often happy as compared to when they could physically receive visitors. Despite the high impact of the lockdown on residents' affect, few relatives reported seeing a resident be *more* frequently happy. In addition, some relatives reported improvements, particularly in disinterest, fear and anger. As compared to before the visitor ban, care staff, practitioners and relatives reported in general less negative affect among residents with cognitive impairment than among other residents (see Figure 10.3).

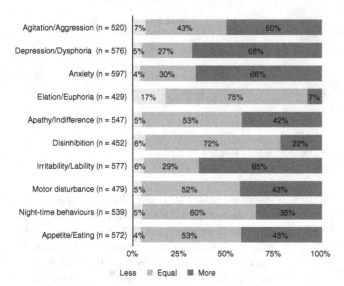

Figure 10.3 Staff perspective on changes in affect and behaviour of residents in their nursing home unit during the visitor ban as compared to before the visitor ban [39, 40].

3.3 Impact on Behaviour

Up to 70–80% of nursing home residents have dementia, while approximately five out of six people living with dementia have behaviour that is challenging for themselves and/or their environment (e.g. agitation, delusions, wandering) [47]. Anti-pandemic measures in nursing homes may accelerate or trigger these behaviours in residents with dementia as they may not understand the necessity of quarantine and may need additional external restrictions that can result in irritability and aggression [44].

Indeed, the two Dutch studies showed more than half of the participants thought restlessness occurred more often in residents during the lockdown. Interestingly, as was the case with affect, almost all practitioners noticed changes in distress behaviour. However, some people appeared less distressed whilst others appeared more so.

> When an increase in distress behaviour is seen, this seems to be due to the disappearance of a regular structure (visits, daytime activities) for some residents.
> *(Psychologist)*

> I noticed that residents on the psychogeriatric unit have become calmer since there are no visitors allowed. There is one resident who always loved to sing but stopped several months ago. Now she has started to sing again.
> *(Care staff member)*

Lastly, newly admitted residents were particularly negatively affected. As their transition from community-based living to institutional living took place under lockdown measures, they could not be adequately supported by their loved ones during this time.

> We got several new residents who came here in crisis. Especially in these new clients I saw more aggression and night-time disturbances.
> *(Care staff member)*

Whilst it is difficult to draw conclusions about cause and effect, the majority of study participants (more than 70%) cited the ban on visitors, being unable to go outside, being unable to leave one's room and the decrease in organized activities as instrumental in changing the mood and behaviour of residents.

3.4 Lessons Learned

In both studies, participants made suggestions for future care based on their experiences during COVID-19. According to several psychologists, a new task for them was to offer (individual) support to nursing staff. They considered this also relevant for the post-pandemic period.

> We became more involved in the well-being of health care providers. We provided individual support and gained a personal connection with them. It is very important to pay attention to their well-being and it should not be forgotten … I noticed that the well-being of health care providers is also important for residents. When [caregivers] radiate happiness, this will be noticed by residents and influence them positively [37].
> *(Psychologist)*

To limit the effects of the lockdown, several strategies had been applied, such as video calls, arranging specific areas where residents could meet their loved ones, adjusting activities to fit with the new regime and limiting exposure to news programmes on TV. The usefulness of electronic communication technologies varied. For some residents these technologies were considered effective, even stimulating more contact than usual with their relatives. However, for many residents with cognitive impairments these technologies proved challenging.

> One resident has a tablet and has used this very frequently to stay in contact with family. Other residents need help to use these devices.
> *(Care staff member)*

> There is a difference between residents with and without cognitive impairment. Residents with cognitive impairment almost always need support in contact with their family. Residents without cognitive impairment can use the telephone independently to call or text their family.
> *(Care staff member)*

The interviewees suggested several strategies that had been applied during the lockdown could be retained in future daily practice (see Box 1).

Suggestions were made for how to reduce the number of stimuli in the future, such as a limit to the number of visitors, volunteers and professionals – especially in shared spaces.

Using the resident's own room for visits instead of the living room was also suggested.

> The fact that an issue can provide both improvement and deterioration is about balance. Before the corona crisis, there were often too many and too long visits, too many volunteers and other people who came to visit, many activities outside the living room. Now there is another extreme, namely no visitors, no volunteers, only activities in the living room. A middle way after the corona crisis is certainly desirable. *(Psychologist)*

Finally, residents, relatives and staff understood the measures but many found them too rigid. It was often reported that residents were not consulted and that their autonomy was compromised over choices within the COVID 19 restrictions. There was a tension between the risk of infection and quality of life. Many residents were thought to prefer visits from loved ones, despite the risk of infection. Yet the dilemma was clear since many residents, relatives and care staff were unable to choose between quality of life and safety. The reality was that with the implementation of the visitor ban, the choice for safety was made for the residents. And because of their disabilities and dependence on the care provided by the facility, residents and their relatives had no choice to escape from or alleviate these measures. Importantly, person-tailored solutions and a partial closure of the nursing home instead of a complete lockdown were suggested in case of future infections.

Box 1 Possible changes in nursing home life

- (More) small-scale activities or activities in small groups
- (More) activities in the living room
- (More) individual activities
- Individual reconsideration of the number of activities offered to a resident
- (Spontaneous) activities outdoors
- (Spontaneous) activities in the hallway
- Digital activities (e.g. physical exercise, virtual excursion, games)
- Social robots or robotic stuffed animals
- Creating environments that are low in stimuli
- Not using corridors for delivery and facility services
- Having specific time slots for deliveries
- Not performing care tasks in the living room
- No visitors in the living room
- Setting up visiting hours

I think we should reconsider the consequences of closing institutions completely and banning visitors. Some residents are very frightened, though others say, 'just allow me to have visitors, even when I become infected' [37].

(Elderly care physician)

You take away the ability from autonomous people to make their own choices about protection of their physical health or their quality of life to protect the other clients. There could have been more tailored measures. *(Care staff member)*

4 Concluding Remarks

In this chapter we focussed on the impact of the COVID-19 pandemic on people living with dementia and their carers both in the community and in nursing homes, and on the impact of the pandemic on the care and support they were provided during the lockdown and the period thereafter. We did not discuss the consequences for people living with dementia in other care settings such as hospitals and psychiatric clinics [48].

From clinical practice and the first scientific studies conducted, it has become clear that the pandemic, especially the social distancing measures, greatly impacted the lives of many people living with dementia both in the community and in residential care settings, resulting in an increase of distress behaviour, such as apathy, anxiety and agitation, albeit with large differences between individuals. Many activities were undertaken by professional caregivers in the community to stay in touch with their clients and to provide them at a distance with, for example, meaningful activities, and to also provide telephone and/or video call support to their families [3].

Evidence for the benefits of video conferencing in addition to telephone calls, resulting in improved resilience and well-being both for persons with dementia and family carers already after four weeks, were shown in a study of Lai et al. [49]. They suggest telehealth should therefore be considered beyond the context of the pandemic. Also in residential care settings various activities were undertaken to compensate for the social distancing and social isolation, to provide people with meaningful activities and to support them staying in touch with their families on a distance. Nevertheless, despite all of these activities it was clear that, in practice, the actual support provided was much

less than people were used to. Also, when most community-based services such as day care centres and meeting centres restarted after the lockdown many restrictions were in place. This of course not only impacted the people with dementia but also their family carers.

Because of the enormous impact of the social isolation on the well-being of nursing home residents during the first lockdown, a guideline to cautiously open nursing homes for visitors during the COVID-19 pandemic was developed in the Netherlands. First findings on a study into the application of this guideline in 26 nursing homes showed compliance to local measures based on the guideline was sufficient to good, all nursing homes noticed the added value of real and personal contact between residents and their loved ones and indicated a positive impact on well-being, and no new COVID-19 infections were reported [36].

Partly based on these study results, the Dutch government decided to allow all nursing homes in the Netherlands to cautiously open their homes again using the guideline (see Box 2). In other countries, such as the UK [50] and Belgium [51], comparable guidelines have been developed. The dilemma between complete social isolation and less risk of infection on one hand, and maintaining social contact and thus quality of life but with more risk of infection on the other, painfully imposed itself on care, especially during the first lockdown. This was the case not only in nursing homes and hospitals, where the risk of infection and mortality was high, but also in group-oriented activities for people with dementia living at home, which aim to maintain the social health of people living with dementia and their family carers. The lessons learned during the COVID-19 pandemic, especially during the first and following lockdowns in 2020 and thereafter, hopefully will prevent such extreme restrictive measures from being taken again.

Although there may be an ethical and legal basis for social isolation, the potential for unintended harm with such interventions is high, especially when there is little guidance on how to keep people with dementia in social isolation while preserving their human dignity and personhood [34]. Training of care staff, implementing appropriate guidelines and taking into account the lessons learned, including suggestions from professional caregivers to maintain some of the changes in nursing home life based on the

---

Box 2 Elements from the first Dutch Guideline for Visitation in Nursing Homes During COVID-19 [36]

Preconditions for visitors
- Make agreements with the nursing home on frequency and duration of the visit
- One designated visitor is allowed per resident
- Take personal hygiene measures (use of hand sanitizer at entrance, temperature check)
- Visitors are spread throughout the day and week
- Visits take place at least 1.5 meters (i.e. 5 feet) distance, including from staff and other residents
- Visitors should be free from COVID-19 symptoms
- Visitors are obliged to wear a protective mouth mask for visiting residents who are difficult to instruct (e.g. people with dementia)

Preconditions for organizations
- Should observe the regulations and keep in perspective the well-being of residents and family
- Sufficient personal protective equipment, thermometer assessment and appropriate application of this
- Strict hygiene protocol
- Sufficient staffing
- Sufficient test capacity by Local Health Authority

---

experiences during the pandemic, are therefore of utmost importance.

Of course, only large-scale vaccinations started worldwide in the spring of 2021, and giving priority to residents of residential care settings will provide the prospect of the protection needed to fully resume group-oriented and social activities for people with dementia and to bring the quality of care back to the level it was before the introduction of the coronavirus, and perhaps even to a higher level thanks to the lessons learned. The virus has taught us what the essence of good care is. Social contact really matters, also for people with dementia, and with creativity, cooperation and initiative alternative ways of good care and support can be used to achieve this.

References

1. Alzheimer Europe. *Dementia in Europe Magazine: The Alzheimer Europe Magazine*. 2021 Feb;**35**. Luxembourg. Alzheimer Europe Office. www.alzheimer-europe.org/Publications/Dementia-in-Europe-magazines. (Accessed 15 March 2021)

2. Tilvis RS, Routasalo P, Karppinen H, Strandberg TE, Kautiainen H, Pitkala KH. Social isolation, social activity and loneliness as survival indicators in old age: A nationwide survey with a 7-year follow-up. *Eur Geriatr Med.* 2012; **3**: 18–22.

3. Simonetti A, Pais C, Jones M, Cipriani MC, Janiri D, Monti L, et al. Neuropsychiatric symptoms in elderly with dementia during COVID-19 pandemic: Definition, treatment, and future directions. *Front Psychiatry* 2020; **11**: 579842.

4. Roach P, Zwiers A, Cox E, Fischer K, Charlton A, Josephson CB, et al. Understanding the impact of the COVID-19 pandemic on well-being and virtual care for people living with dementia and care partners living in the community. *Dementia* (London) 2021 Jan 1; **20**(6): 2007–23. 1471301220977639

5. Thyrian JR, Kracht F, Nikelski A, Boekholt M, Schumacher-Schonert F, Radke A, et al. The situation of elderly with cognitive impairment living at home during lockdown in the corona-pandemic in Germany. *BMC Geriatr.* 2020 Dec 29; **20**: 540.

6. Van der Heide I, de Veer A, van den Buuse S, Francke AL. *Dementiemonitor mantelzorg*. Utrecht, Nivel, 2020. www.nivel.nl/en/project/dementiemonitor-mantelzorg-2020. Dutch. (Accessed 15 March 2021)

7. Huber M, Knottnerus JA, Green L, van der Horst H, Jadad AR, Kromhout D, et al. How should we define health? *BMJ* 2011 Jul 26; **343**:d4163.

8. Dröes RM, Chattat R, Diaz A, Gove D, Graff M, Murphy K, et al. Social health and dementia: A European consensus on the operationalization of the concept and directions for research and practice. *Aging Ment Health* 2017 Jan; **21**(1): 4–17.

9. Miranda-Castillo C, Woods B, Galboda K, Oomman S, Olojugba C, Orrell M. Unmet needs, quality of life and support networks of people with dementia living at home. *Health Qual Life Outcomes* 2010 Nov 12; **8**: 132.

10. Van der Roest HG, Meiland FJ, Comijs HC, Derksen E, Jansen AP, van Hout HP, et al. What do community-dwelling people with dementia need? A survey of those who are known to care and welfare services. *Int Psychogeriatr*. 2009 Oct; **21**(5): 949–65.

11. Cohen G, Russo MJ, Campos JA, Allegri RF. COVID-19 epidemic in Argentina: Worsening of behavioral symptoms in elderly subjects with dementia living in the community. *Front Psychiatry* 2020; **11**: 866.

12. Van der Heide I, van den Buuse S, Francke AL. *Dementiemonitor mantelzorg*. Utrecht, Nivel; 2018. www.nivel.nl/nl/nieuws/dementiemonitor-mantelzorg-2018-de-uitkomsten. Dutch. (Accessed 15 March 2021)

13. Van Maurik IS, Bakker ED, van den Buuse S, Gillissen F, van de Beek M, Lemstra E, et al. Psychosocial effects of corona measures on patients with dementia, mild cognitive impairment and subjective cognitive decline. *Front Psychiatry* 2020; **11**: 585686.

14. Pongan E, Dorey JM, Borg C, Getenet JC, Bachelet R, Lourioux C, et al. COVID-19: Association between increase of behavioral and psychological symptoms of dementia during lockdown and caregivers' poor mental health. *J Alzheimers Dis*. 2021 Feb 23. Epub ahead of print.

15. Morrisby C, Joosten A, Ciccarelli M. Do services meet the needs of people with dementia and carers living in the community? A scoping review of the international literature. *Int Psychogeriatr*. 2018 Jan; **30**(1): 5–14.

16. Alzheimer's Research UK. Dementia Statistics Hub 2020. Cambridge: Alzheimer's Research UK. www.dementiastatistics.org/statistics/impact-on-carers. (Accessed 15 March 2021)

17. Lindeza P, Rodrigues M, Costa J, Guerreiro M, Rosa MM. Impact of dementia on informal care: A systematic review of family caregivers' perceptions. *BMJ Support Palliat Care* 2020 Oct 14. bmjspcare-2020–002242. Epub ahead of print.

18. Wilson RS, Krueger KR, Arnold SE, Schneider JA, Kelly JF, Barnes LL, et al. Loneliness and risk of Alzheimer disease. *Arch Gen Psychiatry* 2007 Feb; **64**(2): 234–40.

19. Courtin E, Knapp M. Social isolation, loneliness and health in old age: A scoping review. *Health Soc Care Community* 2017 May; **25**(3): 799–812.

20. National Academies of Sciences Engineering and Medicine. *Social Isolation and Loneliness in Older Adults: Opportunities for the Health Care System*. Washington, DC, National Academies Press, 2020.

21. Tretteteig S, Vatne S, Rokstad AM. The influence of day care centres designed for people with dementia on family caregivers: A qualitative study. *BMC Geriatr*. 2017 Jan 5; **17**(1): 5.

22. MeetingDem Network. *Newsletter December 2020*. Amsterdam, Department of Psychiatry, VU University Medical Center, 2020.

23. Evans SB, Bray J, Brooker D. How Meeting Centres continue to support people affected by dementia: Report on UK COVID-19 impact. *Working with Older People* 2021; **25**(4): 283–93.

24. Dröes RM. *In Beweging, over psychosociale hulpverlening aan demente ouderen*. Academic thesis. VU University, Amsterdam. Nijkerk, Intro, 1991. Dutch.

25. Dröes RM, Breebaart E, Ettema TP, van Tilburg W, Mellenbergh GJ. Effect of integrated family support versus day care only on behavior and mood of patients with dementia. *Int Psychogeriatr*. 2000 Mar; **12**(1): 99–115.

26. Dröes RM, Meiland FJM, van Tilburg W. The Meeting Centres Support Programme for persons with dementia and their carers: From development to implementation. In Miesen B, Jones G, eds. *Caregiving in Dementia IV*. London, Routledge, 2006; 315–39.

27. Dröes RM, van Mierlo LD, van der Roest HG, Meiland FJM. Focus and effectiveness of psychosocial interventions for people with dementia in institutional care settings from the perspective of coping with the disease. *Non-pharmacological Therapies in Dementia* 2010; **1**(2): 139–61.

28. Brooker D, Droes R, Evans SB. Framing outcomes of post-diagnostic psychosocial interventions in dementia: The adaptation-coping model and adjusting to change. *Work Older People* 2017; **21**(1): 13–21.

29. Danis K, Fonteneau L, Georges S, Daniau C, Bernard-Stoecklin S, Domegan L, et al. High impact of COVID-19 in long-term care facilities, suggestion for monitoring in the EU/EEA, May 2020. *Euro Surveill*. 2020 Jun; **25**(22). pii=2000956.

30. Dichter MN, Sander M, Seismann-Petersen S, Kopke S. COVID-19: It is time to balance infection management and person-centered care to maintain mental health of people living in German nursing homes. *Int Psychogeriatr*. 2020 Oct; **32**(10): 1157–60.

31. Wang L, He W, Yu X, Hu D, Bao M, Liu H, et al. Coronavirus disease 2019 in elderly patients:

Characteristics and prognostic factors based on 4-week follow-up. *J Infect.* 2020 Jun; **80**(6): 639–45.

32. Ayalon L, Zisberg A, Cohn-Schwartz E, Cohen-Mansfield J, Perel-Levin S, Bar Asher-Sigal E. Long term care settings in the times of COVID-19: Challenges and future directions. *Int Psychogeriatr.* 2020 Jul; 1: 1–14. www.ncbi.nlm.nih.gov/pmc/articles/PMC7373829. (Accessed 15 March 2021)

33. Gardner W, States D, Bagley N. The coronavirus and the risks to the elderly in long-term care. *J Aging Soc Policy* 2020 Jul–Oct; **32**(4–5): 310–15.

34. Laboni A, Cockburn A, Marcil, M, Rodrigues, K, Marshall, C, Garcia, MA, et al. Achieving safe, effective, and compassionate quarantine or isolation of older adults with dementia in nursing homes. *Am J Geriatr Psychiatry.* 2020; **28**(8): 835–8.

35. Kruse F, Abma I, Jeurissen P. The impact of COVID-19 on long-term care in the Netherlands. LTCcovid, International Long-Term Care Policy Network, CPEC-LSE. 2020 May 26; https://ltccovid.org/wp-content/uploads/2020/05/COVID19-Long-Term-Care-situation-in-the-Netherlands-25-May-2020-1.pdf. (Accessed 15 March 2021)

36. Verbeek H, Gerritsen DL, Backhaus R, de Boer BS, Koopmans R, Hamers JPH. Allowing visitors back in the nursing home during the COVID-19 crisis: A Dutch national study into first experiences and impact on well-being. *J Am Med Dir Assoc.* 2020 Jul; **21**(7): 900–4.

37. Leontjevas R, Knippenberg IAH, Smalbrugge M, Plouvier AOA, Teunisse S, Bakker C, et al. Challenging behavior of nursing home residents during COVID-19 measures in the Netherlands. *Aging Ment Health* 2020 Dec; 9: 1–6.

38. O'Caoimh R, O'Donovan MR, Monahan MP, Dalton O'Connor C, Buckley C, Kilty C, et al. Psychosocial impact of COVID-19 nursing home restrictions on visitors of residents with cognitive impairment: A cross-sectional study as part of the Engaging Remotely in Care (ERiC) Project. *Front Psychiatry* 2020; **11**: 585373.

39. Van der Roest HG, Prins M, van der Velden C, Steinmetz S, Stolte E, van Tilburg TG, et al. The impact of COVID-19 measures on well-being of older long-term care facility residents in the Netherlands [Research Letter]. *J Am Med Dir Assoc.* 2020 Sep 10; **21**(11): 1569.

40. Van der Roest HG, Prins M, van der Velden C, Steinmetz S, Stolte E, van Tilburg TG, et al. *De impact van sociale isolatie onder bewoners van verpleeg- en verzorgingshuizen ten tijde van het nieuwe coronavirus.* Utrecht: Trimbos-instituut, 2020. www.trimbos.nl/aanbod/webwinkel/product/af1789-de-impact-van-sociale-isolatie-onder-bewoners-van-verpleeg-en-verzorgingshuizen-ten-tijde-van-het-nieuwe-coronavirus. Dutch. (Accessed 15 March 2021)

41. Benzinger P, Kuru S, Keilhauer A, Hoch J, Prestel P, Bauer JM, et al. [Psychosocial effects of the pandemic on staff and residents of nursing homes as well as their relatives: A systematic review]. *Z Gerontol Geriatr.* 2021; **23**: 1–5. German.

42. Van der Ploeg ES, Bax D, Boorsma M, Nijpels G, van Hout HP. A cross-sectional study to compare care needs of individuals with and without dementia in residential homes in the Netherlands. *BMC Geriatr.* 2013 May 24; **13**: 51.

43. Brooks SK, Webster RK, Smith LE, Woodland L, Wessely S, Greenberg N, et al. The psychological impact of quarantine and how to reduce it: Rapid review of the evidence. *Lancet.* 2020 Mar 14; **395**(10227): 912–20.

44. Gerritsen DL, Oude Voshaar RC. The effects of the COVID-19 virus on mental healthcare for older people in the Netherlands. *Int Psychogeriatr.* 2020 Jun 3; 1–4. www.ncbi.nlm.nih.gov/pmc/articles/PMC7300185. (Accessed 15 March 2021)

45. Klomp C, van Houwelingen H, van der Mee T. Sterfte onder bewoners verpleeghuizen en instellingen bijna verdubbeld. *Algemeen Dagblad.* 2020. www.ad.nl/binnenland/sterfte-onder-bewoners-verpleeghuizen-en-instellingen-bijna-verdubbeld~a5c411d2. Dutch. (Accessed 15 March 2021)

46. Dubey S, Biswas P, Ghosh R, Chatterjee S, Dubey MJ, Chatterjee S, et al. Psychosocial impact of COVID-19. *Diabetes Metab Syndr.* 2020 May 27; **14**(5):779–88.

47. Abraha I, Rimland JM, Trotta FM, Dell'Aquila G, Cruz-Jentoft A, Petrovic M, et al. Systematic review of systematic reviews of non-pharmacological interventions to treat behavioural disturbances in older patients with dementia: The SENATOR-OnTop series. *BMJ Open* 2017 Mar 16; **7**(3): e012759.

48. Livingston G, Rostamipour H, Gallagher P, Kalafatis C, Shastri A, Huzzey L, et al. Prevalence, management, and outcomes of SARS-CoV-2 infections in older people and those with dementia in mental health wards in London, UK: A retrospective observational study. *Lancet Psych.* 2020 Dec; **7**(12): 1054–63.

49. Lai FH, Yan EW, Yu KK, Tsui WS, Chan DT, Yee BK. The protective impact of telemedicine on persons with dementia and their caregivers during the COVID-19 pandemic. *Am J Geriatr Psychiatry* 2020 Nov; **28**(11): 1175–84.

50. British Geriatrics Society. *COVID-19: Managing the COVID-19 Pandemic in Care Homes for Older People*. London, British Geriatrics Society, 2020. www.bgs.org.uk/resources/covid-19-managing-the-covid-19-pandemic-in-care-homes. (Accessed 15 March 2021)

51. Agentschap Zorg en Gezondheid. *Algemene principes voor de bezoekregeling in woonzorgcentra, centra voor kort verblijf type-1, centra voor herstelverblijf en groepen van assistentiewoningen en serviceflatgebouwen infrastructureel gelinkt aan een woonzorgcentrum*. Brussels, Vlaamse overheid, 2020. www.zorg-en-gezondheid.be/sites/default/files/atoms/files/kaderrichtlijn_bezoek_WZC_sjabloonVAZG_metlinksdef(003).pdf.Dutch. (Accessed 15 March 2021)

My Brother's Eyes

Pia Tafdrup

– You're not going to kill me, are you?
says my father.
With my brother I wait
for my mother and sister
behind the shockwave's seconds.
My father sits in the chair of the crater,
                        stone cold.
I have lifted his feet up
on my knees
try with my hands
to rub them warm
under the threadbare hospital socks.
We look at each other,
           my ten years younger brother and I.
Bone-dry silence.
What is there to say to that question
that is boring its way
from misty atmospheres?
My father is dressed in the hospital's
chemical white clothes.
My brother's eyes
          are blue, blue.
And then filled with tears:
Total kidney failure combined
with more or less
total memory loss
          produces an astronomical sum
which does not offer the best prospects.
Should we follow my father's will
from a proud moment?
Avoid life-prolonging treatment?
– It's not difficult, says the doctor,
he's already decided for you...
Each year my father's fields bore new stones
fallen from the sky
or sprung up from the earth
          like flowers sown without plan.
We try to listen,
then decide to follow my father's wish
from long ago –
       but isn't that going to kill him?

'My Brother's Eyes' by Pia Tafdrup, *from* Tarkovsky's Horses and Other Poems, *trans. David McDuff (Bloodaxe Books, 2009). Reproduced with permission of Bloodaxe Books.*

Care Planning and the Lived Experience of Dementia

Establishing Real Will and Preferences beyond Mental Capacity

Tim Opgenhaffen, Johan Put, Jan De Lepeleire, John Keady and Aagje Swinnen

1 Introduction

In the journey of a person who lives with dementia, decision-making requires special attention as it no longer becomes self-evident. The decrease of mental capacity impacts both the ability to take decisions of any kind and the ability to participate in the decision-making process. Legal and medical disciplines traditionally apply a cognitive approach and rely on 'mental capacity' as the main criterion for decision-making. This criterion makes high demands regarding autonomous decision-making. Once beyond the point of mental incapacity, actual expression of will of a person who lives with dementia is often deemed unreliable, so that in everyday life others decide for the person.

For many years this cognitive approach has been criticized by adherents of the social model of disability; mental capacity is considered too demanding and the will of those who lack mental capacity is insufficiently protected [1]. The cognitive approach should make way for a broader and more versatile approach with a focus on advance care planning (ACP), supported decision-making, a policy based on values and emotions [2, 3], goal setting [4] and needs and preferences.

In 2006, this criticism and the proposed shift was supported by the UN Convention on the Rights of Persons with Disabilities (CRPD). Article 12 of the CRPD promotes a right for persons with disabilities to take decisions on an equal basis with others. As such, this levelling of the playing field has the potential to cause a paradigm shift [5, 6, 7] as, if fully implemented, this binding right has a massive impact on decision-making and people living with

dementia. The ultimate aim of Article 12 CRPD is to do more justice to the will and autonomy of a person who lives with dementia; to respect autonomy, even when cognitive abilities decline. However, the transposition of this right into a practice that is workable and provides adequate protection against abuse is presently not self-evident [8–10].

While most will agree that being recognized as a decision maker is a part of human dignity, it is not fully clear how to implement this in the lives of a person who lives with dementia. The implementation of Article 12 CRPD indeed raises many questions, especially on how to think beyond the cognitive approach and substituted decisions. Even if the CRPD brought about a paradigm shift, it may not cause a revolution as there is no clear-cut answer ready to be implemented. Instead, dozens of potentially useful new and yet-existing approaches are to be evaluated and pieced together.

In this exploratory contribution we aim to outline two promising, yet-existing approaches in dementia care, and examine whether they could be part of a solution on decision-making with dementia: firstly, advance care plans and secondly, holistic hermeneutic and 'in the moment' frameworks to understand the lived experiences of persons with dementia. To do so, we first elaborate on the approach of Article 12 CRPD and its challenges. Secondly the potential of ACP is discussed. Thirdly, we reflect on whether such holistic hermeneutic and 'in the moment' frameworks could be applied to discover a person living with dementia's real will and preferences.

2 Article 12 of the Convention on the Rights of Persons with Disabilities and Its impact on Decision-Making with Dementia

2.1 The Traditional Approach to Decision-Making with Dementia

Traditionally, care planning and participation go hand in hand with autonomous decision-making and a capacity-based approach to dementia. Whether a person who lives with dementia may autonomously decide on their treatment and care depends on whether they have the mental capacity to do so. Autonomous decision-making requires the ability to understand the given information, to reason that information, to value that information and finally to express a choice [11–15].

Whether current expressions are considered a person's real will depends on a person who lives with dementia's mental capacity. Mental capacity is key to decision-making and the main criterion for legal capacity. Those who lack mental capacity should not be recognized as decision makers, but have to be protected instead, for example by a legal representative [16, 17]. It is commonly accepted that this representative should intervene as little as possible, that they should take into account the interests of the person who lives with dementia as much as possible and that they should act in accordance with what the person who lives with dementia would have wanted. Yet mental incapacity leaves a person who lives with dementia legally incapacitated and dependent on others.

Despite clear theoretical criteria, the distinction between mental capacity and mental incapacity is a minefield in practice. It is full of blurred lines, room for misinterpretation, and under- and overprotection. Moreover, since the 1990s there is a tendency to question the purely rational approach to mental capacity. As humans are not only rational but also emotional beings, a role was sought for emotions when assessing mental capacity [18, 19]. Yet, even then, mental and legal capacity remain communicating vessels.

2.2 The Convention on the Rights of Persons with Disabilities as a Paradigm Shift

The capacity-based model on decision-making with dementia is radically questioned by the social model of disability and the CRPD. In this convention, persons with disabilities include those who have long-term physical, mental, intellectual or sensory impairments which, in interaction with various barriers, may hinder their full and effective participation in society on an equal basis with others (Article 1 CRPD). As disability is approached broadly, it is generally accepted that this convention applies to most – if not all – persons who live with dementia [20, 21].

Article 12 CRPD requires persons who live with dementia to be equally recognized before the law. This implies not only that they *have* the same rights as others but also that they may execute them in the same way [22]. This requires that persons who live with dementia are recognized as decision makers (Article 12.1 CRPD) and that they may exercise their right to take decisions in the same way as others (Articles 12.2 and 12.5 CRPD). That a person has dementia is in itself no justification for a difference in treatment. It is up to the CRPD member states to support persons who live with dementia when taking decisions (Article 12.3 CRPD) and to protect them against abuse (Article 12.4 CRPD).

That the CRPD strives for equal recognition of persons who live with dementia as decision makers is not surprising given its normative point of departure. The CRPD endorses the social model of disability. According to this model, a disability is not an impairment that can be medically assessed and responded to. Instead, a disability results from the inaptness of society to adapt to an impairment. The social model strives to remove barriers that stand in the way of societal participation. Not being allowed to take decisions because society believes mental capacity should be the criterion for legal capacity is such a barrier [23, 24].

In the logic of the CRPD, especially as it is interpreted by the United Nations Committee on the Rights of Persons with Disabilities (CRPD Committee), a disability does not bring about insurmountable internal barriers. For the CRPD Committee, support can solve anything. Doing so, the CRPD Committee radicalizes the principles of the biopsychosocial approach to disability. These principles itself though are not new; in 2001 the World Health Organization had already put forward that healthcare and social care should consider citizens as individuals with a right to a maximal participation. This was published as the 'International Classification of Functioning' (ICF) [25]. Welfare and healthcare have to mention that both environmental and personal elements influence the impact of dysfunctions, activities and participation in general.

2.3 Disentangling Legal from Mental Capacity: What Next?

According to the CRPD, legal capacity must be disentangled from mental capacity. The traditional cognitive approach to decision-making has a discriminatory effect, as it disproportionately affects persons with psychosocial disabilities [22]. In a way, for the CRPD, it is comparable, for example, to physical barriers wheelchair users have to deal with to access buildings or shops that have stepped entrances [23]. Like wheelchair users, persons who live with dementia should be supported to get over this barrier. Nevertheless, despite best intentions, in the Western context where power and language are deeply entwined, this comparison is flawed insofar as the ability of people who live with dementia to express themselves through language is part of the consequences of the condition [26].

According to the CRPD Committee, legal capacity must not be based on mental capacity but must be based instead on a person who lives with dementia's 'will and preferences'. As the underlying rationale is that anyone in any situation has a will and preferences, the CRPD Committee claims that anyone in any situation should have the legal capacity to decide for themselves [27]. Persons who live with dementia may be supported in exercising this legal capacity, but may not be substituted [22].

The CRPD Committee's approach is misunderstood by many, mainly due to its vagueness. Some believe that, according to the CRPD Committee, every preference should be respected. Others state that as substituted decision-making is prohibited, persons who live with dementia will be abandoned to their fate [8, 28, 29]. This raises a number of questions. What to do, for example,

with a person who lives with dementia physically and verbally refusing to take a bath? Must we abolish the door secured with a numeric code that prevents persons who live with dementia from leaving a care home? If legal incapacity may no longer be based on mental capacity, and if the will and preferences of a person who lives with dementia may no longer be set aside by a substituted decision of a medical professional, a guardian or a family member, how can we achieve a fair balance between autonomy and protection? Similarly, how do we enhance autonomous and reliable decision-making (even) when mental competences are affected, without losing sight of the vulnerability of persons who live with dementia?

Although neither the CRPD nor the CRPD Committee gives a comprehensive answer, part of these questions and the criticism that come along with them are based on misconceptions. First, not every preference should lead to a valid decision. A 'real' will is still needed [5, 29, 30]. Really wanting, however, no longer fully depends on the ability to understand and appreciate. Also, beyond mental capacity there is a real will, yet support of others is needed to retrieve and communicate it. Here, there is a role for communication tools and decision aids (infra).

Second, the CRPD has a broad understanding of support. In severe stages of dementia support goes as far as what we traditionally consider substitute decision-making: a third party deciding for a person who lives with dementia. For the CRPD Committee, this is support and not substituted decision as long as the surrogate translates the 'real' will of a person who lives with dementia (what they would have wanted) into a decision.

Third, as long as a decision is in agreement with a person who lives with dementia's 'real' will, one has legal capacity. Legal incapacity only arises from the moment a decision does not reflect a person's real will, which, according to the CRPD Committee, is prohibited if there is a direct or indirect link with dementia [17].

That the critique on the CRPD Committee is partly based on misconceptions does not mean its approach is unproblematic. We do not aim to list all problems raised by the CRPD approach. Instead, we share one very clear example: even if the link between mental capacity testing and decision-making would be cut, it is hard to see how to avoid third-party interference. If the basic assumption is that a decision should be based on a real will, a third-party judgement is unavoidable. Even though this judgement does not need to be a mental capacity test, every alternative to it is a comparable interference. One could of course step away from the assumption that a decision should reflect a person's real will. Yet then it is hard to see how persons who live with dementia can still take decisions in later stages of the disease and how they can still be protected. This relates to a more general critique that the CRPD Committee pays little attention to the protection of persons who live with dementia against unjust interferences.

2.4 The Convention on the Rights of Persons with Disabilities as an Opportunity?

Despite the important open questions that remain, a major virtue of the CRPD today is that having a will is an inherent part of being human and that being recognized as a decision maker is part of human dignity. It is indeed true that everyday expressions might be easily neglected *because* a person has dementia or lacks mental capacity ('What am I doing here?' 'Has it been good?'), or might be set aside because expression leads to a result that is deemed undesirable. Article 12 CRPD needs much more research, debate and legislative changes to be fully operational.

In this chapter it is not our aim to solve all the challenges and problems posed by the CRPD, nor to defend the most radical approach of the CRPD Committee. Instead, we want to reflect on to what extent two promising ways of dealing with dementia we already know today are apt to do justice to a person who lives with dementia's 'real will'. First, we look at ACP. As a process that foreshadows future choices it has major potential within a CRPD-based model. Second, we shift to a somewhat less self-evident practice; dementia care literature's increasing quests for frameworks to understand the lived experiences of persons living with dementia. By looking at both a holistic hermeneutic approach and an 'in the moment' frame, we question whether these frameworks currently applied for understanding lived experiences of persons living with dementia could be applied to disclose a person's real will and can therewith be a footing for decision-making.

3 Planning Care in Advance

3.1 The Process: Advance Care Planning

Looking for opportunities to uncover the real will of persons living with dementia, we first deal with ACP. The process of ACP has to be embedded in the whole diagnostic journey we made explicit in Textbox 1. According to the CRPD Committee, 'the ability to plan in advance is an important form of support whereby they can state their will and preferences which should be followed at a time when they may not be in a position to communicate their wishes to others' [22].

Advance care planning enables individuals to define goals and preferences for future medical treatment and care, to discuss these goals and preferences with family and healthcare providers and to record and review these preferences if appropriate [45]. Advance care planning is a phased process started by healthcare professionals, without forcing the patient and his environment, based on a respectful, personalized attitude. It is a continuous process initiated by professionals who in an interdisciplinary way can take part in that process. Rather than phases or steps, eight domains have to be covered (see Textbox 2).

Advance care planning takes time. Furthermore, it assumes a continuing, personalized, therapeutic relationship and excellent communication skills. It also requires good notifications in the (electronic) patient data file in a way other healthcare professionals understand what the real content and context was. Advanced directives (AD), eventually a 'Do Not Resuscitate' code (DNR) and other documents can be some of the 'results' of ACP, but are ultimately not sufficient.

Advance care planning in dementia is not self-evident. However, in general a systematic review demonstrated its positive effect [46]. Advance care planning was often found to decrease life-sustaining treatment, increase use of hospice and palliative care and prevent hospitalization. Complex ACP interventions seem to increase compliance with patients' end-of-life wishes. Nonetheless, findings underscore both the challenge and need to find ways to routinely incorporate ACP in clinical settings where multiple and competing demands impact practice. Interventions most likely to meet with success

Textbox 1 Diagnosing Dementia as the Key to Advance Care Planning and Decision Aids

'Diagnosing Dementia, No Easy Job' was the title of a paper explaining that this diagnosis is a stepwise process [31]. The first step is the growing suspicion of an upcoming cognitive problem, hampered by many pitfalls, like stigma negative framing and the assumption that people with dementia are unable to take meaningful decisions [32–34]. The negative stigma that surrounds 'losing your mind' is for patients, their carers and professionals an important barrier to think about and to bring it into the consultation [33].

In the second step, the suspicion leads to exploration by the general practitioner (GP). According to recent national and international guidelines, the GP can explore the situation of the patient and his context with an important attention for the global and actual functioning [35]. This is in accordance with the ICF. A cognitive assessment will be performed, for example, using the Mini Mental State Examination or equivalent instruments [36]. A low cognitive performance should always prompt a thorough examination by a specialist. As long as these tests have no impact on the patient's legal capacity (i.e. whether their decisions are still recognized) there is no CRPD inconformity.

In the third step, confirmation is sought by involving a specialist. An in-depth examination is important, not only to value the non-pharmacological and pharmacological treatment options but also exclude treatable conditions causing cognitive disturbance and to get insight into the reactions and performance of the patient.

However, apart from the fact that incipient symptoms of dementia can be caused by treatable conditions like depression, a diagnosis is a facilitator for care planning. Actually and according to guidelines, disclosing a diagnosis of dementia is a crucial step in the process of care planning [37–39]. Getting grip on a person's will and preferences in early stage of dementia through care planning is moreover essential given the CRPD Committee's approach to legal capacity. As a consequence, the diagnosis is not a finishing point but a starting point: post-diagnostic care is essential for coping with dementia and is the gateway to ACP [40–44].

Textbox 2 Recommendations (adapted from Piers et al. [52])

Domain 1 Initiation of Advance Care Planning

1. Start ACP as early as possible and integrate ACP into the daily care of people living with dementia. Specific key moments might be:
   a. the period around the diagnosis of dementia
   b. when discussing the general care plan
   c. when changes occur in the health status, place of residence or financial situation
2. Be alert for triggers and opportunities to start ACP and make use of any opportunity to talk about ACP.
3. The healthcare professional should initiate ACP conversations if the person living with dementia and/or those close to them do not do this themselves.
4. Consider the person as an individual and consider their specific situation when starting ACP conversation.

Domain 2 Evaluation of Mental Capacity

5. Always assume maximal mental capacity.
6. Consider mental capacity as a fluctuating rather than a static condition and stay alert for signs of loss of capacity.
7. Judge mental capacity tasks specifically – that is, for a certain decision at a particular moment in time.
8. Always stay in contact with the person him/herself and ensure his/her maximum participation.
9. Assess mental capacity through formal clinical assessment:
   a. where there is doubt or disagreement between healthcare professionals and/or family
   b. when the decisions can have far-reaching consequences
   c. preferably by a multidisciplinary or interdisciplinary team with experience in dementia

Domain 3 Performing Advance Care Conversations

10. Adjust conversation style and content to the person's level and rhythm.

11. Explore who the significant people in their life are and who can be involved in the ACP conversations, and explore who can become their legal representative.

12. Lead the conversation but do not force it to become too formulaic or phased.

13. Explore the person's disease awareness and their expectations, ideas and possible misconceptions concerning the disease trajectory.

14. Where someone lacks disease awareness or is reluctant to talk about ACP, do not insist.

15. Advance care planning conversations can best be held on several occasions and over a longer period of time and cover several different topics such as the broader values of the person, his/her experience of the present and fears about the future and the end of life, future care goals, specific advance decisions about the end of life and advance directives.

16. Try to understand the whole person living with dementia; explore his/her life story, important values, norms, beliefs and preferences.

17. Explore the person's current experiences; ask what is the perception of the person living with dementia of his or her own quality of life? What are his/her fears and concerns?

18. Explore the person's fears and concerns for the future and for the end of life.

19. If possible and desirable, guide the person in formulating care goals.

20. If possible and desirable, guide the person in formulating specific wishes concerning specific end-of-life decisions.

21. Explore whether the person would like to have a written advance directive or if they have made one in the past.

Domain 4 The Role and Importance of Those Close to Them

22. Involve family or significant others as early as possible in the ACP process and inform them about the role of a surrogate decision maker.

23. Evaluate their disease awareness and inform them about the expected disease trajectory and possible end-of-life decisions.

24. Pay attention to their perceptions during the ACP process.

Domain 5 Advance Care Planning When It Is Difficult or No Longer Possible to Communicate Verbally

25. Keep connected with the person living with dementia and ensure his/her maximum participation: respond to emotions, attend to non-verbal communication and observe behaviour to learn more about current quality of life, fears and desires.

26. Actively involve family and others close to the patient in the ACP process and the expression of care goals and wishes concerning end-of-life decisions.

Domain 6 Documentation of Wishes and Preferences, Including Information Transfer

27. Write down in the medical/care files of the person with dementia the outcomes of the ACP process, values, preferences and care goals, and if applicable, the advance directive and legal representative.

28. Regularly re-evaluate as part of the ACP process; decisions can be revised at all times.

29. Communicate the outcomes of the ACP process with the care team – that is, values, preferences and care goals, and, if applicable, advance directives or legal representatives, especially in the case of transfer to another care setting.

Domain 7 End-of-Life Decision-Making

30. Carefully weigh the wishes (expressed and/or written down earlier) against the current best interest of the person living with dementia, in consultation with those close to him/her and the healthcare professionals involved.

Domain 8 Preconditions for Optimal Implementation of Advance Care Planning

31. Provide enough training opportunities for healthcare professionals to learn how to conduct ACP conversations. Adequate support is essential in making healthcare professionals confident about engaging in ACP.

32. Integrate ACP into the mission and policy of the organization and embed it in the organizational culture.

are those that make elements of ACP workable within complex and time-pressured clinical workflows [47].

A study with persons with dementia supports the need for greater ACP discussions between patients and proxies. Discussions regarding goals of care are likely to benefit patients through delivery of care congruent with their wishes and to benefit healthcare professionals through greater acceptance of patients' illness [48]. It is clear that for patients with cognitive impairment the barriers are higher to start ACP [49]. A cross-sectional study demonstrated that residents with dementia are grateful when being involved in discussing their care, but find it difficult to report what is discussed during the conversations [50]. To bridge the gap between the model and daily practice, a group of experts developed recommendations as a guideline, validated by the Belgian branch of the Cochrane collaboration [51]. From a traditional and currently still predominant point of view, ACP gives a person with dementia the possibility to express his/her will before losing mental capacity. Accordingly, an evaluation of the person's mental capacity is the starting point of the recommendations. This is either done freehand or through formal clinical assessment (cf. domain 2). Moreover, involved third parties are considered 'surrogate' decision makers (cf. domain 5). The process of surrogate decision-making is defined as 'the process whereby a person with disability is enabled to make and communicate decisions with respect to personal or legal matters' [52, 53]. The predominant point of view raises questions in terms of CRPD conformity; as discussed earlier, both mental capacity and substituted decision-making are under siege from the CRPD Committee (supra 2, 3).

3.2 The Result: Advance Directives

Advance care planning as a dynamic process often ends up with 'static documents': advance directives, negative or positive, of which some are – depending on the country – legally enforceable. They often have an undeserved connotation with negative choices on a person who lives with dementia's end-of-life care. However, advance directives have far more potential; they could deal with any positive or negative choice regarding any aspect of a person's future life. In Belgium, for example, in 2014, the concept of 'care proxy' (*zorgvolmacht/mandat de protection*) was introduced in the Civil Code as an alternative for guardianship.

With a care proxy a person who lives with dementia appoints someone to take decisions about goods and person when he/she is no longer mentally capable of taking decisions. The care proxy can be phrased in an open way, confined to a list of mandates, but also be expressed in a very specific way, focussing on the basic values of the person who lives with dementia and how to put them into practice. For example, in a care proxy a person who lives with dementia might indicate that he/she wants to remain at home as long as possible and that all reasonable options should be considered before admission to a residential care facility.

Although important, advance care directives are 'static' documents that only cover certain aspects of the will of persons with dementia. In fact, ACP is a 'continuing process', which is somewhat at odds with advance directives, and depends largely on a continuing and qualitative relationship between a person with dementia and a healthcare professional. This approach assumes active engagement with persons with dementia and their support network [53], which is hard to formalize or control.

3.3 Executing Advance Care Plans and Advance Directives

Up to now we have substantiated that although care plans and advance directives are currently linked to a model based on mental capacity, care planning – if unlinked from a mental capacity based approach – has great potential in the CRPD approach. However, the sting in the tail is that the main challenges of ACP and advance directives do not arise when care is planned (which we discussed up to now), but when the plan is to be executed (what we are about to discuss). At this point the discussion on what is a person's real will culminates. We identify two aspects of that discussion.

The first is when to stop planning in advance and to start executing the advance directive. Given the aim to document a person's with dementia real will in advance, therewith foreshadowing the moment he lacks the actual will to take a decision, there is the assumption one day ACP will end.

Traditionally, this is the moment when a person who lives with dementia due to a lack of mental capacity is no longer able to decide on future choices in a fully informed way. At that moment advance directives should be finalized and can no longer be developed, supplemented or withdrawn. From that moment onwards advance directives enter into force, if relevant issues arise. Whilst this is easy to say on paper, in practice it is hard to determine when to stop planning in advance. Given the known fluctuation of mental capacity, the various consequences of the decisions (e.g. 'What do you want to eat?' versus 'You don't want to be hospitalized') and the ongoing nature of the process, a relational practice is needed. This is described as a more fluid approach which actively engages with the person with dementia and other members of their support network (typically family members) across the trajectory of their illness [53].

From a CRPD point of view, however, the point at which an advance care directive enters into force should not be based on an assessment that the person lacks mental capacity. Instead 'it should be decided by the person and included in the text of the directive' (General Comment N°1, 2014). Although this might seem self-evident considered that CRPD aims to do justice to disabilities, the approach of the CRPD Committee is problematic. By stating that the fate of ACP should be decided upon by the persons himself or herself in the early stages of dementia, the CRPD Committee suggests that the preferences of the (non-disabled) 'then-self' constitute the 'real will' and that the preferences of the (disabled) 'now-self' are no longer relevant [54].

This links up with the second aspect – that is, whether the real will of the person who lives with dementia is by definition represented in the advanced care plan, and what weight is given to current preferences. Although the CRPD

Committee seems to suggest that the advance care plan embodies a person's real will, we would rather expect that – if one aims to do justice to the autonomy of a person with dementia – an advance directive is a testimony of a person's prior preferences before he or she was disabled. These could coincide as well as conflict with a person's current preferences now he/she is disabled [55], or, as Guy Widdershoven and Ron Berghmans stated in 2001:

> Advance directives are often regarded as instructions to the doctor about future care. This view is problematic, in that it obliterates that decisions about treatment and care always take place in a concrete situation, and require interpretation and communication. From a hermeneutic perspective, advance directives can be regarded as instruments which do not replace interpretation and communication, but sustain joint decision-making about treatment and care, including the patient and the family in a process of meaning-making. [56]

4 From Lived Experiences to Decision-Making

4.1 The 'Real Will' of Persons Living with Dementia: Towards New Approaches

As this chapter has so far explained, in order to operationalize Article 12 of the CRPD, it will become necessary to find new ways to ascertain a person living with dementia's 'real will' and to ensure that this is grounded in the person's 'preferences'. This task will undoubtedly become more challenging for people living with advanced dementia when the cumulative and temporal impacts of cognitive and other sensory impairments will make articulating and indicating an everyday decision increasingly challenging, both to do and for others to interpret. If there are advance care directives, they could be of help in such circumstances.

As explained earlier, they are not to be applied as objective and static records of the prior wishes of a person living with dementia. Instead, as Widdershoven and Berghmans suggest, we should think of them as 'vehicles for joint meaning-making before and during the experience of dementia' ([56], p. 190). However, how can we understand 'joint meaning-making' when the parties involved differ in cognitive abilities?

There are some basic rules when dealing with persons who live with dementia: one should be respectful, open to their story, show understanding, solace and support, be patient and use non-verbal communication [58]. Communication is preferably based on the concept of person-centred care, defined as follows:

> Person-centred care means that individuals' values and preferences are elicited and, once expressed, guide all aspects of their health care, supporting their realistic health and life goals. Person-centred care is achieved through a dynamic relationship among individuals, others who are important to them, and all relevant providers. This collaboration informs decision-making to the extent that the individual desires. [59]

Unlike in earlier days, anyone will agree that persons who live with dementia should be approached as autonomous decision makers. The diagnosis of dementia is not a diagnosis of mental incapacity. Moreover, even if a person lacks the mental capacity to decide on things autonomously, the remaining capacities and 'real' will of persons who live with dementia should be traced, explored and valued as important elements in the decision-making process. The concept of 'best interest', decision aids and the process of shared decision-making (SDM) may be helpful.

Shared decision-making implies a process in which physicians and patients share in the decision-making process, which is conducted through one or more face-to-face encounters. As to SDM, one should notice that there is a spectrum starting at 'autonomous decision-making over supported autonomous decisions, joint decisions, delegated decisions, adopted decisions, pseudo-autonomous decisions to no involvement in decisions' [60]. The aim of SDM is to empower the patient but also to comply with legal and ethical patient rights, provide patient-centred care, be responsive to patients' desire to be involved, remain accountable for screening and treatments used, improve patient satisfaction with the decision-making process, and potentially improve patient health outcomes [61].

Over the years, research and public policy reports have upheld the professional need to ensure that people living with advanced dementia are supported to make their own choices and decisions, with such an act fundamental to supporting personhood and successfully conducting person-centred care practices [62–64]. Despite all changes, a systematic review concludes that people living with dementia value opportunities to be involved in every day decision-making about their care, as is in general the case for people with intellectual disabilities. [65]

Another systematic review identified 10 out of 3,618 studies to conclude that:

> Decision aids offer a promising approach for providing support for decision-making in dementia care. People are often faced with more than one decision, and decisions are often interrelated. The decision aids identified in this review focus on single topics. There is a need for decision aids that cover multiple topics in one aid to reflect this complexity and better support caregivers. [66]

As an illustration of this latter point, Alzheimer Scotland [67] has written passionately about the need for practitioners to support the person living with dementia's decision-making and to do so via a broad range of interpersonal techniques, such as keeping communication straightforward; being clear about the decision in hand; using props, including biographical photographs, to support the personalization of decision-making; taking as much time as needed during an encounter; and drawing upon what has previously influenced a person's decision-making to contrast and compare to what is being indicated in the present. Similarly, keeping distractions in the environment down to a minimum was also seen as helpful technique, as was closely observing the person living with dementia's body language [67, 68].

To try and move beyond these mainly structural indicators of choice and capacity to uncover a person living with advanced dementia's 'real will and preferences', it might become necessary to look more deeply at the person's everyday decision-making and how decisions are made and enacted. To do so, we propose two approaches: arts as pathways to a holistic and hermeneutic approach to dementia care, and 'in the moment' as a pathway for everyday decision-making for people living with advanced dementia.

4.2 Exploring Arts as Pathways to a Holistic and Hermeneutic Approach to Dementia Care

4.2.1 The Holistic and Hermeneutic Approach as a Frame for Understanding Lived Experiences

First, we explore how the arts are applied to understand the lived experiences of people with dementia and next, how they could be applied to discover a person's real will and preferences. Several scholars in the domain of critical dementia studies argue that successful joint meaning-making requires 'whole sight' and 'a hermeneutic approach' [57, 69]. 'Whole sight' means that persons who live with dementia are not to be reduced to brain disease and patient role. Independent of the stage of the illness, they are subjects of their own – with intentions, desires, preferences and feelings – which emerge in interactions with other people and non-human partners (such as architectural and natural environments, technologies, and animals).

The fact that disease symptoms profoundly change these interactions does not relieve caregivers from the moral duty to approach people who live with dementia as equal partners in the exchange. Hughes et al. state that 'there is an evaluative and interactive core to the type of thing that dementia is' ([69], p. 4). This brings us to the notion of the 'hermeneutic circle' that can be a source of inspiration to improve interactions with people who live with dementia. A hermeneutic approach comprises a reiterative process of discovering diverging perspectives, reconsidering one's initial position and attempting to jointly arrive at new common ground. Such a process is still possible in the exchange with people who live with dementia but requires a special effort and *empathic* listening and communication skills on the part of the person who is cognitively stronger.

Steven R. Sabat, a renowned social psychologist and representative of the personhood movement in dementia research, describes what such *empathic* listening and communication skills entail in his landmark publication *The Experience of Alzheimer's Disease: Life through a Tangled Veil* [70]. By means of ethnographic vignettes, he reveals the meaning-making processes behind his exchange with several persons who live with dementia in a day care setting.

For Sabat, the starting point of successful communication lies in the recognition that people who live with dementia are 'semiotic subjects' or 'individuals who can act intentionally given their interpretations of the circumstances in which they find themselves; they are people who can evaluate their own behavior and the behavior of others in accordance with socially agreed-upon standards of propriety and reason' ([71], p. 171). As such, in his conversations with the visitors at the day care centre, he consistently and explicitly showed his collocutors that he took their speech (whatever truncated) and their feelings (whatever strong) seriously and that he was committed to earning their trust and trying to understand them.

In the communication process, he did not only attempt to piece together disparate language utterances but also connected them to gestures and comportment. After all, speech actions are always situated and embodied, and conversations are often more about social mediation (signalling approval, interest, compassion etc.) than about conveying content.

In a similar vein, Widdershoven and Berghmans demonstrate what linguistic and non-linguistic signals got lost in the communication between professional caregivers and a woman who lives with dementia when trying to detect how she now feels about her advance care directive [56]. Their example painfully shows the negative impact on well-being when caregivers – unintentionally – fail to become *empathic* listeners and communicators and stop to see people living with dementia as 'semiotic subjects'.

How good listeners and communicators are we usually in day-to-day interactions? How sensitive are we to non-verbal cues, including the pitch of the voice, the look, body posture etc., when entering into dialogue? Many would agree that it depends on different factors, including the time we have available, the way we feel in the moment (stress certainly does not help) and how familiar we are with a person's communicative repertoire. Artistic representations of exchanges with people who live with dementia can be valuable sources to – safely – reflect on and practice *empathic* communication skills.

The documentary *Mum* (2009) by the Dutch artist Adelheid Roosen is an example of such a source [72]. In a series of staged scenes, the main character, Mum (the on-screen persona of the director's mother who lives with Alzheimer's disease), interacts with two daughters, her son-in-law and her sister. What is so remarkable about this film production is – amongst other things – that Mum's fragmented and unconventional speech (e.g. 'No I don't have to be on the leg, on the dove ... or on the breaking, but I do want to be free ... because I want beautiful bite and together and with her ... I want that just fine ... and then I place you with the ... and then you floated with ... with me between ... but it doesn't have to ... you don't have to ... you can ... but don't have to.') dominates the soundtrack. It is even subtitled so that the viewer is both visually and aurally drawn to her words.

In doing so, the documentary explicitly invites viewers to engage with mum's speech and to try to understand what she is communicating on screen. Viewers can watch the documentary over and over again to apply the principles of the 'hermeneutic circle' and 'the semiotic subject' to become part of the meaning-making process that is evolving right before their eyes. As Mum's family members diligently listen to the mother's speech and are accepting of its unusual nature, they function as exemplary figures. They listen attentively so as to assure the viewers that there is intention and meaning behind Mum's words and they never reciprocate her speech with baby talk.

Several scenes of the documentary *Mum* further reveal the importance of physicality in addition to the linguistic aspects of communication. In one of them, Mum is held by her son-in-law and together they eat chocolates. When Mum discovers that the chocolates are filled with liquor, the discovery sparks shared amusement. Mum's son-in-law attunes to the main character's mood and playful desire to put the chocolates into his mouth but not without gently refusing more chocolates than he wants to eat.

Scenes like this one beautifully illustrate that language is 'not just a matter of argumentation and discursive deliberation ... Dialogue is first and foremost a process of *play* between parties, based upon rituals. Conscious forms of interaction are dependent upon such preconscious ways of aligning and tuning' ([56], p. 188). Feeding and being fed is a deeply ingrained practice that does not take much intellectual deliberation. Knowing how to unwrap chocolate candy and feed it to a relative constitutes embodied ways of knowing.

Such practical embodied knowledge is probably as essential as discursive knowledge when interacting with a person who lives with dementia, Pia Kontos argues ([73], pp. 206–7). Inspired by Maurice Merleau-Ponty's notion of the 'body-subject', Kontos turns to the body as source of 'practical intentionality' and 'index for meaning' to improve our understanding of the continued abilities of people who live with dementia. Kontos draws on Pierre Bourdieu's concept of 'habitus' to add that bodies assume their embodied significance in a specific social context. While doing participant observations in a Canadian Orthodox Jewish care facility, for instance, Kontos discovered residents were capable of enacting ritual gestures connected to holidays like Hanukkah. Such capabilities are typically developed over a lifetime in a specific community and have become continuous tacit knowledge manifested through the body.

The participatory arts are increasingly called upon in dementia care because they ultimately facilitate *empathic* communication, building on play, ritual and embodied knowledge. Indeed, some art professionals turn out to be great allies in the quest for deconstructing the hierarchical dichotomy between the person who is ill and the person who is not (which we earlier referred to as cognitively stronger/frailer) by assigning a creative (rather than patient) role to the latter.

The participatory arts are not be confused with medical interventions whose longer-term efficiency can be measured by randomized controlled trials. The methods behind the collaborative arts facilitate first and foremost the quality of the exchange in the here and now of the encounter between people who live with dementia and trained professionals. Participatory art programming in dementia care incorporates many art disciplines, ranging from dance, music and fine arts to storytelling and oral poetry. Since the latter is the most counter-intuitive because it heavily relies on putting thoughts or feelings into language, it is worth having a look at the Alzheimer's Poetry Project (APP) by Gary Glazner and TimeSlips by Anne Davis Basting [74, 75], two methods specially aimed at people living in the mid to advanced stages of dementia.

The APP consists of joint poetry recitation by means of call and response as well as collaborative poetry improvisation. TimeSlips is a collective storytelling technique in which participants come up with answers to open questions related to a surprising image. Neither method requires the systematic exposure of the participant's past or excellent linguistic performance. The emphasis is on any creative input in the here and now of the fictional world.

Ethnographic research has shown that even in improvisational storytelling and poetry exercises, the participants often share what preoccupies them in real life and do so in a rather systematic manner over the course of 10 weeks. For instance, poetry recitation and improvisation around the topic of love prompted a participant in a Dutch nursing home to share her sadness and embarrassment over not immediately having recognized a visitor and having refused his kiss (while he supposedly was a close family member) – a theme other participants could relate to all too well.

4.2.2 The Holistic and Hermeneutic Approach as a Frame for Decision-Making: Detour through Fiction

The process of aligning and attuning that characterizes the participatory arts in dementia care has not yet spilled over to other domains of exchange with people who live with dementia. Often people assume that the step from creativity as practised under the lead of an art professional to everyday creative solutions and expressions is too big a leap [76]. This is not only a misunderstanding but also a missed opportunity. What if we would apply some of the imaginative techniques developed by professional artists to continuously work on ACP, especially when the predominantly discursive abilities of the person in question are diminishing?

To conclude this section, we make a first and modest exploration of what this could entail, especially in relation to the strategies that people who are cognitively stronger can rely on to improve their communication skills when trying to identify and negotiate the goals and preferences (the 'real will') of people who live with dementia. Several of the recommendations adapted from Piers et al., especially in domain 3, 'Performing ACP Conversations', can be reconceived when turning to creative approaches to care. Examples include 10. to adjust conversation style and content to the person's level and rhythm, 16. to try to understand the whole person living with dementia and 17. to explore the person's current experiences [51].

In contrast to reminiscence and life story work, participatory arts interventions stimulate people who live with dementia to step into an imaginary world they co-create with the workshop facilitator and other participants with similar capacities to themselves. It is the facilitator's responsibility to create a stimulating non-clinical and non-stigmatizing environment and to assure the participants that entering this world in which anything goes is a safe and comforting endeavour.

A fictional world typically consists of characters around whom actions/events evolve and whose feelings and motivations are expressed. Coming up with and sharing fictional characters and narrative scenarios through a visual (a photograph, a painting, a sculpture) or a literary cue (a poem, a song, a saying) in the third person (in the form of a child, a husband, a bird, a hippo, an astronaut etc.) enables participants not only to indicate preferable types and storylines but to do so in relation to other participants' contributions.

This type of improvisational play of give and take is intrinsically polyphonic as it does not intend to arrive at a consensus between the participants [75]. The idea is that every contribution has value of its own (cf. the person who lives with dementia as a semiotic subject), which reinforces the 'narrative agency' of the participant [77]. Accordingly, many collaborative arts approaches to dementia care are based on a ritualized form of repetition and echoing [72].

In TimeSlips, for instance, all of the replies of the participants to open questions (e.g. 'Where could this be?' 'Who could these characters be?' 'How would they feel?') are collected on a flip chart and told back to the audience by the facilitator at regular intervals. In the poetry recitations of the APP, the same lines are echoed/recited by the group a dozen times. As such, the fact that many people who live with dementia repeat certain linguistic and behavioural patterns (their individual repertoire) over and over again is turned into a strength rather than a nuisance.

Let us stress once more that practical embodied knowledge is valued as much as discursive knowledge (even though the latter seems to predominate in the spoken word interventions TimeSlips and the APP) in collaborative art activities in dementia care. Just like words, actions (including comportment and gestures) can carry narrative meaning [78]. Especially creative interventions that build on the performance arts (theatre and dance) support 'the body's potentiality for ... telling one's story' ([78], pp. 361–2). Improvisational acting and dancing offer people who live with dementia the opportunity to become who they never were, to act out personalities, undertakings and emotions that may be as surprising to them as to others.

Although the collaborative arts are meant to serve as pleasant distractions from the often-ugly reality of the illness – next to affirming the personhood of the participants and honouring their remaining strengths – imaginative play offers room for the expression of both positive and negative affects. Indeed, a wide range of emotions are usually part of co-creation. Occasionally, fiction bleeds over into reality (real and imaginary life getting blurred) and the here and now of the story world merge with past and current experiences, as mentioned earlier. This has potential for future experiments with and explorations of collaborative arts approaches to discussing ACP.

A detour through fiction may be a less confrontational way to provoke responses to important topics (such as what a loving relationship entails, what it entails to care well for someone or for oneself, what it means to relocate, how one can cope with disappointments and anxieties etc.) than directly asking urgent instrumental care-related questions to a specific individual. If the arts activities take place at regular intervals over a longer period of time, the contributions will eventually reveal the core values and 'real will' of the participants at that point in their lives.

Translating and adapting some of the approaches behind professional collaborative arts activities tailored to people who live in the mid to advanced stages of dementia does not first and foremost require a background in the professional arts but rather a holistic and hermeneutic mindset as described earlier. This mindset can only be developed through ongoing reflection on one's own role in the relational power dynamics with a person who is cognitively more vulnerable. It compels an effort to deconstruct taken-for-granted assumptions about selfhood and the quality of interpersonal relationships. Most importantly, it involves taking risks and sharing vulnerabilities on the part of the person who is cognitively stronger.

4.3 Exploring 'in the Moment' as a Pathway for Everyday Decision-Making for People Living with Advanced Dementia

4.3.1 'In the Moment' as a Frame for Understanding Lived Experiences

Next to arts, we uncover whether the 'in the moment' frame as a way to understand the lived experiences of people with dementia could be applied to discover a person's real will and preferences. Applying the 'in the moment' frame of reference to a decision-making process would follow the general philosophy of positive psychology in dementia studies where the focus is on upholding the social context of well-being and maintaining the importance of resilience-promoting factors – that is, the personal right to take risks and to try alternative solutions if the first approach did not get the desired result [79]. Moreover, the findings of two recent systematic reviews of the literature in dementia studies that were focussed, separately, on reminiscence activities and life story work [80, 81] have both concluded that finding more creative ways to integrate and record 'in the moment' experiences within care practices and research reporting would provide a more authentic account of what it is like to live with more advanced dementia.

However, whilst these are important developments, reaching a consensus about what constitutes 'being in the moment' has, until relatively recently, been missing from the literature. Working to address this knowledge deficit, Keady and his colleagues have recently (2020) generated the first definition of 'being in the moment' by performing secondary data analysis on a number of qualitative studies undertaken by members of the Dementia and Ageing Research Team at the University of Manchester in the UK [82]. Based on a comparative synthesis of their qualitative data sets, the authors defined the experience as follows:

> Being in the moment is a relational, embodied and multi-sensory human experience. It is both situational and autobiographical and can exist in a fleeting moment or for longer periods of time. All moments are considered to have personal significance, meaning and worth. *(p. 7)*

When considering how everyday decisions are taken by people living with advanced dementia 'in the moment', this definition showcases the importance of the autobiographical and relational context built from a position of resilience and life experience.

Interestingly, the authors went on to place 'being in the moment' within a continuum of moments that they argued revolved around: creating the moment; being in the moment; ending the moment; and reliving the moment, with the opportunity to relive moments being a spark to ignite creating the moment once again. This cyclical continuum suggests that being in the moment is not a once-only, stand-alone event and that a range of factors will be needed to explore and contextualize what it is to be 'in the moment', such as time, place and environment.

4.3.2 'In the Moment' as a Frame for Decision-Making?

Whilst 'being in the moment', and an appreciation of moments in general in dementia studies, is steadily gaining momentum as a frame of reference for better understanding the lived experience of dementia, especially for those living in its later stages, applying this emergent understanding to a decision-making model that could better communicate a person's 'real will and preferences' is not straightforward [82]. This is because an 'in the moment' everyday decision-making model is not currently available/written about in the decision-making literature. Indeed, the nearest model that we could locate and craft onto this positioning is the 'recognition-primed decision model' of rapid decision-making [83, 84].

In the recognition-primed decision model, a central tenet is that people (not just people with dementia of course) use experience – generated from their life script – to avoid some of the limitations of analytical strategies and that decisions can be taken without having to compare options. This immediacy of thought and action relies on two interlinked processes; first a situation assessment to generate a plausible course of action and then cognitive simulation to evaluate that course of action [83].

The recognition-primed decision model has been used in various emergency situations such as to better understand firefighters' rapid decision-making processes when faced with a real-time, life-threatening event, such as responding to a house fire [85]. It has also been applied by military strategists to find out how battlefield commanders make intuitive decisions when faced with the changing tactics of the enemy that require an immediate response. In this battlefield work a conclusion was reached that 'the key to a good solution lies in the ability to correctly assess the situation, since that assessment will guide the judgement about what is a good course of action' ([83], p. 9). This also suggests that plans can be rapidly changed should the circumstances continue to call for it.

When considering the implementation of the recognition-primed decision model for people with more advanced dementia, it will become necessary to better understand such instinctive and intuitive rapid decision-making and the place where those decision are coming from/being taken. Consider, for example, a person with advanced dementia's anguish in wanting to leave the place they are in order to meet their young children from school as they are already 'late' to pick them up. Whilst 'we' may reasonably conclude that such an event is not happening in 'real time', for the person living with dementia all decisions and actions will be made to meet this situational assessment/motivation that *is* happening in real time.

The ability/inability to be physically present at the school gate is a cognitive simulation that will subsequently drive all immediate decisions and actions and trigger a number of responses from those in the presence of the person with advanced dementia – which could, of course, include restraint. Therefore, we would suggest that in advanced dementia, the recognition-primed decision model will need to be adapted in order to provide a situational context for such 'in the moment' situations and meanings and to establish a more rounded profile for the person's 'real will and preferences'. Whilst hypothetical at present, we have illustrated this adapted 'in the moment' recognition-primed decision model in Figure 11.1 and have elaborated on each of its quartile segments.

- The life script is the starting point in the first quartile segment and the starting point in the adapted 'in the moment' recognition-primed decision model. It is a foundational domain as without knowing a person living with advanced dementia, their 'real will and preferences' will be difficult, if not impossible, to ascertain – especially if cognitive and other sensory impairments continue to make verbal communication challenging for the person.

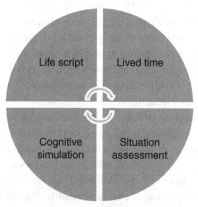

Figure 11.1 'In the moment' everyday decision-making for people living with advanced dementia: establishing 'real will and preference' (adapted from the recognition-primed decision model [83])

Other cues, such as body language, body movement and vocalized sounds, may need to be the connecting point that indicate likes and dislikes, choices, distractions and motivations. This first quartile segment should be considered as being attuned to person-centred care practices and values [62, 63], and underpinned with robust life story work [81].

- Lived time is symbiotic with 'being in the moment' for people living with advanced dementia and thus we consider it also a foundational domain of the recognition-primed decision model as adapted and applied to this specific context. Lived time was first described by the Dutch philosopher Max van Manen, who conceptualized lived time as 'subjective time' as opposed to 'clock time' [86]. Lived time is important for better appreciating the ways people experience the temporal dimensions of their life; again, this formulation is not exclusively applied to people living with dementia, but its connection to the more advanced stages of the condition is heightened given issues of impaired autobiographical memory recall and orientation to time, place and person [87]. Indeed, a recent meta-synthesis by Eriksen et al. on the experience of lived time by people with dementia has reported that people living with dementia experience changes in the self related to all three dimensions of time, namely past, present and future [88]. Therefore, meeting the person living with advanced dementia in their own reality/construction of lived time provides

an opportunity for both illuminating and interpreting the person's 'real will and preferences' [88].

- Situation assessment is seen in our adapted model in an everyday life context and as applied to dementia studies [89]. Moving the frame of reference to the mundane and to the ordinary provides an opportunity for the person with advanced dementia to make vital life choices based on supporting their personal needs and wants and drawing directly from their life script and remembered/automatic behaviours and actions. Here, new and repeated everyday situations will be continually faced and encountered 'in the moment' and decisions will need to be taken quickly to maintain a form of aesthetic presence – for example, the person with advanced dementia suddenly indicating they no longer want to shave, or be shaved, by care home staff after a lifetime of being facially clean-shaven. What is the 'real will and preferences' of the person living with advanced dementia in such a situation and what should the response be?

- Cognitive simulation provides the outcome indicator as to whether the 'in the moment' everyday decision-making has been successfully undertaken and communicated by people living with advanced dementia, or if further interpretation/clarification/care planning is required. Outcome indicators will be different for each person in each different set of circumstances, but applying a life script and personal well-being lens against the consequences of the 'in the moment' everyday decision-making will help to provide an evolving person-centred frame of reference. As intimated in Figure 11.1, these outcomes will be replayed and contrasted to the life script of the person living with advanced dementia, which will give additional authenticity to interpreting and upholding the person's 'real will and preferences'.

If we hold that communication, in whatever form, is the means by which all people indicate choice and decision-making, then for people living with advanced dementia especially, reliable interpretation of that communication approach is crucial to determining real will and preferences [90]. Arguably, this is not a new position to take. For example, for people with more complex presentations of dementia, a need to interpret the meaning of behaviour, such as excessive walking punctuated by shouting and seemingly aggressive gestures, is a cornerstone of the challenging behaviour literature.

As an illustration, the Newcastle Challenging Behaviour Model is a multifactorial assessment of behaviour using a needs-led approach to support the well-being of a person living with dementia [91]. In this model, exhibited behaviour(s), such as excessive walking, are considered a manifestation of a need or unmet need. Identification and assessment of such challenging behaviour would involve four set approaches, namely (1) gathering background information about the person living with dementia e.g. personal history, physical health, cognition, an in-depth description of the behaviour and when, where and how often it is occurring; (2) developing a formulation (also known as a functional analysis) based on the collation of such background information; (3) conducting an intervention based on the formulation; and (4) documenting the effectiveness of the intervention on a care record/plan. However, what appears missing from such an appraisal is the reality that the excessive walking, to continue with the example, is occurring 'in the moment', in separate moments in time and as a rapid decision by the person living with dementia to deal with the underlying motivation/stressor that is being faced.

In many ways, what constitutes being in the moment for a person living with advanced dementia, how it is enacted and then how it is remembered for the person, if at all, are crucial determinants to establishing a person's real will and preferences. As we have seen earlier in this chapter, arts and creative practices/interventions are beginning to inhabit this space through a focus on embodied and sensory approaches to communication, such as through music and dance, rather than focussing on meaning-making alone through verbal communication and expression.

This is an important step forward as John Killick has argued that being 'in the moment' is the basic unit of creative provision for people with dementia and is closely associated with the concept of 'flow' [92]. In this context, 'flow' is a state linked to the work of Mihaly Csikszentmihalyi and means being totally absorbed in a task or activity where the person has increased well-being and is totally lost in time. As Killick goes on to explain, 'flow' is also 'a dynamic experience

between the person [with dementia] and their social environment' ([93], p. 182). This alignment opens up the possibility of people with advanced dementia being in the moment and in a 'flow' state with everyday mundane activities, much as we are proposing in the situation assessment in Figure 11.1 (third quartile segment).

Perhaps what is needed going forward is to view a person holistically and to accept that ascertaining the real will and preference of a person with advanced dementia will always be an imperfect science. However, by adopting an 'in the moment' lens, much as we have set out in Figure 11.1 and augmented by existing knowledge from the challenging behaviour and creative arts fields, there is an opportunity to provide a more robust and person-centred way of interpreting decision-making in advanced dementia. That said, more work is required to turn these words and thoughts into practical solutions that can be implemented on the ground and in an everyday practice context to satisfy the needs of Article 12 CRPD.

5 Conclusion

5.1 The Potential of Advance Care Planning and Lived Experiences

The aim of this contribution was to explore whether ACP and existing frameworks to understand lived experiences of persons who live with dementia have potential to be integrated into a CRPD approach to decision-making with dementia. This CRPD approach radically questions the capacity-based model on decision-making with dementia that is key to most current decision-making practices. The CRPD requires legal capacity to be disentangled from mental capacity, and calls for legal capacity to be based on a person who lives with dementia's will and preferences instead.

However, a 'real will' is still needed: not every preference should lead to a valid decision. Really wanting however, does no longer fully depend on the ability to understand and appreciate. Also beyond mental capacity there is a real will, yet support of others is needed to retrieve and communicate it. Here the potential for ACP and lived experiences is to be found.

First, regarding ACP, this is proposed as a solution by the CRPD Committee itself. Indeed, planning care in advance is a way to overcome ruptures in the lives of persons living with dementia. Yet the textbook way of ACP is not necessarily in line with the CRPD's approach to decision-making. In particular the basic assumption that ACP foreshadows a future of mental incapacity wherein the preferences of the 'then-self', uttered in times of mental capacity, takes precedence over the preferences of a mentally incapacitated 'now-self', is problematic.

The solution the CRPD Committee suggests – it is up for the person with dementia himself/herself to decide upon this – does not help us any further. If the then-self decides on how an advance directive is to be executed, the preferences of the now-self could be overlooked. Consequently, in order to keep in touch with the now-self and overcome the mental incapacity trap, ACP should be a process that never stops. There is no divide between planning and executing an care plan: a real will cannot be established in advance. In a way, there is even no 'advance' in ACP.

Second, if a real will cannot be established in advance, the currently lived experiences of a person with dementia are an essential support or counterweight for the preferences of the then-self. We maintain that exploratory frameworks to understand the lived experiences of people with dementia – for example, a framework based on arts and/or the 'in the moment' frame – could and should play a role in discovering a person's real will and preferences. Both arts and the 'in the moment' frame would offer an opportunity to provide a more robust and person-centred way of interpreting decision-making. Despite this confident claim, our thoughts are just exploratory. Much work is required to turn these thoughts into practical solutions that can be implemented on the ground and in an everyday practice context to satisfy the needs of Article 12 CRPD.

5.2 Is There a Future for Best Interests?

The main focus of this exploratory contribution was to find out whether ACP and lived experiences could a play role in retrieving a person's real will beyond mental capacity. Our answer was mainly positive; although there are questions, both have a large potential. What we did not deal with is the more fundamental question of what is a real will; even though the CRPD Committee guides in a certain direction by forcing us beyond the traditional mental capacity approach, the highly normative question on how to weigh (up) preferences of the then-self and the now-self lies ahead.

As explained, agreeing on what makes a will real is the first step to respecting a real will. In this regard, even if we agree on what makes a will 'real', there is a last question: if we know what a person who lives with dementia really wants, are we obliged to respect this?

Traditionally *best interests* play a part in decision-making with dementia by surrogate decision makers. On this point Smith et al. note that:

> Rising use of advance directives has made surrogate decision-making both easier and harder. In many cases, these directives help guide decision-making for patients who have lost decision-making capacity. In some cases, however, directives may conflict with what physicians or surrogates view as what is in the patient's best interest. These conflicts can place substantial emotional and moral burdens on physicians and surrogates, and there is little practical guidance for how to address them. [94]

A framework of 'best interest' is used, for example, to overcome a conflict of the 'now-self' versus the 'then-self [94]. In this framework questions are raised for weighing previously expressed preferences and best interests. 'Is the clinical situation an emergency that allows no time for deliberation?' 'In view of the person's values and goals, how likely is it that the benefits of the intervention outweigh the burdens?' 'To what degree does the advance directive fit the situation at hand?' 'How much leeway did the patient allow the surrogate in overriding the advance directive?' 'How well does the surrogate represent the patient's best interests?'

In a CRPD approach, this type of comparative assessment between a prior preference and a current best interest is no longer self-evident. If there is something to be comparatively assessed, it is the prior and the current preference. Either one of both or a combination constitutes a person's real will. It is indeed a major virtue of the CRPD that it recognizes that any person with dementia in any situation has a real will, that this real will should be retrieved and that current preferences, even if in later stages of dementia, play a role. This approach makes it easier to recognize coercion in dementia care. In the capacity approach, beyond mental incapacity the concept of coercion is vague. Can we speak of coercion if there is a lack of mental capacity? The CRPD approach instead forces us to make a clear distinction between two questions: 'What does the person who lives with dementia really wants in this situation?' and 'Are we able and willing to execute that will?' [17]

This raises the question whether there is room for best interests at all. While it is clear that under a CRPD approach not every 'real' will has to be executed – for example, the will of a person with dementia can still be in conflict with rights of others – disregarding what a person really wants because it is deemed highly undesirable for themselves becomes dubious, especially if these best-interest considerations would not be made if a person without dementia has the same real will.

Nonetheless, a person who lives with dementia really wanting to stay home until the end of their life can end up in a situation where this is reasonably impossible. Despite all efforts, they can refuse to take a bath for weeks, therewith being an unreasonable burden for others. Although the CRPD Committee rejects any coercion related to a disability, it seems reasonable to strike a fair balance in these cases. However, this should never be taken for granted.

References

1. Traustodóttir R. Disability studies, the social model and legal developments. In Arnodóttir O, Quunn G, eds. *The UN Convention on the Rights of Persons with Disabilities: European and Scandinavian Perspectives*. Leiden, Brill, 2009; 1–16.

2. De Hert M, Wampers M. Juridische aspecten in België. In Hein I, Hondius A, eds. Wilsbekwaamheid in de medische praktijk. Utrecht, De Tijdstroom, 2018; 18–28.

3. Ruissen A, Meynen G, Widdershoven GA. [Perspectives on patient competence in psychiatry: Cognitive functions, emotions and values]. *Tijdschrift voor Psychiatrie* 2011; 53(7): 405–14.

4. Halpern SD. Goal-concordant care: Searching for the Holy Grail. *New England Journal of Medicine* 2019; 381(17): 1603–6.

5. Bach M, Kernzer L. *A New Paradigm for Protecting Autonomy and the Right to Legal Capacity*. Ontario, Law Commission of Ontario, 2010.

6. Booth Glen K. Changing paradigms: Mental capacity, legal capacity, guardianship and beyond. *Columbia Human Rights Law Review* 2012; 44: 94–5.

7. De Bhailis C, Flynn M. Recognising legal capacity: Commentary and analysis of article 12 CRPD.

International Journal of Law in Context 2017; 13 (1): 6–11.

8. Appelbaum P. Protecting the rights of persons with disabilities: An international convention and its problems. *Psychiatric Services* 2016; 67 (4): 366–8.

9. Scholten M, Gather J. Adverse consequences of Article 12 of the UN Convention on the Rights of Persons with Disabilities for persons with mental disabilities and an alternative way forward. *Journal of Medical Ethics* 2018; 44(4): 226–33.

10. Freeman M, Kolappa K, Caldas de Almeida JM, Kleinman A, Makhashvili N, Phakathi S, et al. Reversing hard won victories in the name of human rights: A critique of the General Comment on Article 12 of the UN Convention of the Rights of Persons with Disabilities. *Lancet Psychiatry* 2015; 2(9): 844–50.

11. Appelbaum PS, Grisso T. Assessing patients' capacities to consent to treatment. *New England Journal of Medicine* 1988; 319(25): 1635–8.

12. Appelbaum PS, Grisso T. The MacArthur Treatment Competences Study I: Mental illness and competence to consent to treatment. *Law and Human Behavior* 1995; 19(2): 105–26.

13. Grisso T, Appelbaum PS. The MacArthur Treatment Competence Study III: Abilities of patients to consent to psychiatric and medical treatments. *Law and Human Behavior* 1995; 19(2): 149–74.

14. Grisso T, Appelbaum PS, Mulvey EP, Fletcher K. The MacArthur Treatment Competence Study II: Measures of abilities related to competence to consent to treatment. *Law and Human Behavior* 1995; 19(2): 127–48.

15. Hein I, Hondius A. *Wilsbekwaamheid in de medische praktijk*. Utrecht, De Tijdstroom, 2018.

16. Council of Europe. Recommendation on principles concerning the legal protection of incapable adults, 1999.

17. Opgenhaffen T. *Vrijheidsbeperkingen in de zorg*. Mortsel, Intersentia, 2020.

18. White B. *Competence to Consent*. Washington, DC, Georgetown University Press, 1994.

19. Haekens A. *Beslissingsbekwaamheid in de gerontopsychiatrische context*. Leuven, Faculteit Geneeskunde KU Leuven, 1998.

20. Donnelly M. A legal overview. In Foster C, Herring J, Doron I, eds. *The Law and Ethics of Dementia*. London, Hart, 2014; 271–82.

21. De Sabbata K. Dementia, treatment decisions, and the UN Convention on the Rights of Persons with Disabilities: A new framework for old problems. *Frontiers in Psychiatry* 2020; 11: 1–16.

22. Committee on the Rights of Persons with Disabilities. General Comment N°1 of the Committee on the Rights of Persons with Disabilities on Article 12 (Equal Recognition before the Law) (19 May 2014). UN Doc. CRPD/C/GC/1 (2014), 2014.

23. Arstein-Kerslake A, Flynn E. The General Comment on Article 12 of the Convention on the Rights of Persons with Disabilities: A roadmap for equality before the law. *International Journal of Human Rights* 2016; **20**(4): 471–90.

24. Gooding P. Navigating the 'flashing amber lights' of the right to legal capacity in the United Nations Convention on the Rights of Persons with Disabilities: Responding to major concerns. *Human Rights Law Review* 2015; **15**(1): 45–71.

25. World Health Organization. *International Classification of Functioning, Disability and Health.* Geneva, World Health Organization, 2001.

26. Hendriks R, Hendrikx A, Kamphof D, Swinnen A. Goede verstaanders: Wederzijdse articulatie en de stem van mensen met dementie. in Van Hove G, Schippers A, Cardol M, De Schauwer E, eds. *Disability Studies in de Lage Landen.* Antwerpen, Garant, 2016; 81–99.

27. Dhanda A. Universal legal capacity as a universal human right. In Dudley M, Silove D, Gale F, eds. *Mental Health and Human Rights: Vision, Courage and Practice.* Oxford, Oxford University Press, 2012.

28. Bartlett P. The United Nations Convention on the Rights of Persons with Disabilities and the future of mental health law. *Psychiatry* 2009; **8**(12): 496–8.

29. Szmukler G. The UN Convention on the Rights of Persons with Disabilities and UK mental health legislation. *British Journal of Psychiatry* 2014; **205**(1): 76.

30. Slobogin C. Eliminating mental disability as a legal criterion in deprivation of liberty cases: The impact of the Convention on the Rights of Persons with Disabilities on the insanity defense, civil commitment, and competency law. *International Journal of Law and Psychiatry* 2015; **40**: 36–42.

31. Buntinx F, De Lepeleire J, Paquay L, Iliffe S, Schoenmakers B. Diagnosing dementia: No easy job. *BMC Family Practice* 2011; **12**(1): 60.

32. Swinnen A, Schweda AM, eds. *Popularizing Dementia: Public Expressions and Representations of Forgetfulness.* Bielefeld, Transcript, 2015.

33. Van Gorp B, Vercruysse T. Frames and counter-frames giving meaning to dementia: A framing analysis of media content. *Social Science & Medicine* 2012; **74**: 1274–81.

34. Iliffe S, De Lepeleire J, Van Hout H, Kenny G, Lewis A, Vernooij-Dassen M. Understanding obstacles to the recognition of and response to dementia in different European countries: A modified focus group approach using multinational, multi-disciplinary expert groups. *Aging and Mental Health* 2005; **9**(1): 1–6.

35. De Brandt M, Bakker S, Felrackers S, Stulens T, Verschraegen J, De Lepeleire J. *Richtlijn diagnostiek van dementie in de huisartsenpraktijk.* Leuven, Academisch Centrum Huisartsgeneeskunde, KU Leuven/Expertisecentrum Dementie Vlaanderen, 2020.

36. Folstein M, Folstein S, McHugh P. 'Mini mental state': A practical method for grading the cognitive state of patients for the clinician? *Journal of Psychiatric Research* 1975; **12**: 189–98.

37. Fahy M, Wald C, Walker Z, Livingston G. Secrets and lies: The dilemma of disclosing the diagnosis to an adult with dementia. *Age and Ageing* 2003; **32**: 439–41.

38. Iliffe S, Wilcock J, Haworth D. Obstacles to shared care for patients with dementia: A qualitative study. *Family Practice* 2006; **23**(3): 353–62.

39. Vanderschaeghe G, Schaeverbeke J, Bruffaerts R, Vandenberghe R, Dierickx K. From information to follow-up: Ethical recommendations to facilitate the disclosure of amyloid PET scan results in a research setting. *Alzheimer's and Dementia (NY)* 2018; **4**: 243–51.

40. Piercy H, Fowler-Davis S, Dunham M, Cooper C. Evaluation of an integrated service delivering post diagnostic care and support for people living with dementia and their families. *Health & Social Care in the Community* 2018; **26**(6): 819–28.

41. Vermandere M. *Zorgdiagnose bij thuiswonende dementerenden: Een nieuw concept?* Leuven, KU Leuven, 2009.

42. NHS Information Services Division. Dementia post-diagnostic support. NHS Board performance 2015/2016, NHS, 2018.

43. Scottish Action on Dementia. *Five Pillars of Post-diagnostic Care.* Edinburgh, Scottish Action on Dementia, 2018.

44. Vermandere M, Decloedt P, De Lepeleire J. Zorgdiagnose bij thuiswonende, dementerende patiënten. Een nieuw concept? *Tijdschrift voor Gerontologie en Geriatrie* 2012; **43**: 25–32.

45. Rietjens JAC, Sudore RL, Connolly M, Van Delden JJ, Drickamer MA, Droger M, et al. European Association for Palliative Care: Definition and recommendations for advance care planning: An international consensus supported by the European Association for Palliative Care. *Lancet Oncology* 2017; **18**(9): e543–e551.

46. Brinkman-Stoppelenburg A, Rietjens JA, Van der Heide A. The effects of advance care planning on end-of-life care: A systematic review. *Palliative Medicine* 2014; **28**(8): 1000–25.

47. Lund S, Richardson A, May C. Barriers to advance care planning at the end of life: An explanatory systematic review of implementation studies. *PLoS One* 2015; **10**(2): e0116629.

48. Givens JL, Sudore RL, Marshall GA, Dufour AB, Kopits I, Mitchell SL. Advance care planning in community-dwelling patients with dementia. *Journal of Pain Symptom Management* 2018; **55**(4): 1105–12.

49. deLima Thomas J, Sanchez-Reilly S, Bernacki R, O'Neill L, Morrison LJ, Kapo J, et al. Advance care planning in cognitively impaired older adults. *Journal of the American Geriatrics Society* 2018; **66**(8): 1469–74.

50. Goossens B, Sevenants A, Declercq A, Van Audenhove C. Shared decision-making in advance care planning for persons with dementia in nursing homes: A cross-sectional study. *BMC Geriatrics* 2020; **20**(1): 381.

51. Piers RD, Albers G, Gilissen J, De Lepeleire J, Steyaert J, Van Mechelen W, et al. Advance care planning in dementia: Recommendations for healthcare professionals. *BMC Palliative Care* 2018; **17**(1): 88.

52. United Nations Office of the High Commissioner on Human Rights. Thematic study by the office of the United Nations High Commissioner for Human Rights on enhancing awareness and understanding of the Convention on the Rights of Persons with Disabilities, 2009. www.un.org/dis abilities/documents/reports/ohchr/A.HRC.10.48 AEV.pdf

53. Sinclair C, Bajic-Smith J, Gresham M, Blake M, Bucks RS, Field R, et al. Professionals' views and experiences in supporting decision-making involvement for people living with dementia. *Dementia* (London) 2019; **20**(1): 84–105. doi:1471301219864849

54. Bianchi D. Advance directives: Addressing the obligations of support as part of the right of a person with disabilities to equal recognition before the law? *International Journal of Law and Psychiatry* 2020; **70**: 101561.

55. Donnelly M. Deciding in dementia: The possibilities and limits of supported decision-making. *International Journal of Law and Psychiatry* 2019; **66**: 101466.

56. Widdershoven GA, Berghmans RL. Advance directives in dementia care: From instructions to instruments. *Patient Education and Counseling* 2001; **44**(2): 179–86.

57. Widdershoven GAM, Berghmans RLP. Meaning-making in dementia: A hermeneutic perspective. In Hughes J, Louw S, Sabat S, eds. *Dementia: Mind, Meaning and the Person*. Oxford, Oxford University Press, 2006; 179–91.

58. Van de Ven L, Vandenbulcke M. Personen met Dementie. In De Lepeleire J, Keirse M, eds. *Wegwijzer naar bijzondere noden: Over kwaliteit van zorg en communicatie*. Leuven, Acco, 2013; 131–44.

59. American Geriatric Society. Person-centered care: A definition and essential elements. *Journal of the American Geriatric Society* 2016; **64**(1): 15–18.

60. Van Bosseghem R, Desmet V, Cornelis E, De Vriendt P. [*Taking Decisions Together with Residents with Dementia*]. Ghent, Artevelde Hogeschool, 2019.

61. Stacey D, Murray MA, Legare F, Sandy D, Menard P, O'Connor A. Decision coaching to support shared decision making: A framework, evidence, and implications for nursing practice, education, and policy. *Worldviews on Evidence-Based Nursing* 2008; **5**(1): 25–35.

62. Kitwood T. *Dementia Reconsidered: The Person Comes First*. Buckinghamshire, Open University Press, 1997.

63. Kitwood T, Brooker D, eds. *Dementia Reconsidered, Revisited: The Person Still Comes First*. London, Open University Press, 2019.

64. Voss H, Vogel A, Wagemans AMA, Francke AL, Metsemakers JFM, Courtens AM, de Veer AJE. Advance care planning in palliative care for people with intellectual disabilities: A systematic review. *Journal of Pain Symptom Management* 2017; **54**(6): 938–60 e1.

65. Daly RL, Bunn F, Goodman C. Shared decision-making for people living with dementia in extended care settings: A systematic review. *BMJ Open* 2018; **8**(6): e018977.

66. Davies N, Schiowitz B, Rait G, Vickerstaff V, Sampson EL. Decision aids to support decision-making in dementia care: A systematic review. *International Psychogeriatrics* 2019; **31**(10): 1403–19.

67. Alzheimer Scotland Action on Dementia. *Dementia. Making Decisions: A Practical Guide for Family Members, Partners and Friends with Powers of Attorney, Guardianship or Deputyship*. Edinburgh, Alzheimer Scotland Action on Dementia2012.

68. O'Connor D, Purves B, eds. *Decision-Making, Personhood and Dementia: Exploring the Interface*. London, Jessica Kingsley, 2016.

69. Hughes J, Louw S, Sabat N. *Dementia: Mind, Meaning and the Person.* Oxford, Oxford Medical, 2006.

70. Sabat S. *The Experience of Alzheimer's Disease: Life through a Tangled Veil.* Oxford, Blackwell, 2001.

71. Sabat S, Harré R. The Alzheimer's disease sufferer as a semiotic subject. *Philosophy, Psychiatry & Psychology* 1994; **1**(3): 145–60.

72. Swinnen A. Dementia in documentary film: *Mum* by Adelheid Roosen. *Gerontologist* 2013; **53**(1): 113–22.

73. Kontos P. Embodied selfhood: An ethnographic exploration of Alzheimer's disease. In Leibing A, Cohen L, eds. *Thinking about Dementia: Culture, Loss, and the Anthropology of Senility.* New Brunswick, NJ, Rutgers University Press, 2003.

74. Swinnen AM. Healing words: A study of poetry interventions in dementia care. *Dementia* (London) 2016; **15**(6): 1377–1404.

75. Swinnen A, de Medeiros K. 'Play' and people living with dementia: A humanities-based inquiry of TimeSlips and the Alzheimer's Poetry Project. *Gerontologist* 2018; **58**(2): 261–9.

76. Bellass S, Balmer A, May V, Keady J, Buse C, Capstick A, et al. Broadening the debate on creativity and dementia: A critical approach. *Dementia* (London) 2019; **18**(7–8): 2799–2820.

77. Baldwin C. Narrative, citizenship and dementia: The personal and the political. *Journal of Aging Studies* 2008; **22**: 222–8.

78. Dupuis SL, Kontos P, Mitchell G, Jonas-Simpson C, Gray S. Re-claiming citizenship through the arts. *Dementia* (London) 2016; **15**(3): 358–80.

79. Clarke C, Wolverson E. *Positive Psychology Approaches to Dementia: Exploring the Interface.* London, Jessica Kingsley, 2016.

80. Woods B, O'Philbin L, Farrell EM, Spector AE, Orrell S. Reminiscence therapy for dementia. *Cochrane Database System Review* 2018; **3**: CD001120.

81. Gridley K, Brooks J, Birks Y, Baxter K, Parker G. *Improving Care for People with Dementia: Development and Initial Feasibility Study for Evaluation of Life Story Work in Dementia Care.* Southampton, NIHR Journals Library, 2016.

82. Keady JD, Campbell S, Clark A, Dowlen R, Elvish R, Jones L, et al. Re-thinking and re-positioning 'being in the moment' within a continuum of moments: Introducing a new conceptual framework for dementia studies. *Ageing and Society* 2020; 1–22. doi: 10.1017/S0144686X20001014

83. Ross KG, Klein G, Thunholm P, Schmitt J, Baxter H. The recognition-primed decision model. *Military Review* 2004; **6**: 6–10.

84. Zsambok C, Klein G, eds. *Naturalistic Decision Making.* New York, Psychology Press, 2014.

85. Klein G, Calderwood R, Clinton–Cirocco A. Rapid decision making on the fire ground: Technical Report 796. In K Associates, ed. *Research Institute for the Behavioral and Social Sciences.* Alexandria, VA, US Army, 1988.

86. Van Manen M. *Researching Lived Experience: Human Science for an Action Sensitive Pedagogy.* Second edition. London, Routledge, 2016.

87. National Institute for Health and Care Excellence. Dementia, assessment, management and support for people living with dementia and their carers. Nice guideline, 2018. www.nice.org.uk/guidance/ng97

88. Eriksen SB, Grove RLE, Ibsen T, Telenius ER. The experience of lived time in people with dementia: A systematic meta-synthesis. *Dementia and Cognitive Disorders* 2020; **49**: 435–55.

89. Nedlund C, Barlett R, Calarke C. *Everyday Citizenship and People with Dementia.* Edinburgh, Dundein Academic Press, 2019.

90. Moniz-Cook E, Hart CH, Woods B, Whitaker C, James I, Russell I, et al. Challenge Demcare: Management of challenging behaviour in dementia at home and in care homes: Development, evaluation and implementation of an online individualised intervention for care homes and a cohort study of specialist community mental health care for families. *NIHR Programme Grants for Applied Research* 2017; **5**(15). www.ncbi.nlm.nih.gov/books/NBK447072

91. James I, Jackman L. *Understanding Behaviour in Dementia That Challenges: A Guide to Assessment and Treatment.* Second edition. London, Jessica Kingsley, 2017.

92. Killick J. *Creativity and Dementia: Positive Psychology Approaches to Dementia.* London, Jessica Kingsley, 2016.

93. Csikszentmihalyi M. *Creativity: Flow and the Psychology of Discovery and Invention.* New York, Harper Collins, 1996.

94. Smith AK, Lo B, Sudore R. When previously expressed wishes conflict with best interests. *JAMA Internal Medicine* 2013; **173**(13): 1241–5.

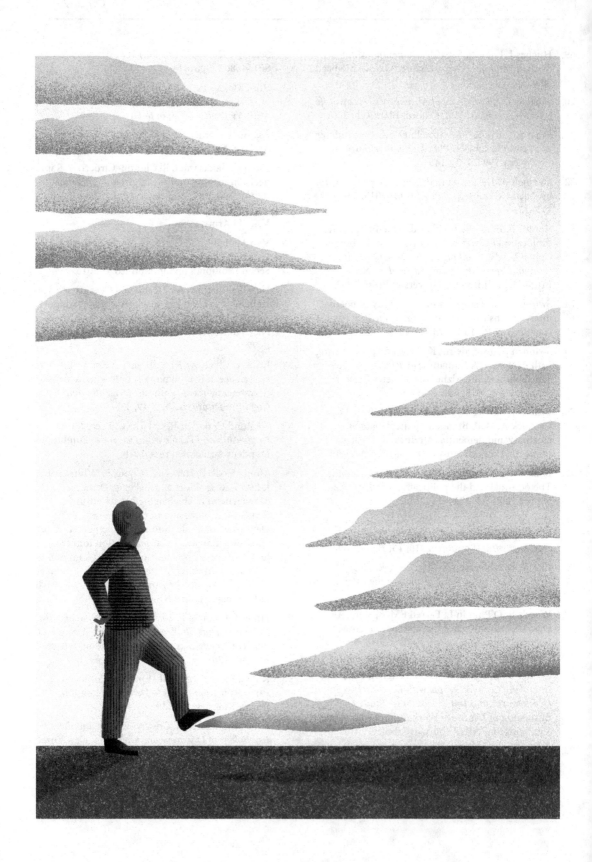

Chapter 12

Societal and Ethical Views on End-of-Life Decisions in Dementia

Chris Gastmans, Jenny van der Steen and Wilco Achterberg

1 End-of-Life Decisions

Most people in contemporary Western societies do not die suddenly, but from organ failure or dementia after a period with declining health due to chronic-progressive disease. With increasing options for care and treatment, decisions about useful or desirable treatment and care are made in the last phase of life of most people. In case of dementia, in a representative sample of deaths in Flanders in 2013, at least one end-of-life decision was made in 57% of persons who died with dementia [1]. In the Netherlands, in persons with dementia who died in nursing homes, which represents the great majority of persons with dementia, such decisions were taken in 72% of cases [2].

End-of-life decisions can be classified by the nature of the treatment (starting, withholding, stopping treatment) and by any intention with regard to hastening death [3, 4]. In this chapter, we pragmatically report on three categories of decisions. First is decisions primarily aimed at alleviating pain and other symptoms or improving quality of life in other ways, while possible effects on length of life are deemed irrelevant compared to that aim. Second is decisions around life-sustaining treatment or treatment to cure acute or comorbid conditions which may or may not affect length and quality of life. Third is decisions around terminating life.

2 First Category: Decisions on Alleviating Pain and Other Symptoms and on Palliative Care in General

2.1 Palliative Care and Improving Quality of Life

The first group of decisions addressed in this chapter includes whether to alleviate pain and other symptoms with, for example, opioids, benzodiazepines or barbiturates, but also about palliative care more generally. Palliative care offers holistic, highly multidisciplinary care developed initially to improve quality of life in the terminal phase of those with incurable cancer. However, it has shown benefits for more people when there is no cure for progressive disease, and this includes dementia. It aims to alleviate suffering due to severe illness, and although not limited to the terminal phase, still it aims to alleviate suffering, 'especially of those near the end of life' [5].

The suffering can be physical, psychological, social or spiritual (existential) in nature. Spiritual care being part of palliative care is a distinctive feature compared with other holistic- or person-centred care approaches, which is relevant to existential questions that may play a role in a wish to hasten death (the third category of decisions addressed later in this chapter). Palliative care also explicitly includes care for family and other relatives. This aspect is even more important in dementia than in other incurable diseases given the elevated caregiver burden along with fewer positive caregiving experiences with dementia [6, 7] and complexities in decision-making [8].

Decisions on palliative care refer to what can be done as much as about what is not being done (treatment withheld as part of the second category of decisions). Palliative care decisions consider a focus on improving quality of life in terms of comfort and functioning, *regardless* of any effects on length of life (Figure 12.1; [6]). Such focus implies goals of care are prioritized while there may be more goals at a time. Goals, or a mixture of goals, can also shift over time and therefore re-evaluation is needed, such as in advance care planning conversations. Shared decision-making approaches are preferred [6], but the amount of input in decision-making differs between jurisdictions and cultures, for example, with a more

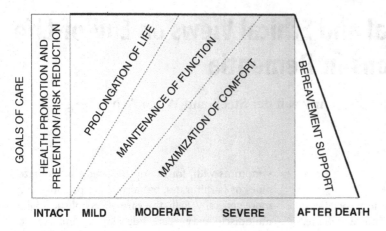

Figure 12.1 Dementia progression and suggested prioritizing of care goals. (Reproduced from [6])

pronounced role for family as proxy decision makers in the United States versus more directive input from specialist elderly care physicians in the Netherlands [9].

Regarding other societal issues, palliative care as a broader concept than terminal care, and dementia being a disease you can die from are two conceptualizations that are still rather unknown. Studies have shown limited awareness and knowledge on dementia being a life-shortening illness among the general public, among family caregivers of nursing home residents with dementia and among nursing staff caring for nursing home residents with dementia in the Netherlands and other Western countries [10–12].

Palliative care decisions do not necessarily imply referral to specialist palliative care [6]. For example, regarding decisions to treat behavioural symptoms which most persons with dementia and caregivers encounter at some point during the course of the disease, specialized dementia care consultation may be indicated when such symptoms are severe [13]. Further, a palliative approach applied by generalists is being implemented upstream with an orientation towards addressing needs [14]. It requires societies to build capacity and partnership between specialists for referral, consultation and addressing generalists' educational needs. Palliative care may thus be integrated and perceived as a standard for good care, and therefore become 'mainstream'.

Indeed, the quality of palliative care for persons with dementia has improved in the Netherlands (from the perspective of bereaved family; [15]) and

in Flanders (from the perspective of nursing home staff; [16]). Yet symptom burden has remained substantial in both countries. Perhaps this relates to the inability to prevent all symptoms from developing towards the end of life or to higher expectations among clinicians, patients, family or perhaps society at large of effects of management of pain and other symptoms.

2.2 Pain Prevalence at the End of Life

Towards the end of life, pain often persists or emerges and pain and shortness of breath increase in persons with dementia towards the end of life while agitation is more likely to decrease [17]. Pain is an important symptom that strongly influences quality of life and of dying. As people grow older, they accumulate chronic illnesses associated with pain and functional impairment. In the terminal phase, people are often bedridden, which may lead to even more pain-related conditions such as stiffness, contractures or pressure ulcers. Unfortunately, pain is therefore a very common feature in dying patients, which physicians generally recognize in patients with a terminal oncological disease.

However, many physicians are surprised to learn that in patients dying with dementia pain is almost just as prevalent. In a recent prospective study in the UK, 85 persons with advanced dementia were followed for nine months, 31 of them until death [18]. It was found that more than half of people with advanced dementia had pain during movement, and 1 in 9 also had pain when in rest, and this persisted throughout the study.

Also in Flanders high symptom burden was found in patients with advanced dementia until the end of life [19]. In the Netherlands, pain was found in between 47% and 68% of nursing home residents with dementia, and in the last week of life even in 78% of nursing home residents [17].

2.3 Pain Assessment at the End of Life

Decisions regarding pain management are complicated by barriers in communication and assessment. Dementia leads to progressive impairment in verbal communication and in an ability to communicate about more abstract issues. Most nursing home residents with dementia can still self-report pain [20], but for others, recognition and monitoring of treatment is more complicated. Over the past decades, several observational instruments have been developed to overcome this problem; examples include the Pain Assessment Checklist for Seniors with Limited Ability to Communicate (PACSLAC), Pain Assessment in Advanced Dementia (PAINAD) and the recently developed Pain Assessment in Impaired Cognition-15 (PAIC15).

One review describes 15 studies that made use of instruments that can be seen as appropriate for people with dementia at the end of life [21]. However, many of these tools lack sound psychometric evaluations. A systematic review that only included studies if they evaluated reliability, validity or clinical feasibility of instruments, selected only four observational instruments for the end of life (Abby Pain scale, Critical-care Pain Observation Tool (CPOT), Multidimensional Objective Pain Assessment Tool (MOPAT) and PAINAD) [22]. However, quality assessment with the Consensus-Based Standards for the Selection of Health Status Measurement Instruments (COSMIN) criteria made the authors conclude it is not possible yet to give evidence-based recommendations about which tool should be used. Given the lack of sound psychometric evidence for the end-of-life situation, the use of observational instruments for the detection of pain in dementia has received more attention. In many guidelines that refer to pain in older persons or persons with cognitive impairment, the use of an observational pain instrument such as the Dutch guideline for pain in vulnerable older persons is advised [23].

However, implementation in everyday practice is not easy, often because of a lack of ongoing training and multidisciplinary transfer of knowledge [24]. Nurses have difficulties recognizing pain in dementia as a result of a lack of training in this subject [25]. They particularly find it difficult to classify the discomfort they may observe and, for instance, to differentiate between anxiety and pain [26]. They also report a feeling of inadequacy because they cannot connect with the patient and problems in getting prescriptions from physicians for adequate pain management [27]. Physicians also struggle with pain in dementia at the end of life. They find it hard to make a good diagnosis in the absence of self-report, to make a choice in type of painkiller (because of side effects) and administration route (because of swallowing difficulties) [28]. Physicians indicate they need more training, consultation and mentoring. A study that evaluated telementoring for pain assessment and management in end-stage dementia has shown beneficial effects on knowledge and self-efficacy in healthcare workers, including physicians and nurses [29].

2.4 Pain Management at the End of Life

Pain control (with medication) refers to 'the intentional administration of analgesics and/or other drugs in dosages and combinations required to adequately relieve pain' ([4], pp. 32–3). Not all patients receive the same amount of pain control; one of the explanatory factors is the primary diagnosis. Patients with cancer generally receive the most and best pain control [30]. In 2013, intensified alleviation of pain and/or symptoms was performed in 43% of persons with dementia [1], and in the Netherlands from 2007 to 2011, this was performed in 49% of nursing home residents who died with dementia [2]. Generally, people with dementia receive less pain medication than people with intact cognition [31, 32]. However, several studies show a hesitance to use morphine seems to disappear when persons approach the end of life. A prospective observation study in 24 dying nursing home patients showed good pain control [33], and also in a hospice study pain control in persons with dementia was appropriate [30].

Sometimes the dying process is accompanied by very distressing symptoms, such as severe dyspnoea or intractable pain, for which intensive medical and palliative treatment cannot alleviate those symptoms. As a last resort, palliative sedation can be used to induce a state of unconsciousness in order to end these refractory symptoms. Broeckaert in 2002 defined palliative sedation as 'the intentional administration of sedative drugs in dosages and combinations required to reduce the consciousness of a terminal patient as much as necessary to adequately relieve one or more refractory symptoms' ([34], p. 246).

A special form is continuous palliative sedation, in which unconsciousness is deliberately continued until death, and this is mostly what is meant when the term *palliative sedation* is used. In the Netherlands, 1 in 5 persons who died with dementia received palliative sedation [35]. In Flanders, a retrospective case series in nursing homes suggested about 1 in 10 patients with dementia received palliative sedation, and 1 in 7 patients with advanced dementia received it [36]. The same study showed sedation does not always lead to total symptom control.

Surely, the decision to start palliative sedation should not be taken lightly, and the communication impairments that accompany the course of dementia hamper this decision-making process. In many countries such as the Netherlands and Belgium, most patients with dementia die in nursing or residential homes which are generally less equipped for technical medical procedures. However, recently a practice protocol has been developed to assist physicians in both the decision-making process and the technical procedures for palliative sedation in nursing homes that address the aforementioned issues [37].

3 Second Category: Decisions around Life-Sustaining Treatment and Cure of Acute or Comorbid Conditions

The second category of decisions contains whether to initiate or withhold, continue or withdraw life-sustaining treatment such as cardiopulmonary resuscitation (CPR) in case of cardiac arrest. It also comprises treatment of conditions that can be viewed as life-threatening comorbid conditions or conditions related to the dementia such as food and fluid intake problems, and acute conditions that can be life-threatening and often occur in frail persons. For example, mortality from lower respiratory tract infections, in particular pneumonia, is high among nursing home residents, as shown by studies from the United

States [38], the Netherlands [39] and other European countries [40].

Therefore, for persons with dementia, decisions about antibiotic treatment and artificial nutrition and hydration (ANH) commonly need to be taken. In Western countries, this often concerns a *non*-treatment decision with regard to CPR and ANH. Non-treatment refers to 'withdrawing or withholding a curative or life-sustaining treatment, because in the given situation this treatment is deemed to be no longer meaningful or effective' ([4], pp. 30–2). In Flanders in 2013, treatment was withheld in 31% and withdrawn in 33% of persons with dementia [1]. In the Netherlands, in nursing homes, where as mentioned before the great majority of Dutch persons with dementia die, these percentages were 42% and 54%, respectively (nationally representative study 2007–11 [41]).

3.1 Cardiopulmonary Resuscitation

Cardiopulmonary resuscitation is an invasive intervention in case of cardiac arrest. While it is rarely effective in terms of survival, quality of life in persons with dementia may decrease because of worsened pre-existing brain damage. Indeed, in a study on in-hospital CPR of persons aged 70 and older, 12% survived, but among the 45 persons with dementia, there were no survivors [42]. Older studies had already confirmed dementia as a risk factor for not surviving CPR [43].

Physicians have long warned not to attempt CPR as the default in persons with dementia (e.g. [44, 45]). The Dutch professional organization for elderly care physicians Verenso advises discussing preferences for CPR as part of advance care planning, but physicians can decide on a do-not-resuscitate (DNR) order in individual cases when they believe CPR to be medically futile, with no specific advice for dementia [46]. A subsequent Dutch study showed DNR decisions in case of dementia are often (two-thirds of persons) made only when the person is incompetent [47].

This proportion hardly changed from 1990 to 2010. This might have changed through the COVID-19 pandemic when Dutch general practitioners (GPs) called older persons to document preferences for acute situations. However, in a Dutch study, the GPs probably referred to decisions about hospital or intensive care unit (ICU) admission, not in particular to DNR [48]. Studies in institutional settings from Ireland (hospital, one-third with cognitive impairment or dementia [49]) and the United States (nursing homes, including discussions with family [50]) did show the pandemic prompted earlier discussion of preferences around resuscitation.

Before the pandemic, nursing homes in the Netherlands and elsewhere often recorded preference for CPR ('code status') and hospitalization soon after admission in the context of advance care planning as these are the two decisions that typically need to be taken acutely or in a crisis situation [51]. In the Netherlands, resuscitation is rarely attempted in nursing home residents with dementia (2 of 330 deaths in 2007–11) [41].

However, a number of persons with dementia and family caregivers do want resuscitation performed. That is, vignette and interview studies have shown individuals with dementia and family caregivers in Western and non-Western countries vary substantially in their preference for resuscitation in case of cardiac arrest (e.g. [52, 53]). This may in part relate to being ill informed on prognosis or to little understanding of how a goal of care to not prolong life relates to a DNR decision, or to family not knowing the preferences of the person with dementia well enough [45, 52, 53].

3.2 Antibiotics

Most persons with dementia and family caregivers in Western and non-Western countries prefer use of antibiotics in case of infection [52–54]. Indeed, antibiotics might prolong life, but they might also relieve symptoms such as when achieving a fast cure of a urinary tract infection. Such infections can be burdensome but not fatal: antibiotic use for urinary tract infection was unrelated to survival in an observational study in the United States [55].

However, in particular regarding life-threatening lower respiratory tract infections including pneumonia, potential effects on both survival and symptom burden complicate decision-making. Evidence from research is sparse. Observational studies have shown associations with mortality and symptom relief in opposite directions [56–58], which probably depends on incomplete adjustment

for antibiotics used in more severe acute illness (in the United States) or withheld in more severe illness (in the Netherlands [54]).

A newer Dutch study [59] showed no association between comfort and antibiotics used to treat pneumonia, perhaps due to trends of improved symptom-relieving treatment in persons with pneumonia and dementia. Antibiotics are often provided empirically because with dementia, symptoms may be unclear or communicated with difficulty and diagnostic workup may be complicated (e.g. inability to produce sputum [60]). In persons with severe dementia and pneumonia, antibiotics may prolong the dying process rather than prolong life substantially [61]. Apart from possible side effects of antibiotics, this indicates just trying antibiotics is not a neutral decision with no risk of harm.

After all, however, in case of pneumonia, mortality may be affected more by decisions not to rehydrate than by decisions to withhold antibiotics [61]. Another interesting finding from research is that it makes more sense to regard pneumonia as a marker of frailty more generally rather than inherent to the dementia disease, while dehydration and malnutrition are more closely related to the dementia. Therefore, it is common in end-stage dementia and at the end of life with dementia [39, 40, 62]. Regardless, or perhaps because of sparse evidence of its effects, treatment with or without antibiotics, and with or without invasive rehydration in case of pneumonia varies widely across countries; withholding is more common in the Netherlands than in Italy, the United States and Israel [63, 64].

3.3 Artificial Nutrition and Hydration

In Italian nursing homes, half of persons with dementia and pneumonia received intravenous rehydration therapy, mostly to reduce suffering or symptoms and therefore with a palliative intent [64]. The therapy was provided in the nursing home, avoiding potentially burdensome hospitalization which was facilitated by on-site physicians. Decisions to withhold fluids or food, whether taken by mouth or artificially, are particularly sensitive decisions that are heavily influenced by the particular medical traditions and a broader cultural context [65].

In a study in the UK, persons with mild dementia valued the ability to eat and drink as it represented quality of life, sense of identity and agency [66]. This was found in family caregivers as well [67]; they did not recognize a relationship between problems with eating and drinking and the dementia. Even though some expressed unease with eating less because of difficulty using utensils, they were not willing to discuss it in advance and would leave future decisions to others. However, considering case vignettes and asked about tube feeding, the persons with dementia perceived ANH as unnatural. It would not bring them enjoyment and quality of life. Indeed, an early ethnographic study in nursing homes in the Netherlands showed interpretation of the person's quality of life, rather than any advance document or care planning, was the main consideration in the decision to not provide ANH [68].

However, eating and drinking problems and any intervening may be perceived differently outside north-west Europe. Views of ANH as part of basic human care are related to social, religious, racial and professional values of sanctity of life and foster hope among family and professional caregivers, especially in countries such as Japan, the United States and Israel [65]. Indeed, in a Canadian family booklet on comfort care adapted for use in Italy, Japan, the Netherlands and, more recently, for use in other countries, sections on tube feeding were among the most revised along with sections on euthanasia and spirituality [69, 70].

Concerns voiced in the Netherlands and the UK related to the mere mention of tube feeding even though recommending against it, as it would create expectations among families that it is after all an option and thus would increase demand [70, 71]. Indeed, also in Western countries, the decision whether to offer food and fluids and whether to use artificial means can be highly sensitive [72].

The European Association for Palliative Care (EAPC) recommends that 'hydration, preferably subcutaneous, may be provided if appropriate, such as in case of infection; it is inappropriate in the dying phase', as, for example, it increases death rattle and other secretions while mouth care can resolve dry mouth in the dying phase [6]. However, the EAPC expert panel with experts from 23 countries was unable to reach a full consensus on the topic mostly because of concerns about cultural and religious sensitivities and subcutaneous hydration not being routine practice in some countries.

Similarly, only moderate consensus was achieved on the recommendation that 'permanent enteral tube nutrition may not be beneficial and should as a rule be avoided in dementia; skillful hand feeding is preferred'. Some experts felt general rules were inappropriate and would decide on a case-by-case basis. Regardless, time should be taken for careful and skilful hand feeding or comfort feeding with small amounts of food for pleasure. This is indicated if dementia is the cause of the eating or swallowing problems, according to the first item in a practice set of decision rules and heuristics, developed by Davies et al. [73]. Comfort feeding is also indicated if there is no other reversible cause which is considered in the next step of these heuristics.

Accumulating evidence from observational studies indicates that in persons with advanced dementia, tube feeding probably does not prolong life, although incomplete adjustment for factors related to the decision remains an issue [74]. Causes of food and fluid intake problems can be multiple and cognitive or physical in origin. Some are treatable while swallowing problems may also relate to the dementia with few treatment options as summarized in recent reviews [74, 67].

Further, no appetite is common in dying persons. Gradual dehydration in the dying phase does not usually induce discomfort [75]. Indeed, observational studies in persons dying with dementia in the Netherlands [56, 35, 33] and other European countries [40] have consistently observed low discomfort in persons with advanced dementia dying after food and fluid intake problems, and such a dying process to be more comfortable than dying from a pneumonia.

A recent development in advance decision-making around food and fluid intake problems potentially increases these dilemmas: when persons state in an advance directive that they refuse food and fluids in a certain stage or condition with dementia, such an advance directive implies discontinuing help with eating and drinking [76]. However, if it also includes an order that an active request from the person for food or assistance should be honoured, some ethical dilemmas may be avoided. Nevertheless, the Ethics Committee of the US Society for Post-Acute and Long-Term

Care Medicine (AMDA) does not accept this type of advance decision-making.

In contrast, Davies et al. [8], based on studies in the UK, recommend a non-linear shared decision-making process for persons with dementia that takes into account that outcomes of decision-making may influence future decisions or advance care planning. They also included 'managing and considering emotions' of family caregivers as one of the important steps in decision-making for persons with dementia. Further, this decision-making model was specific to dementia in considering and reconsidering capacity and social support and role clarity throughout a cyclic process of decision-making. This model may help navigate the sensitivities in decision-making, which can be strong as it regards meaningful life and death with dementia.

4 Third Category: Decisions around Terminating Life

The third group contains decisions concerning whether to administer purposefully lethal medication. Voluntary euthanasia – intentionally terminating the life of a patient by someone other than the patient at the patient's request – did occur in 1.2% of persons with dementia in Flanders in 2013 [1]. In the Netherlands, it occurred in 0.9% of persons with dementia, with 2.1% of persons with dementia requesting it [77].

Non-voluntary euthanasia is intentionally terminating the life of a patient by someone other than the patient and not at the patient's request. This illegal practice occurred in 2013 in 2.9% of persons with dementia in Flanders [1]. It is important to stress that non-voluntary euthanasia differs radically from palliative interventions such as palliative sedation in its intentionality, with the former aiming to terminate life and the latter aiming for alleviation of refractory symptoms regardless of its effects on length of life (see earlier in this chapter).

4.1 Euthanasia in Persons with Dementia: Societal Views and Attitudes

Since the early 1990s, an intense societal debate about euthanasia in persons with dementia has existed in the Netherlands. Research into the practice of euthanasia in persons with dementia shows 6% of Dutch older adults (61–92 years old) have an advance euthanasia directive [78]. They

were more likely to have an advance euthanasia directive if they were single, did not adhere to a specific faith, did not trust their physician to carry out their end-of-life wishes, suffered from a chronic disorder or experienced functional restrictions.

Only a few cases of euthanasia in persons with dementia based on an advance euthanasia directive have been reported in the Netherlands [79, 80]. Twenty-nine per cent of Dutch physicians (GPs and nursing home physicians) stated that they have already treated a person with dementia who had an advance euthanasia directive [81]. Three per cent of these physicians stated that they have performed euthanasia in a person with dementia based on an advance directive. Forty-four per cent stated that, although they had not performed euthanasia in these patients to date, they did not rule out performing euthanasia in the future. Fifty-four per cent of the physicians ruled out performing euthanasia on persons with dementia in the future. The latter considered euthanasia in persons with dementia unacceptable. Furthermore, they did not view an advance euthanasia directive as a valid request.

In more recent empirical studies, the negative attitudes of Dutch physicians towards euthanasia in advanced dementia were confirmed [82–87]. Crucial in the reticent attitudes of physicians appears to be the impossibility of patient–physician communication at the time of decision-making as well as the impossibility to receive confirmation of the unbearableness of suffering. A 2019 survey among dementia specialists in Belgium reported a majority (65%) of them disapproved of a change in the law allowing euthanasia in advanced dementia [88].

The study of Rurup et al. [89] showed patients' relatives often adopt a more tolerant attitude towards life-terminating behaviour in persons with dementia than nurses and physicians do. Ninety per cent of relatives, 57% of nurses and 16% of physicians agreed with the statement that euthanasia based on an advance directive in persons with dementia is acceptable. However, in more recent studies, also some relatives and members of the general public were reluctant to adhere to advance euthanasia directives in case of dementia [84, 86].

A similar trend was reported in other countries [90]. In Finland, 8% of physicians are in favour of euthanasia in persons with dementia [91]. Canada, Finland and the Netherlands report approximately a third (or just under) of nurses support euthanasia in persons with dementia [89, 91–93]. Studies in Finland, the Netherlands and the UK examining general public attitudes towards euthanasia in severe dementia found around 50% were in favour [94, 91, 95]. Brinkman-Stoppelburg et al. [82] and Kouwenhoven et al. [85] reported respectively 60% and 77% of the Dutch sample in favour.

4.2 Euthanasia in Persons with Severe Dementia: Ethical Approaches

Although, to our knowledge, no official ethical documents on euthanasia for persons with dementia exist, some philosophical ethical studies [96–108] have been conducted. The topic of advance euthanasia directives for patients with dementia enables us to present two influential ethical approaches to end-of-life care in persons with dementia; the principles-oriented autonomy approach that generally favours the use of advance euthanasia directives on one hand, and the care-oriented relational approach that mostly criticizes advance euthanasia directives on the other.

4.2.1 Principles-Oriented Autonomy Approach

Older people often associate dignity with autonomy, independence and preserving one's intellectual powers. Losing one's autonomy and cognitive capacities are reasons for requesting euthanasia via an advance euthanasia directive in a timely way [100]. These advance directives rely on the authority of the competent pre-dementia person (the 'then' self) to govern the welfare of the incompetent person with dementia (the 'now' self) [106, 109, 110]. Proponents of this 'precedent autonomy or critical interest' approach underline the stewardship responsibility of the 'then' self for the journey into forgetfulness [111, 109, 110]. As a consequence, post-dementia decisions should be based on historical lifetime values and beliefs. De Boer et al. [112] clarify:

> The former decisions of a person with dementia, laid down in an advance directive, remain in force because the person now lacks the necessary

capacity to exercise autonomy, and because the critical interests of the formerly competent person (the 'then' self) prevail over the actual preferences or experiences of the person who is now in a state of dementia (the 'now' self). The experiences of the demented person are not part of the autonomous decision-making.

An important presupposition of this approach is that individuals are perfectly capable of determining their wishes concerning future end-of-life care individually and cognitively, and in such a way that advance directives unambiguously tell caregivers what to do. Persons are, in this approach, mainly considered as beings with thoughts, intelligence, reason, reflection and consciousness [113]. In order to facilitate the development of advance directives, decision aids are presented. These aids help people by providing neutral information about the dementia process so they can take an informed decision [114].

Respect for autonomy largely covers moral reasoning on advance euthanasia directives. Within the included literature, autonomy is mainly described as the right to self-determination and individual choice [100]. Respect for autonomy is founded upon the ideal of the autonomous agent. As an autonomous person, one is entitled to act in accordance with a freely self-chosen and informed plan. Within this anthropological viewpoint, advance euthanasia directives are considered instruments that enable older adults their autonomous wishes concerning a dignified end of life to be respected.

4.2.2 Care-Oriented Relational Approach

While the principle of respect for autonomy generally leads to an argument in favour of advance euthanasia directives, questions arise about its applicability to cases in which dementia patients are involved. Because dementia is marked by progressive deterioration affecting both the memory and reasoning capabilities, dementia patients fall short of the ideal of the autonomous agent that grounds the principle of respect for autonomy. Hence – according to the proponents of the care-oriented relational approach – ethical reflection on the end of life of persons with dementia should not start from the ideal of the autonomous agent, but from the relational context in which dementia care practices are embedded [115].

By providing care, caregivers enter as persons into a relationship with a vulnerable fellow human being – a person with dementia – who is in need of care. However, it is not clear from the beginning what can be considered the most adequate and appropriate answer to the care needs of a particular person with dementia. Finding the right answer is not the result of a general and abstract balancing of principles or of logical deduction. It is reached through a shared dialogical process of communication, interpretation and understanding that takes place within the care relationship [116].

4.3 Problems Associated with Advance Euthanasia Directives

Based on the relational approach to dementia care, some clusters of problems associated with the use of advance euthanasia directives according to the aforementioned autonomy approach have been formulated [99, 105, 107, 108, 117].

The first group of problems is related to the interpretation of a patient's wishes. As many authors have already pointed out, clearly expressing one's wishes and thoughts can be difficult. But interpreting the meaning of a patient's wishes is also a difficult task for fellow human beings such as relatives and caregivers. A patient's wishes cannot be considered a given whose contents can easily be deduced from an advance directive and which clarifies for all those involved what must be done for the patient throughout the consecutive stages of his or her care. What a patient would have wanted under specific circumstances needs to be constructed through fairly elaborated interpretative processes based on what we know of his or her life, previous pronouncements (e.g. as reported in advance directives) and the patient's actual reactions to concrete proposals [118].

Even if persons with dementia might be incompetent, they still have the capacity to experience their life and the context wherein it is embedded [112]. Hence contemporary preferences, needs and desires and the present well-being of the person with dementia cannot be ignored when taking decisions. This perspective on the relationship between the 'then' self that existed prior to the onset of dementia and the 'now' self is known as the

so-called experiential interest approach [106, 119].

Even if, as in advance euthanasia directives, the medical decision to be performed – euthanasia – is very clear, communication and interpretation are still needed. The specific difficulty resides in having to determine the moment when euthanasia should be performed. Suppose, for instance, that a person with an early dementia diagnosis has been able to clearly state that he or she wants euthanasia from the moment he or she no longer recognizes his or her child.

The physician has to determine whether this person's actual situation does indeed match the circumstances specified by him or her in the advance directive calling for euthanasia to be performed. This is very difficult, for even carefully formulated specifications about the chosen moment of death require interpretation [108, 116]. For instance, how should one determine the act of recognition? There are many ways of recognizing a person. Where should the line be drawn [116]?

This brings us to the category of problems with future forecasting. They refer to the fact that a person's preferences and values can change, to the fact that people's ability to constructively adapt to even the most severe debilities and to the fact that previously communicated wishes may not reflect a change of heart [117]. The issue of irreversibility is much stronger in persons with dementia. It may be that the aforementioned person with an advance euthanasia directive offers resistance when the action is performed. How is such resistance to be interpreted? Hence the dilemma faced by physicians and proxies: how to balance the actual preferences and experiences of the person with dementia against the patient's earlier opinions laid down in a now-forgotten advance directive [107, 112, 108, 116].

Following the 'experiential interest approach', the well-being and interests of the 'now' self are of moral significance and the absolute primacy of precedent autonomy seems wrong [111]. Goering clarifies:

> This does not mean that we should never make plans for our future-selves; rather, it means that we should take care to provide for flexibility in any advance directive, with the recognition that our values or priorities may change, and due to

declining decisional capacities, those judgements may need to be made by others in conjunction with our future-selves, rather than solely and individually by our presently competent selves. [120, p. 63]

A third group of problems is situated on the level of the patient's autonomy versus the patient being related to other people such as relatives, friends and caregivers. It seems that, in the case of advance euthanasia directives, supporting the respect for autonomy principle is much more complicated. People's wishes and values are very often of a pre-reflexive and emotional kind. Without sufficient attention to emotions, feelings of grief, or even resistance, within an ongoing, interpersonal face-to-face dialogue between the patient and other people, one risks entering a situation in which people can easily draft an advance euthanasia directive while in a state of panic or depression, or having little or unclear information about the course of dementia. In this case, advance euthanasia directives could even increase the vulnerability of the patient, as they do not reflect a well-informed wish of the patient [107].

Finally, a patient's decision to write an advance euthanasia directive has important implications for all parties involved in the patient's care [108]. The decision to perform euthanasia at a certain moment in time has to be made by someone (e.g. the physician) other than the patient himself or herself. This raises questions around autonomy of the other person. To what extent can our fellow man be given the responsibility to ensure our right of self-determination is respected?

These critiques bring us to the basic problem in the use of advance euthanasia directives: insufficient communication and shared understanding between the person with dementia on one hand, and the caregivers on the other. This is confirmed by studies from the Netherlands where, despite the legal recognition of advance euthanasia directives for persons with dementia, euthanasia occurs rarely in this patient group [86, 87, 78, 89]. The Dutch researchers concluded that:

> Communication and interpretation are crucial in determining the circumstances as well as the exact moment of performing euthanasia and this cannot be captured in or replaced by advance euthanasia directives. This is precisely what seems to cause the fundamental problem of complying with advance euthanasia directives in cases of severe dementia. [87, p. 261]

4.4 Dialogue and Interpretation in Ethical Decision-Making on Advance Euthanasia Directives

Given the aforementioned difficulties that arise from advance euthanasia directives when conceptualized within a principles-oriented autonomy approach, some authors suggest a care-oriented relational approach to deal with advance euthanasia directives [112, 107, 108]. According to them, taking into account the dialogical and interpretative nature of ethical decision-making should be a standard and indispensable element of good dementia care. As Moody says: 'The heart of the matter is not to be found in the legal instrument as much as in the process of communication and negotiation which leads up to the result' [121, p. 92].

In the care-oriented relational approach, the search for what is best for the patient should not solely focus on the patient's wishes as an isolated individual, but should always start with listening to the concerns expressed by the patient, his or her close relatives, his or her caregivers etc. because they outline the rich relational context in which the person's care has to take shape. Understanding persons implies an understanding of the relational stories in which they are embedded [115, 122, 113].

If preferred, decision-making can be shared among all people involved. There will never be a legal instrument or a brief or simple paper process that provides an escape from this demanding process of communication and interpretation among parties to a decision. Therefore, these authors suggest that advance euthanasia directives may be helpful, for example, to facilitate the ethical dialogue and the interpretation process among all people involved. However, such directives cannot replace communication and interpretation [123, 116].

References

1. Wendrich-van Dael A, Pivodic L, Cohen J, Deliens L, Van den Block L, Chambaere K. End-of-life decision making for people who died of dementia: A mortality follow-back study comparing 1998, 2007, and 2013 in Flanders, Belgium. *J Am Med Dir Assoc.* 2019; **20**: 1344–50.

2. Van der Steen JT, Deliens L, Koopmans RTCM, Onwuteaka-Philipsen BD. Physicians' perceptions of suffering in people with dementia at the end of life. *Palliat Support Care* 2017 Oct; **15**(5): 587–99. doi: 10.1017/S147895151600098

3. Van der Steen JT, van der Wal G, Mehr DR, Ooms ME, Ribbe MW. End-of-life decision making in nursing home residents with dementia and pneumonia: Dutch physicians' intentions regarding hastening death. *Alzheimer Dis Assoc Disord*. 2005 Jul–Sep; **19**(3): 148–55. doi: 10.1097/01.wad.0000175525.99104.b7

4. Broeckaert B, Flemish Palliative Care Federation. Treatment decisions in advanced disease: A conceptual framework. *Indian J Palliat Care* 2009; **15**: 30–6.

5. Radbruch L, De Lima L, Knaul F, Wenk R, Ali Z, Bhatnaghar S, et al. Redefining palliative care: A new consensus-based definition. *J Pain Symptom Manage*. 2020 Oct; **60**(4): 754–64. doi: 10.1016/j.jpainsymman.2020.04.027

6. Van der Steen JT, Radbruch L, Hertogh CM, de Boer ME, Hughes JC, Larkin P, et al. White paper defining optimal palliative care in older people with dementia: A Delphi study and recommendations from the European Association for Palliative Care. *Palliat Med*. 2014 Mar; **28**(3): 197–209. doi: 10.1177/0269216313493685

7. Boogaard JA, van der Steen JT, de Boer AH, van Groenou MIB. How is end-of-life care with and without dementia associated with informal caregivers' outcomes? *Am J Hosp Palliat Care* 2019 Nov; **36**(11): 1008–15. doi: 10.1177/1049909119836932

8. Davies N, De Souza T, Rait G, Meehan J, Sampson EL. Developing an applied model for making decisions towards the end of life about care for someone with dementia. *PLoS One* 2021 May 27; **16**(5): e0252464. doi: 10.1371/journal.pone.0252464. eCollection 2021

9. Helton MR, van der Steen JT, Daaleman TP, Gamble GR, Ribbe MW. A cross-cultural study of physician treatment decisions for demented nursing home patients who develop pneumonia. *Ann Fam Med*. 2006 May–Jun; **4**(3): 221–7. doi: 10.1370/afm.536

10. Van der Steen JT, Onwuteaka-Philipsen BD, Knol DL, Ribbe MW, Deliens L. Caregivers' understanding of dementia predicts patients' comfort at death: A prospective observational study. *BMC Med*. 2013 Apr 11; **11**: 105. doi: 10.1186/1741-7015-11-105

11. Robinson A, Eccleston C, Annear M, Elliott KE, Andrews S, Stirling C, et al. Who knows, who cares? Dementia knowledge among nurses, care workers, and family members of people living with dementia. *J Palliat Care*. 2014 Autumn; **30**(3): 158–65.

12. McInerney F, Doherty K, Bindoff A, Robinson A, Vickers J. How is palliative care understood in the context of dementia? Results from a massive open online course. *Palliat Med*. 2018 Mar; **32**(3): 594–602. doi: 10.1177/0269216317743433. Epub 2017 Dec 13

13. Macfarlane S, Atee M, Morris T, Whiting D, Healy M, Alford M, Cunningham C. Evaluating the clinical impact of national dementia behaviour support programs on neuropsychiatric outcomes in Australia. *Front Psychiatry* 2021 Apr 13; **12**: 652254. doi: 10.3389/fpsyt.2021.652254

14. Sawatzky R, Porterfield P, Lee J, Dixon D, Lounsbury K, Pesut B, et al. Conceptual foundations of a palliative approach: A knowledge synthesis. *BMC Palliat Care* 2016 Jan 15; **15**: 5. doi: 10.1186/s12904-016-0076-9

15. Klapwijk MS, Bolt SR, Boogaard JA, ten Koppel M, Gijsberts M-JHE, van Leussen C, et al. Trends in quality of care and dying perceived by family caregivers of nursing home residents with dementia 2005–2019. *Palliat Med*. 2021 Dec; **35**(10): 1951–60. doi:10.1177/02692163211030831. Epub 2021 Aug 28.

16. Miranda R, Smets T, Van den Noortgate N, Deliens L, Van den Block L. Higher prevalence of dementia but no change in total comfort while dying among nursing home residents with dementia between 2010 and 2015: Results from two retrospective epidemiological studies. *Int J Environ Res Public Health* 2021; **18**: 2160. https://doi.org/10.3390/ijerph18042160

17. Hendriks SA, Smalbrugge M, Galindo-Garre F, et al. From admission to death: Prevalence and course of pain, agitation, and shortness of breath, and treatment of these symptoms in nursing home residents with dementia. *J Am Med Dir Assoc*. 2015; **16**: 475–81.

18. Sampson EL, Candy B, Davis S, Gola AB, Harrington J, King M, et al. Living and dying with advanced dementia: A prospective cohort study of symptoms, service use and care at the end of life. *Palliat Med*. 2018 Mar; **32**(3): 668–81. doi: 10.1177/0269216317726443. Epub 2017 Sep 18. PMID: 28922625; PMCID: PMC5987852

19. Vandervoort A, Van den Block L, Van der Steen JT, Volicer L, Vander Stichele R, Houttekier D, et al. Nursing home residents dying with dementia in Flanders, Belgium: A nationwide postmortem study on clinical characteristics and quality of dying. *J Am Med Dir Assoc*. 2013; **14**: 485–92.

20. Van der Steen JT, Westzaan A, Hanemaayer K, Muhamad M, de Waal MWM, Achterberg WP. Probable pain on the Pain Assessment in Impaired Cognition (PAIC15) instrument: Assessing sensitivity and specificity of cut-offs against three standards. *Brain Sci.* 2021 Jun 29; 11(7): 869. doi: 10.3390/brainsci11070869

21. McAnee G, Norwood K, Rosato M, Leavey G. Assessment of pain in people living with dementia at the end of life: A systematic review. *Int J Palliat Nurs.* 2021 Apr 2; 27(2): 72–85. doi: 10.12968/ijpn.2021.27.2.72. PMID: 33886358

22. Tapp D, Chenacher S, Gérard NPA, Bérubé-Mercier P, Gelinas C, Douville F, Desbiens JF. Observational pain assessment instruments for use with nonverbal patients at the end of life: A systematic review. *J Palliat Care* 2019 Oct; 34(4): 255–66. doi: 10.1177/0825859718816073. Epub 2019 Jan 13. PMID: 30638134

23. Achterberg WP, de Ruiter CM, de Weerd-Spaetgens CM, Geels P, Horikx A, Verduijn M, et al. Multidisciplinaire richtlijn 'Herkenning en behandeling van chronische pijn bij kwetsbare ouderen' [Multidisciplinary guideline 'Recognition and treatment of chronic pain in vulnerable elderly people']. *Ned Tijdschr Geneeskd.* 2012; 155(35): A4606. Dutch. PMID: 22929749.

24. De Witt Jansen B, Brazil K, Passmore P, Buchanan H, Maxwell D, McIlfatrick S, et al. 'A tool doesn't add anything.' The importance of added value: Use of observational pain tools with patients with advanced dementia approaching the end of life – a qualitative study of physician and nurse experiences and perspectives. *Int J Geriatr Psychiatry* 2018 Oct; 33(10): 1346–54. doi: 10.1002/gps.4931. Epub 2018 Jul 1. PMID: 29961948.

25. May K, Scammell J. Nurses' experiences of pain management in end-of-life dementia care: A literature review. *Int J Palliat Nurs.* 2020 Mar 2; 26(3): 110–18. doi: 10.12968/ijpn.2020.26.3.110. PMID: 32275475

26. Lundin E, Godskesen TE. End-of-life care for people with advanced dementia and pain: A qualitative study in Swedish nursing homes. *BMC Nurs.* 2021 Mar 20; 20(1): 48. doi: 10.1186/s12912-021-00566-7. PMID: 33743691; PMCID: PMC7981921

27. Brorson H, Plymoth H, Örmon K, Bolmsjö I. Pain relief at the end of life: Nurses' experiences regarding end-of-life pain relief in patients with dementia. *Pain Manag Nurs.* 2014 Mar; 15(1): 315–23. doi: 10.1016/j.pmn.2012.10.005. Epub 2013 Feb 28. PMID: 23453467

28. De Witt Jansen B, Brazil K, Passmore P, Buchanan H, Maxwell D, McIlfatrick SJ, et al. 'There's a Catch-22.' The complexities of pain management for people with advanced dementia nearing the end of life: A qualitative exploration of physicians' perspectives. *Palliat Med.* 2017 Sep; 31(8): 734–42. doi: 10.1177/0269216316673549. Epub 2016 Oct 26. PMID: 28659013

29. De Witt Jansen B, Brazil K, Passmore P, Buchanan H, Maxwell D, McIlfatrick SJ, et al. Evaluation of the impact of telementoring using ECHO© technology on healthcare professionals' knowledge and self-efficacy in assessing and managing pain for people with advanced dementia nearing the end of life. *BMC Health Serv Res.* 2018 Apr 2; 18(1): 228. doi: 10.1186/s12913-018-3032-y. PMID: 29606132; PMCID: PMC5879835

30. Romem A, Tom SE, Beauchene M, Babington L, Scharf SM, Romem A. Pain management at the end of life: A comparative study of cancer, dementia, and chronic obstructive pulmonary disease patients. *Palliat Med.* 2015 May; 29(5): 464–9. doi: 10.1177/0269216315570411. Epub 2015 Feb 13. PMID: 25680377

31. Achterberg WP, Erdal A, Husebo BS, Kunz M, Lautenbacher S. Are chronic pain patients with dementia being undermedicated? *J Pain Res.* 2021 Feb 15; 14: 431–9. doi: 10.2147/JPR.S239321. PMID: 33623425; PMCID: PMC7894836

32. Griffioen C, Willems EG, Husebo BS, Achterberg WP. Prevalence of the use of opioids for treatment of pain in persons with a cognitive impairment compared with cognitively intact persons: A systematic review. *Curr Alzheimer Res.* 2017; 14(5): 512–22. doi: 10.2174/1567205013666160629080735. PMID: 27357646

33. Klapwijk MS, Caljouw MA, van Soest-Poortvliet MC, van der Steen JT, Achterberg WP. Symptoms and treatment when death is expected in dementia patients in long-term care facilities. *BMC Geriatr.* 2014 Sep 2; 14: 99. doi: 10.1186/1471-2318-14-99. PMID: 25181947. PMCID: PMC4158395

34. Broeckaert B. Palliative sedation: Ethical aspects. In Gastmans C, ed. *Between Technology and Humanity: The Impact of Technology on Health Care Ethics.* Leuven, Leuven University Press, 2002; 239–55.

35. Hendriks SA, Smalbrugge M, Hertogh CM, van der Steen JT. Dying with dementia: Symptoms, treatment, and quality of life in the last week of life. *J Pain Symptom Manage.* 2014 Apr; 47(4): 710–20. doi: 10.1016/j.jpainsymman.2013.05.015

36. Anquinet L, Rietjens JA, Vandervoort A, van der Steen JT, Vander Stichele R, Deliens L, Van den Block L. Continuous deep sedation until death in nursing home residents with dementia: A case series. *J Am Geriatr Soc.* 2013 Oct; 61

(10): 1768–76. doi: 10.1111/jgs.12447. Epub 2013 Sep 3. PMID: 24000974

37. Robijn L, Gijsberts MJ, Pype P, Rietjens J, Deliens L, Chambaere K. Continuous palliative sedation until death: The development of a practice protocol for nursing homes. *J Am Med Dir Assoc.* 2021 Apr 28: S1525-8610(21)00304-2. doi: 10.1016/j.jamda.2021.03.008. Epub ahead of print. PMID: 33930319

38. Mitchell SL, Teno JM, Kiely DK, Shaffer ML, Jones RN, Prigerson HG, et al. The clinical course of advanced dementia. *N Engl J Med.* 2009 Oct 15; 361(16): 1529–38. doi: 10.1056/NEJMoa0902234

39. Hendriks SA, Smalbrugge M, van Gageldonk-Lafeber AB, Galindo-Garre F, Schipper M, Hertogh CMPM, van der Steen JT. Pneumonia, intake problems, and survival among nursing home residents with variable stages of dementia in the Netherlands: Results from a prospective observational study. *Alzheimer Dis Assoc Disord.* 2017 Jul–Sep; 31(3): 200–8. doi: 10.1097/WAD.0000000000000171

40. Miranda R, van der Steen JT, Smets T, Van den Noortgate N, Deliens L, Payne S, et al. Comfort and clinical events at the end of life of nursing home residents with and without dementia: The six-country epidemiological PACE study. *Int J Geriatr Psychiatry* 2020 Jul; 35(7): 719–27. doi: 10.1002/gps.5290

41. Hendriks SA, Smalbrugge M, Deliens L, Koopmans RTCM, Onwuteaka-Philipsen BD, Hertogh CMPM, van der Steen JT. End-of-life treatment decisions in nursing home residents dying with dementia in the Netherlands. *Int J Geriatr Psychiatry* 2017 Dec; 32(12): e43–e49. doi: 10.1002/gps.4650

42. Beesems SG, Blom MT, van der Pas MH, Hulleman M, van de Glind EM, van Munster BC, et al. Comorbidity and favorable neurologic outcome after out-of-hospital cardiac arrest in patients of 70 years and older. *Resuscitation* 2015 Sep; 94: 33–9. doi: 10.1016/j.resuscitation.2015.06.01

43. Ebell MH, Becker LA, Barry HC, Hagen M. Survival after in-hospital cardiopulmonary resuscitation. A meta-analysis. *J Gen Intern Med.* 1998 Dec; 13(12): 805–16. doi: 10.1046/j.1525-1497.1998.00244.x

44. Volandes AE, Abbo ED. Flipping the default: A novel approach to cardiopulmonary resuscitation in end-stage dementia. *J Clin Ethics* Summer 2007; 18(2): 122–39.

45. Arcand M. End-of-life issues in advanced dementia. Part 1: Goals of care, decision-making

46. Verenso, the Dutch Association of Elderly Care Physicians. *Multidisciplinaire richtlijn besluitvorming over reanimatie: Anticiperende besluitvorming over reanimatie bij kwetsbare ouderen. Deel 1 Samenvatting en aanbevelingen.* Utrecht, Verenso, 2013.

47. Geijteman EC, Brinkman-Stoppelenburg A, Onwuteaka-Philipsen BD, van der Heide A, van Delden JJ. Two decades of do-not-resuscitate decisions in the Netherlands. *Resuscitation* 2015 Sep; 94: e7–e8. doi: 10.1016/j.resuscitation.2015.06.028. Epub 2015 Jul 17

48. Dujardin J, Schuurmans J, Westerduin D, Wichmann AB, Engels Y. The COVID-19 pandemic: A tipping point for advance care planning? Experiences of general practitioners. *Palliat Med.* 2021 Jul; 35(7): 1238–48. doi: 10.1177/02692163211016979. Epub 2021 May 27

49. Connellan D, Diffley K, McCabe J, Cotter A, McGinty T, Sheehan G, et al. Documentation of do-not-attempt-cardiopulmonary-resuscitation orders amid the COVID-19 pandemic. *Age Ageing* 2021 Jun 28; 50(4): 1048–51. doi: 10.1093/ageing/afab075

50. Ye P, Fry L, Champion JD. Changes in advance care planning for nursing home residents during the COVID-19 pandemic. *J Am Med Dir Assoc.* 2021 Jan; 22(1): 209–14. doi: 10.1016/j.jamda.2020.11.011. Epub 2020 Nov 19

51. Hendriks SA, Smalbrugge M, Hertogh CMPM, van der Steen JT. Changes in care goals and treatment orders around the occurrence of health problems and hospital transfers in dementia: A prospective study. *J Am Geriatr Soc.* 2017 Apr; 65(4): 769–76. doi: 10.1111/jgs.14667

52. Harrison-Dening K., King M, Jones L, Vickerstaff V, Sampson EL. Advance care planning in dementia: Do family carers know the treatment preferences of people with early dementia? *PLoS One.* 2016 Jul 13; 11(7): e0159056. doi: 10.1371/journal.pone.0159056

53. Malhotra C, Mohamad H, Østbye T, Pollak KI, Balasundaram B, Malhotra R, et al. Discordance between dementia caregivers' goal of care and preference for life-extending treatments. *Age Ageing* 2021 Jun 28; 50(4): 1382–90. doi: 10.1093/ageing/afab04

54. Van der Maaden T, Hendriks SA, de Vet HC, Zomerhuis MT, Smalbrugge M, Jansma EP, et al. Antibiotic use and associated factors in patients with dementia: A systematic review. *Drugs Aging* 2015 Jan; 32(1): 43–56. doi: 10.1007/s40266-014-0223-z

process, and family education. *Can Fam Physician* 2015 Apr; 61(4): 330–4.

55. Dufour AB, Shaffer ML, D'Agata EMC, Habtemariam D, Mitchell SL. Survival after suspected urinary tract infection in individuals with advanced dementia. *J Am Geriatr Soc.* 2015 Dec; **63**(12): 2472–7. doi: 10.1111/jgs.13833

56. Van der Steen JT, Pasman HR, Ribbe MW, van der Wal G, Onwuteaka-Philipsen BD. Discomfort in dementia patients dying from pneumonia and its relief by antibiotics. *Scand J Infect Dis.* 2009; **41**(2): 143–51. doi: 10.1080/00365540802616726

57. Givens JL, Jones RN, Shaffer ML, Kiely DK, Mitchell SL. Survival and comfort after treatment of pneumonia in advanced dementia. *Arch Intern Med.* 2010; **170**(13): 1102–7.

58. Van der Steen JT. Prolonged life and increased symptoms vs prolonged dying and increased comfort after antibiotic treatment in patients with dementia and pneumonia. *Arch Intern Med.* 2011 Jan 10; **171**(1): 93–4. doi: 10.1001/archinternmed.2010.487

59. Van der Maaden T, van der Steen JT, de Vet HC, Hertogh CM, Koopmans RT. Prospective observations of discomfort, pain, and dyspnea in nursing home residents with dementia and pneumonia. *J Am Med Dir Assoc.* 2016 Feb; **17**(2): 128–35. doi: 10.1016/j.jamda.2015.08.010. Epub 2015 Sep 26

60. Parsons C, van der Steen JT. Antimicrobial use in patients with dementia: Current concerns and future recommendations. *CNS Drugs* 2017 Jun; **31**(6): 433–8. doi: 10.1007/s40263-017-0427-y

61. Van der Steen JT, Lane P, Kowall NW, Knol DL, Volicer L. Antibiotics and mortality in patients with lower respiratory infection and advanced dementia. *J Am Med Dir Assoc.* 2012 Feb; **13**(2): 156–61. doi: 10.1016/j.jamda.2010.07.001

62. Koopmans RT, van der Sterren KJ, van der Steen JT. The 'natural' endpoint of dementia: Death from cachexia or dehydration following palliative care? *Int J Geriatr Psychiatry* 2007 Apr; **22**(4): 350–5. doi: 10.1002/gps.1680

63. Sternberg SA, Shinan-Altman S, Volicer L, Casarett DJ, van der Steen JT. Palliative care in advanced dementia: Comparison of strategies in three countries. *Geriatrics* (Basel). 2021 Apr 22; **6**(2): 44. doi: 10.3390/geriatrics6020044

64. Van der Steen JT, Di Giulio P, Giunco F, Monti M, Gentile S, Villani D, et al. End of Life Observatory–Prospective Study on Dementia Patients Care (EoLO-PSODEC) Research Group. Pneumonia in nursing home patients with advanced dementia: Decisions, intravenous rehydration therapy, and discomfort. *Am J Hosp Palliat Care* 2018 Mar; **35**(3): 423–30. doi: 10.1177/1049909117709002

65. Anantapong K, Davies N, Chan J, McInnerney D, Sampson EL. Mapping and understanding the decision-making process for providing nutrition and hydration to people living with dementia: A systematic review. *BMC Geriatr.* 2020 Dec 2; **20**(1): 520. doi: 10.1186/s12877-020-01931-y

66. Anantapong K, Barrado-Martín Y, Nair P, Rait G, Smith CH, Moore KJ, et al. How do people living with dementia perceive eating and drinking difficulties? A qualitative study. *Age Ageing* 2021 Jun 11: afab108. doi: 10.1093/ageing/afab108. Online ahead of print

67. Barrado-Martín Y, Nair P, Anantapong K, Aker N, Moore KJ, Smith CH, et al. Family caregivers' and professionals' experiences of supporting people living with dementia's nutrition and hydration needs towards the end of life. *Health Soc Care Community* 2021 May 6. doi: 10.1111/hsc.13404. Online ahead of print

68. The AM, Pasman R, Onwuteaka-Philipsen B, Ribbe M, van der Wal G. Withholding the artificial administration of fluids and food from elderly patients with dementia: Ethnographic study. *BMJ.* 2002 Dec 7; 325(7376): 1326. doi: 10.1136/bmj.325.7376.1326

69. Van der Steen JT, Hertogh CM, de Graas T, Nakanishi M, Toscani F, Arcand M. Translation and cross-cultural adaptation of a family booklet on comfort care in dementia: Sensitive topics revised before implementation. *J Med Ethics* 2013 Feb; **39**(2): 104–9. doi: 10.1136/medethics-2012-100903

70. Bavelaar L, McCann A, Cornally N, et al.; on behalf of the mySupport study group. Guidance for family information about comfort care in dementia: a comparison of an educational booklet adopted in six jurisdictions over a 15 year timespan. [Submitted]

71. Van der Steen JT, Heck S, Juffermans CC, Garvelink MM, Achterberg WP, Clayton J, et al. Practitioners' perceptions of acceptability of a question prompt list about palliative care for advance care planning with people living with dementia and their family caregivers: A mixed-methods evaluation study. *BMJ Open* 2021 Apr 12; **11**(4): e044591. doi: 10.1136/bmjopen-2020-044591

72. Verelst SG, Pasman HR, Onwuteaka-Philipsen BD, Ribbe MW, van der Wal G. Ervaringen van familie met de besluitvorming rond kunstmatige toediening van vocht en voedsel (ktvv) bij mensen met dementie in het verpleeghuis. [Experience of family members with the decision concerning artificial nutrition and hydration in people with

dementia in nursing homes.] *Tijdschr Gerontol Geriatr*. 2006 Apr; **37**(2): 51–8. doi: 10.1007/BF03074766. https://tvgg.nl/artikelen/ervaringen-van-familie-met-de-besluitvorming-rond-kunstmatige-toediening-van-vocht-en-voedsel-ktvv-bij-mensen-met-dementie-in-het-verpleeghuis

73. Davies N, Manthorpe J, Sampson EL, Lamahewa K, Wilcock J, Mathew R, Iliffe S. Guiding practitioners through end of life care for people with dementia: The use of heuristics. *PLoS One* 2018 Nov 14; **13**(11): e0206422. doi: 10.1371/journal.pone.0206422

74. Lee YF, Hsu TW, Liang CS, Yeh TC, Chen TY, Chen NC, Chu CS. The efficacy and safety of tube feeding in advanced dementia patients: A systemic review and meta-analysis study. *J Am Med Dir Assoc*. 2021 Feb; **22**(2): 357–63. doi: 10.1016/j.jamda.2020.06.035

75. Wu CY, Chen PJ, Ho TL, Lin WY, Cheng SY. To hydrate or not to hydrate? The effect of hydration on survival, symptoms and quality of dying among terminally ill cancer patients. *BMC Palliat Care* 2021 Jan 12; **20**(1): 13.

76. Volicer L, Pope TM, Steinberg KE. Assistance with eating and drinking only when requested can prevent living with advanced dementia. *J Am Med Dir Assoc*. 2019 Nov; **20**(11): 1353–5. doi: 10.1016/j.jamda.2019.08.035

77. Evenblij K, Pasman HRW, van der Heide A, Hoekstra T, Onwuteaka-Philipsen BD. Factors associated with requesting and receiving euthanasia: A nationwide mortality follow-back study with a focus on patients with psychiatric disorders, dementia, or an accumulation of health problems related to old age. *BMC Med*. 2019 Feb 19; **17**(1): 39. doi: 10.1186/s12916-019-1276-y

78. Rurup M, Onwuteaka-Philipsen B, van der Heide A, van der Wal G, Deeg G. Frequency and determinants of advance directives concerning end-of-life care in the Netherlands. *Soc Sci Med*. 2006; **62**:1552–63.

79. Mangino D, Nicolini M, De Vries R, Kim S. Euthanasia and assisted suicide of persons with dementia in the Netherlands. *Am J Geriatr Psychiatry* 2020; **28**: 466–77.

80. Regional Euthanasia Review Committees. *Annual Report 2017*. The Hague, 2018.

81. Rurup M, Onwuteaka-Philipsen B, van der Heide A, van der Wal G, van der Maas P, et al. Physicians' experiences with demented patients with advance euthanasia directives in the Netherlands. *J Am Geriatr Soc*. 2005; **53**: 1138–44.

82. Brinkman-Stoppelenburg A, Evenblij K, Pasman R, van Delden J, Onwuteaka-Philipsen B, van der Heide A. Physicians' and public attitudes toward euthanasia in people with advanced dementia. *J Am Geriatr Soc*. 2020; **68**: 2319–28.

83. Bolt E, Snijdewind M, Willems D, van der Heide A, Onwuteaka-Philipsen B. Can physicians conceive of performing euthanasia in case of psychiatric disease, dementia or being tired of living? *J Med Ethics* 2015; **41**: 592–8.

84. Kouwenhoven P., Raijmakers N., van Delden J., Rietjens J., van Tol D., van de Vathorst S, et al. Opinions about euthanasia and advanced dementia: A qualitative study among Dutch physicians and members of the general public. *BMC Med Ethics* 2015; **16**: 7.

85. Kouwenhoven P, Raijmakers N, van Delden J, Rietjens J, Schermer M, van Thiel G, et al. Opinions of health care professionals and the public after eight years of euthanasia legislation in the Netherlands: A mixed method approach. *Palliative Medicine* 2013; **27**: 273–80.

86. De Boer M, Dröes R-M, Jonker C, Eefsting J, Hertogh C. Advance directives for euthanasia in dementia: How do they affect resident care in Dutch nursing homes? Experiences of physicians and relatives. *J Am Geriatr Soc*. 2011; **59**: 989–96.

87. De Boer M, Dröes R-M, Jonker C, Eefsting J, Hertogh C. Advance directives for euthanasia in dementia: Do law-based opportunities lead to more euthanasia? *Health Policy* 2010; **98**: 256–62.

88. Picard G, Bier J-C, Capron I, De Deyn PP, Deryck O, Engelborghs S, et al. Dementia, end of life, and euthanasia: A survey among dementia specialists organized by the Belgian Dementia Council. *J of Alzheimers Dis*. 2019; **69**: 989–1001.

89. Rurup M, Onwuteaka-Philipsen B, Pasman H, Ribbe M, van der Wal G. Attitudes of physicians, nurses and relatives towards end-of-life decisions concerning nursing home patients with dementia. *Patient Educ Couns*. 2006; **61**: 372–80.

90. Tomlinson E, Stott J. Assisted dying in dementia: A systematic review of the international literature on the attitudes of health professionals, patients, carers and the public, and the factors associated with these. *Int J Geriatr Psychiatry* 2015; **30**: 10–20.

91. Ryynänen O-P, Myllykangas M, Viren M, Heino H. Attitudes towards euthanasia among physicians, nurses and the general public in Finland. *Public Health* 2002; **116**: 322–31.

92. Armstrong-Esther C, Browne K, McAffee J. Investigation into nursing staff knowledge and attitude to dementia. *Int J Psychiatr Nurs Res*. 1999; **4**: 489–97.

93. Kitchener B, Jorm A. Conditions required for a law on active voluntary euthanasia: A survey of nurses' opinions in the Australian Capital Territory. *J Med Ethics* 1999; **25**: 25–30.

94. Williams N, Dunford C, Knowles A, Warner J. Public attitudes to life-sustaining treatments and euthanasia in dementia. *Int J Geriatr Psychiatry* 2007; **22**: 1229–34.

95. Van Holsteyn J., Trappenburg M. Citizens' opinions on new forms of euthanasia: A report from the Netherlands. *Patient Educ Couns.* 1998; **35**: 63–73.

96. Gómez-Virseda C, Gastmans C. Euthanasia in persons with advanced dementia: A dignity-enhancing care approach. *J Med Ethics* 2021 May 20. doi: 10.1136/medethics-2021-107308. Online ahead of print

97. Mondragon J, Salame-Khouri L, Kraus-Weisman A, De Deyn PP. Bioethical implications of end-of-life decision-making in patients with dementia: A tale of two societies. *Monash Bioeth Rev.* 2020; **38**: 49–67.

98. Cholbi M. 2015. Kant on euthanasia and the duty to die: Clearing the air. *J Med Ethics* 2015; **41**: 607–10.

99. Gastmans C. Dignity-enhancing care for persons with dementia and its application to advance euthanasia directives. In Denier Y, Gastmans C, Vandevelde A, eds. *Justice, Luck and Responsibility in Health Care: Philosophical Background and Ethical Implications for End-of-Life Care.* Dordrecht, Springer,2013; 145–65.

100. Den Hartogh G. The authority of advance directives. In Denier Y, Gastmans C, Vandevelde A, eds. *Justice, Luck and Responsibility in Health Care: Philosophical Background and Ethical Implications for End-of-Life Care.* Dordrecht, Springer, 2013; 167–88.

101. Nys T. The wreckage of our flesh: Dementia, autonomy and personhood. In Denier Y, Gastmans C, Vandevelde A, eds. *Justice, Luck and Responsibility in Health Care: Philosophical Background and Ethical Implications for End-of-Life Care.* Dordrecht, Springer, 2013; 189–203.

102. Johnstone M. Metaphors, stigma and the 'Alzheimerization' of the euthanasia debate. *Dementia* 2013; **12**: 377–93.

103. Sharp R. The dangers of euthanasia and dementia: How Kantian thinking might be used to support non-voluntary euthanasia in cases of extreme dementia. *Bioethics* 2012; **26**: 231–5.

104. Alvargonzalez D. Alzheimer's disease and euthanasia. *J Aging Stud.* 2012; **26**: 377–85.

105. Gastmans C, De Lepeleire J. Living to the bitter end? A personalist approach to euthanasia in persons with severe dementia. *Bioethics* 2010; **24**: 78–86.

106. Draper B, Peisah C, Snowdon J, Brodaty H. Early dementia diagnosis and the risk of suicide and euthanasia. *Alzheimers Dement.* 2010; **6**: 75–82.

107. Gastmans C, Denier Y. What if patients with dementia use decision aids to make an advance euthanasia request? *Am J Bioeth.* 2010; **10**(4): 25–6.

108. Hertogh C, De Boer M, Dröes RM, Eefsting J. Would we rather lose our life than lose our self? Lessons from the Dutch debate on euthanasia of patients with dementia. *Am J Bioeth.* 2007; **7**(4): 48–56.

109. Dworkin R. *Life's Dominion: An Argument about Abortion and Euthanasia.* London, Harper Collins, 2003.

110. Dworkin R. Life past reason. In Kuhse H, Singer P, eds. *Bioethics: An Anthology.* Malden, Blackwell, 2006; 357–64.

111. Post S. Alzheimer disease and the 'then' self. *Kennedy Inst Ethics J.* 1995; **4**: 307–21.

112. De Boer M, Hertogh C, Dröes R-M, Jonker C, Eefsting J. Advance directives in dementia: Issues of validity and effectiveness. *Int Psychogeriatr.* 2010; **22**: 201–8.

113. Hughes J. Views of the person with dementia. *J Med Ethics* 2001; **27**: 86–91.

114. Levy B, Green M. Too soon to give up: Re-examining the value of advance directives. *Am J Bioeth* 2010; **10**(4): 2–22.

115. Gómez-Virseda C, De Maeseneer Y, Gastmans C. Relational autonomy in end-of-life care ethics: A contextualized approach to real-life complexities. *BMC Med Ethics* 2020; **21**(1): 50.

116. Widdershoven G, Berghmans R. Advance directives in dementia care: From instructions to instruments. *Patient Educ Couns.* 2001; **44**: 179–86.

117. Hertogh C. The role of advance euthanasia directives as an aid to communication and shared decision-making in dementia. *J Med Ethics* 2009; **35**: 100–3.

118. Agich G. *Dependency and Autonomy in Old Age: An Ethical Framework for Long-Term Care.* Cambridge, Cambridge University Press, 2003.

119. Dresser R. Dworkin on dementia: Elegant theory, questionable policy. *Hastings Cent Rep.* 1995; **25** (6): 32–8.

120. Goering S. What makes suffering 'unbearable and hopeless'? Advance directives, dementia and disability. *Am J Bioeth*. 2007; **7**(4): 62–3.

121. Moody H. *Ethics in an Aging Society*. Baltimore, MD, Johns Hopkins University Press, 1992.

122. Gómez-Virseda C, De Maeseneer Y, Gastmans C. Relational autonomy: What does it mean and how is it used in end-of-life care? A systematic review of argument-based ethics literature. *BMC Med Ethics* 2019; **20**(1): 76.

123. Tulsky J. Beyond advance directives: Importance of communication skills at the end of life. *JAMA* 2005; **294**: 359–65.

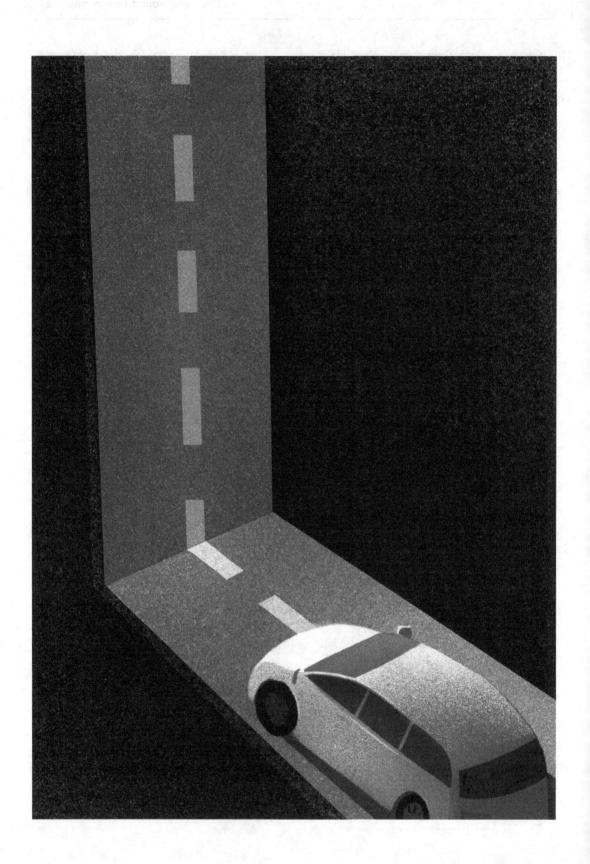

Chapter 13

Driving and Dementia

Catarina Lundberg and Dorota Religa

1 Introduction

In the general population, driving is appreciated as an important condition of independent mobility. In middle- and high-income societies, it is common for young people to look forward to obtaining their driver's licence, not only for practical reasons but also because it is a symbol of freedom and adulthood. During the lifespan, driving and choice of car may be an expression of social status and lifestyle preferences. An inclination towards speed and excitement, family orientation, an interest in advanced technology, environmental concerns, a preference for a particular brand or a perceived interest in supporting the industry of one's own country will all lead to different choices. Driving thus becomes strongly associated with personal identity.

Although driving for professional reasons is less frequent among older adults than in younger age groups, older drivers use their cars to visit relatives and friends, grocery shop, transport heavy items and travel for pleasure and recreation. Private cars are viewed as a necessity when public transportation is unavailable or insufficient, as in some suburbs or in rural areas. Frequently, at least one other older person depends on an individual older driver for transportation. This is the case not only in couples where the wife does not drive but also in groups of older adults where the majority have never driven or have given up driving.

In our clinical experience, one older driver may drive several friends or acquaintances for recreational trips or to social or religious events. Older drivers may also help their adult children with business-related errands and grandparents are often called upon to pick up their grandchildren at school or drive them to different activities. Furthermore, the ongoing COVID-19 pandemic underscores the importance for vulnerable groups of having access to means of transportation that enable physical distancing.

People with diagnoses of mild dementia generally lead independent lives and only gradually relinquish professional activities or political/societal functions. In this respect, their transportation needs do not differ from those of their peers in the general population. Hence a substantial proportion of people with early-stage dementia continue driving after diagnosis (e.g. [1]). In addition, specific community programmes for people living with dementia and their carers may improve their social inclusion. However, participation in many of these programmes requires transportation and people who are eligible benefit more when they are still able to travel by car to the proposed activities.

Placement in a long-term care facility is considered when a person is no longer able to live independently. However, this represents a heavy financial burden on society, individuals and families. It is therefore of great value if this measure can be delayed for as long as possible and the possibility to drive a car may be vital to attaining this goal. Furthermore, being able to live at home is extremely important for a person's well-being and quality of life. Continuing to live in familiar surroundings and maintaining routines and pursuing accustomed activities may also contribute to a slower rate of cognitive and functional deterioration.

Older drivers in general are often perceived as a particularly vulnerable group in traffic, not least because of their increasing representation in the driving population [2], and media as well as the general public express concern about the perceived risk they pose [3]. Very frequently, when an older driver is involved in a traffic incident, media indicate his or her age in a prominent way. This then gives rise to a usually short-lived debate or to comments in the press about the necessity to adopt measures for better control or monitoring of older drivers. For example, letters or emails from newspaper readers will state that the problem is their slowness or insufficient eyesight and call for different examinations or compulsory renewed driving tests. However, with an ageing population in large parts of the world, older drivers are gaining visibility in traffic; other road users are becoming more used to interacting with them and sometimes can adapt to their driving style. In the same way that female drivers, in the past decades, make up an increasing proportion of the driving population and are generally no longer viewed as less skilled and potentially risky exceptions, it is likely older drivers will be considered legitimate road users.

In the 1990s, discussions about older drivers in several countries shifted from a focus on age to a dichotomy between 'sick older drivers' and 'healthy older drivers', with dementia as a prominent example of the former [4]. 'People with dementia experience the double jeopardy of being old and having a cognitive impairment' [5] and are today often automatically considered unfit to drive. This might reflect the fact that knowledge about dementia, especially about different stages of dementia, is not properly communicated in society. Although drivers with dementia are not apparent in the traffic environment in the same way as women and people over a certain age, it is hoped they will be viewed in a more nuanced way in the future.

The present chapter focusses on the impact of dementia on driving behaviour and its consequences for traffic safety. At the same time, it is necessary to recognize that all drivers living with dementia are not affected in the same way and that they do not, as a group, represent a threat to other road users or themselves. Regulatory approaches to medically impaired drivers in different countries are described, as well as assessment methods to determine fitness to drive and communication strategies when driving is no longer advisable.

The issue of driving in dementia can be considered in differing ways, depending on the adopted perspective. The individual's right to autonomous mobility may be opposed to the rights of other road users not to be exposed to the behaviour of an unfit driver. Also, for healthcare professionals, focus may be on reducing the individual patient's risk of injury in traffic. However, for the individual, giving up driving leads to very real personal consequences, while

the reduction in risk of removing a possibly unfit driver from the road is difficult to evaluate and may be very small. Indeed, in view of the risk posed by drivers under the influence of alcohol or other drugs, the increased crash risk of drivers with dementia can hardly be viewed as a public health problem.

2 Driving Behaviour in Dementia

The driving task can be described as a continuous cycle of acquisition and processing of information, decision-making and action. The cognitive impairments associated with dementia (notably impaired eye–hand coordination, memory impairment and poor decision-making and problem-solving skills [6]) are all likely to impact each step in this process.

The topic of driving in dementia emerged as an issue in its own right in the end of the 1980s. Investigations from different memory clinics [7] revealed an awareness that many patients were still driving despite cognitive impairments and difficulties managing activities of daily life, and that they appeared to be over-involved in accidents. Subsequent studies, sometimes with larger groups and with more robust study designs, have elaborated on this issue and addressed topics such as driving behaviour in dementia, involvement in motor vehicle crashes (MVCs) relative to healthy older people and the assessment of fitness to drive.

Comparisons between driving ability in healthy people and those with dementia show the latter, as a group, are more likely to fail an on-road assessment. Specific problem areas are safety behaviours, landmark or sign identification, lane observance and orientation [6]. Structured driving tests conducted in our centre show many drivers with dementia have difficulty dealing with complex situations that require them to simultaneously attend to several features in the environment. Typical examples are complex intersections or motorway entrances, involving interaction with other road users and timely adjustment of vehicle speed.

Drivers with dementia are also less able to flexibly adapt to more unfamiliar circumstances – for example, driving on the pavement when the road surface is being repaired. The traffic environment often provides cues that help the driver to follow an appropriate sequence of behaviours. Our patients sometimes say it is not necessary to recognize or understand the meaning of road signs because they follow the example of other road users. However, when memory impairment becomes more pronounced, the driver may become less receptive to such cues. In some cases, the driver might perceive an acceleration lane or a parking lot as an ordinary road or street.

Most studies of driving behaviour in dementia have focussed on Alzheimer's disease (AD), the most common cause of dementia. It is reasonable to assume dementias affecting other regions of the brain or that have a different rate of progression may have a different impact on driving. Frontotemporal lobar degeneration (FTLD) in particular, which involves more personality and behavioural changes with a more pronounced effect on insight and judgement, is associated with norm-breaking behaviour in general [8]. Compared to patients with AD, those with FTLD show more dangerous driving behaviours [9].

Trajectories in vascular dementia are often characterized by a more stepwise deterioration than in AD and therefore the affected person might maintain a relatively satisfactory level of functioning for a long period of time before being considered unfit to drive. Characteristic features of Lewy body dementia, such as impairments of attention and alertness, of visuospatial functioning and judgement, in combination with visual hallucinations and movement disorders, suggest the affected patient is unfit for driving at an early stage of the disease.

3 Cognitive Impairment or Dementia and the Risk of Motor Vehicle Crashes

It is unclear whether the signs of impaired driving fitness described previously lead to an increased risk of MVCs. Motor vehicle crashes are rare occurrences determined by multiple circumstances and are therefore not an ideal outcome variable to use in statistical analyses. Furthermore, it is not unreasonable to assume at-fault crashes are not the only outcome of interest when studying crash involvement of drivers with dementia. Near misses, where the other party acts appropriately to avoid the crash, are difficult to identify and quantify, but nevertheless represent an aspect of the risk in traffic. Conversely, some crashes are not caused by the driver with dementia, but by the other party, who might be guilty of speeding or rule-breaking. In

these cases, the driver with dementia, due to difficulties in anticipating the hazard, might not be able to avoid the crash and will be seriously injured or killed. Thus, the argument that drivers with dementia should be identified because they might put other road users at risk should be taken seriously but should be completed by the argument that their safety is sometimes compromised by the behaviour of others.

An overview of studies published before the year 2000 concluded the overall crash risk in dementia is moderately high, in the same order as alcohol abuse and dependence [10]. However, these studies were often based on small groups and had other methodological limitations. For example, information on crashes based on reports by informants generally shows higher risks than state reports and is therefore less reliable. Even among more recently published studies of crash risk in dementia [6] few meet sufficiently high scientific standards [2]. Findings are conflicting, with some studies showing a high relative risk of crashes in drivers with dementia and others showing no increased risk at all. There is some indication that people with dementia have an increased MVC risk compared to healthy controls (four times and almost two times higher, respectively) in the three years prior to their diagnosis, but not in the subsequent three years [11, 12].

Thus the period preceding diagnosis might be critical: the driving fitness of the person with incipient dementia might already be affected, although the driver, not yet identified as cognitively impaired or suffering from dementia, has not been assessed by the healthcare system and may not yet have taken any self-restriction measures such as reducing the amount of driving or avoiding more challenging situations.

Some support for this view comes from a large-scale study carried out among older drivers seeking to renew their licences. Results on tests of psychomotor speed, mental flexibility, processing of visual information and attention predicted involvement in crashes during the following three-year period [13]. Moreover, the transition from healthy ageing to dementia is characterized not only by changes in cognition but also by changes in mood states and the presence of neuropsychiatric symptoms [14].

In a group of cognitively normal individuals, such changes (notably irritability, appetite, depression and agitation) interacted with biomarkers of AD to impact driving performance [15]. From a different perspective, a post-mortem investigation of older drivers killed in MVCs (but who were not identified as suffering from dementia) showed one third had neuropathological signs in their brain tissue that make a diagnosis of AD histologically certain. For another 20%, these signs suggested the presence of AD [16].

The type of crash considered typical of older drivers can indicate the nature of the cognitive impairment that played a part in its causation. Crashes in intersections, particularly when an older driver is struck by a vehicle coming from the left, often lead to fatal injuries. As described previously, intersections pose simultaneous demands on visual attention, working memory, speed perception and decision-making. When driving through an intersection, one must perform several actions in parallel and under time pressure, and this may be a task exceeding the capabilities of a person with cognitive deficits.

In conclusion, in older adults, the boundaries between normal functioning, cognitive impairment and dementia are not clear-cut and a diagnosis of dementia does not automatically make a person unfit to drive. Many patients can pass a driving test in the early stage of the disorder and there is no clear-cut evidence that, as a group, they represent a threat to traffic safety. At the same time, drivers with an incipient or non-detected dementia may be involved in traffic incidents because they find themselves in situations where demands exceed their cognitive capacities.

4 Regulations

In most developed countries, legislators recognize motor vehicle drivers must fulfil certain requirements regarding physical fitness and usually a person applying for a licence must therefore show stipulated medical conditions (as a minimum, sufficient visual acuity) are met. The applicant must also have a satisfactory level of knowledge and skill (typically having passed a theoretical examination and a driving test). An overview of regulations for drivers with dementia in the United States, Canada, Australia, the UK, Germany, France, Italy, Japan, China and South Korea states all countries except China and South Korea have more specific medical guidelines [17]. In Japan and China, dementia at any stage precludes licence holding, whereas only advanced dementia leads to licence revocation in all the other countries. In Canada and some states of the United States, there is mandatory reporting by physicians, and in all other countries except Germany the driver has the duty to report his or her condition to the relevant authorities.

Annex III of the European (EU) directive 2006/126/EC on driving licences lays down minimum standards of physical and mental fitness in areas such as vision, locomotor impairments, medical conditions that might lead to a sudden incapacitation or neurological diseases. Dementia is not mentioned explicitly but is covered by conditions such as 'severe mental disturbance, whether congenital or due to disease, trauma or neurosurgical operations' and 'severe behavioural problems due to ageing' (Annex III, 13.1). The Directive states such conditions are obstacles to licence holding unless 'their application is supported by authorized medical opinion and, if necessary, subject to regular medical check-ups'.

European Union member states are free to stipulate more stringent requirements than the Directive minimum. National regulations on licence holding and renewal may vary concerning the frequency of licence renewal for drivers with different medical conditions and may also demand licences be renewed more frequently, in combination with some type of screening or medical check-up, once a licence holder reaches a certain age (the Directive mentions 50 years).

Many countries worldwide have implemented age-related controls of medical fitness to drive. Such controls usually do not aim at identifying dementing processes in particular and may be carried out in many different manners. Some countries rely on the general healthcare system to perform these controls; others have specialized multidisciplinary organizations that issue medical certificates for drivers. When the cost of the examinations is not subsidized by national or private health insurance, there is a potential risk older drivers with insufficient financial means will give up their licence rather than bear the cost related to renewal.

National legislation regarding medical confidentiality also leads to variation in regulations concerning the responsibility of medical practitioners to report unfit drivers. In some countries, there is strict confidentiality and the only option for the physician might be to advise the patient to report himself or herself to the licencing authority. Other countries have mandatory reporting, sometimes with the option (as in Sweden) of refraining from doing so if it is possible to make an agreement with the patient to stop driving. Once a driver has caused a crash or displayed aberrant behaviour in traffic, the licencing authority or insurance company might suspect a medical or cognitive impairment and initiate an opportunistic medical examination.

Age-related screening of the general older population of licence holders is generally not considered to have an effect on traffic safety in terms of lower crash rates. Indeed, it has been argued that such check-ups could be counterproductive. On one hand, they might be too cursory to identify real problems and could therefore encourage overconfidence in the driver and less willingness to take self-restriction measures to increase safety. On the other hand, some drivers could perceive that screening is a signal that society considers them undesirable road users, leading them to give up driving and opting for modes of transportation that provide less protection (e.g. mopeds or bicycles). In recognition of the possible increased risk in traffic of people with cognitive impairment or incipient dementia, a more targeted screening procedure has been introduced in Denmark. However, it has not proved to have a safety effect [18].

5 Assessment of Driving Fitness in Dementia

From the early studies on driving in dementia and onwards, one of the topics of interest has been how to determine whether a patient poses too great a risk to himself or herself and other road users. Ideally, a study design would be prospective, examining a patient group and then following them over time to determine whether there are associations between the results of the clinical examinations and an outcome such as crash involvement. In a retrospective investigation, the researchers attempt to relate *present* cognitive performance to *previous* adverse traffic events. This is not appropriate in cases of progressively deteriorating conditions. However,

prospective studies are difficult to carry out. One reason is that crashes, as mentioned previously, are rare.

Furthermore, many individuals in the study group will voluntarily limit their driving during the course of the study period, thus reducing their exposure in traffic, until they stop driving altogether. Other studies have used surrogate measures of safe driving such as performance on an in-traffic driving test, in simulators or driving status. It is quite possible that small study groups and methodological limitations contribute to the conclusion of a Cochrane review on dementia and driving [19] that the available literature (published until 2012) fails to demonstrate the benefit of driver assessment for either preserving transport mobility or reducing MVCs.

Older persons with possible dementia are often encouraged by family, healthcare providers and the community to seek a cognitive assessment and they do so in good faith. However, many are not properly informed about the disadvantages associated with the outcome of the assessment [20], among these the risk that they might lose their driver's licence after diagnosis. To give them a fair description of the post-assessment situation, one suggestion would be to implement pre-assessment counselling [21].

A structured driving assessment generally consists of off-road psychometric tests, sometimes complemented by an on-road evaluation. In many countries, this is not covered by health insurance. Carr and co-authors [22] indicate only patients who are qualified for vocational rehabilitation can benefit from insurance and that others must bear the cost of USD $300–500, a sum that can be prohibitive for many, especially if the assessment must be repeated (often more than once) during the course of the dementing illness.

5.1 Global Cognitive Measures and Neuropsychological Tests

To test for the presence of cognitive impairment or to grade dementia, global cognitive measures such as rating scales, short screening batteries or single screening tests (e.g. clock drawing) are used in primary care and memory clinics. However, such measures have not been shown to be sufficiently associated with on-road test performance, involvement in MVCs or other measures of driving fitness [23] and there is no consensus on formal cut-off scores to determine whether a patient is unfit to drive [24]. Neuropsychological tests have the advantage of examining selected cognitive domains in more depth and yield fine-graded results that can take into account demographic aspects such as age and sometimes level of educational attainment.

Published studies have used a great variety of neuropsychological tests and there is as yet no consensus on what cognitive areas or particular tests are the most predictive of driving impairment. According to one review [25], visuospatial ability is the most relevant domain. This appears reasonable given the importance of being able to correctly interpret visual information – for example, when positioning the vehicle, at intersections or in roundabouts, or when navigating according to road signs. However, a more recent review [26] has concluded no single cognitive domain is more reliable than others to determine driving fitness.

Frequently, the tests used are the same that are available for ordinary diagnostic purposes. It is interesting to note that patients describe the neuropsychological testing as the most challenging component of the memory workup [20] and they do not perceive them as relevant to the assessment of driving fitness, even when different studies show they are associated with the outcome of a driving test.

There is some agreement that a combination of tests should be preferred to single tests due to the multidimensionality of the driving task. This is also reasonable from a clinical point of view, not least because a stand-alone test is vulnerable to errors related to administration and to patient-related factors such as nervousness or resistive behaviour. Using several different tests can improve patient–examiner rapport and put a single low score into perspective. Simple timed paper-and-pencil tests tapping eye–hand coordination, speed and visual scanning and search have been shown to predict driving performance [27]. In everyday clinical practice, office-based paper-and-pencil tests, sometimes in combination with computerized testing, are frequently used to assign a patient to one of three categories: (a) those who presently fulfil cognitive requirements for licence holding, (b) those who are clearly unfit and (c) borderline cases who need further assessment, usually an on-road test.

Another category of tests or test batteries than those used for standard clinical diagnostic purposes are those that are explicitly designed to examine cognitive fitness to drive (e.g. the Useful Field of View Test [28] or the Stroke Drivers Screening Assessment [29]). Although they are not always necessarily designed with patients with dementia in mind, they have some advantage regarding face validity (visual content may include vehicles, traffic signs or traffic situations and can be perceived by patients as more relevant to driving than more general tests). In addition, most of them have been validated against measures of safe driving (most frequently performance on an on-road test, but also future crash involvement) [13].

As mentioned previously, there is no perfect association between the results of cognitive testing and outcome measures reflecting safe driving. This is true also for the driving-related tests described earlier. Some patients will be categorized as unfit because they obtain low test results, although they pass an on-road test. Conversely, other patients will pass the clinical tests but fail the driving test. Clinical experience gives some insight into factors that might disadvantage a patient who undergoes cognitive testing. A low level of formal education is in itself a risk factor associated with dementia [30] and this, sometimes in combination with low intelligence, leads to difficulties with tests that are perceived as too theoretical, difficulties that are compounded by the patient's anxiety or scepticism.

In our centre, it is not unusual for patients to comment that they are 'too stupid' to understand how to deal with the test. In addition, present-day clinical populations include a non-negligible proportion of people who have grown up outside Western countries and who often have a different educational background than the majority population. They may also not be sufficiently fluent in the language of their country of residence and, due to the dementing process, they may have lost their command of this second language. All of these circumstances lead to the risk that they might wrongly be classified as unfit to continue driving.

There are also protective factors that can delay the point in time when a driver with dementia will be considered unsafe. The most important is probably extensive experience. Often this experience is associated with and may compensate for a low level of educational attainment. The typical patient in this case has left school after the minimum number of years and has then gone on to driving a lorry, bus or taxi professionally or to hold a job that requires driving (e.g. in the delivery or maintenance sector).

For experienced drivers, the driving task is an overlearned activity. They have gained expertise thanks to exposure to a multitude of situations and have a broad behavioural repertoire that does not require conscious decision-making to be activated. Behavioural automatisms and the performance of tasks in parallel rather than serially (e.g. simultaneously checking the environment, signalling shifting gears and adjusting speed when crossing an intersection, rather than performing these actions one at a time) require less of a mental load than for drivers with a lower level of driving expertise. Hence the expert driver needs less cognitive reserve than the less experienced one. In fact, driving errors, mainly due to inattention, that the latter make during a driving test are largely of the same type that can be observed in novice drivers.

Personality factors such as premorbid low impulsivity may also be protective. If the patient has insight and awareness that he or she is not functioning in the same way as before, it should be possible (although this is not certain) to make strategic decisions to refrain from driving under more demanding circumstances (rush hour, bad weather etc.) or to make tactical decisions when driving (e.g. keeping a greater distance from the vehicle in front). In a group of AD patients, a clinical interview related to orientation and judgement as well as the patients' own assessment of driving fitness proved to be important components in predicting the outcome of an on-road test [31].

5.2 The Role of Informants

To determine whether there is a change from a previous level of functioning, clinical assessments rely heavily on information from the patient's family (spouse, partner and/or adult children). Family members can also provide valuable information about the driving capabilities of a driver with dementia. In our clinical experience, however, negative opinions should be taken more seriously than positive ones. The informant may detect a deterioration in driving performance, even if no incidents occur – for instance when other road users react by signalling.

Also, the partner may have been active in encouraging the patient to seek a memory assessment but will then be reluctant to elaborate on cognitive deficits at the driving fitness assessment, either due to the patient's reactions or to the fact that she is dependent on the patient for transportation. Sometimes, the partner may value the patient's continued driving because this is the only domain in which the patient can still function normally: 'He is no longer able to set the table or choose what clothes to wear, but when he is driving I recognize my husband as he used to be.'

Adult children do not always appear reliable either. They may not have an updated knowledge of their parents' driving habits and capabilities, or they may fear the consequences for themselves if the patient can no longer drive. Negative opinions, often formulated as a partner no longer daring to be driven by the patient or an unwillingness on the part of adult children to let the patient drive grandchildren, are very important indicators of a deteriorated capacity.

5.3 On-Road Tests

A practical in-traffic driving test is often viewed as the golden standard against which to evaluate the predictive ability of clinical examinations in scientific studies. In clinical practice, it can be used to determine whether patients with borderline test results still show sufficient skill and appropriate behaviour in traffic. Many clinical facilities have developed their own road tests with a standardized route and scoring of behaviours. Conducting a driving test for patients with dementia in exactly the same manner as for novice drivers is not advisable. Novice drivers are often at the peak of their physical and other abilities, although they lack experience and sometimes risk consciousness. They have a higher risk of crashes than middle-aged drivers per distance driven, despite having passed required licencing tests. Therefore, driving tests with older adults in general should, in some respects, be evaluated more liberally.

One driving examiner has expressed that he would accept some flaws in older drivers but not in novices (e.g. rolling stops) because the foreseeable driving career of the novice driver is much longer than that of the older person. Therefore, it is important to send a message to the young driver that rules of the road must be followed strictly. For a driver with dementia, who may have to give up driving within a few years, other aspects such as vehicle positioning, anticipation and interaction with other road users are worthy of interest. On the other hand, driving examiners and instructors are not always accustomed to the driving style of older people and may therefore be too lenient in their evaluations. Instead, behaviour during the road test should preferably be observed and scored in a standardized way by a healthcare professional (such as an occupational therapist) who can relate observations of aberrant traffic behaviour to manifestations of the patient's disease.

Driving tests, which mostly take place under routine conditions, obviously have the limitation of not being able to capture an inability to deal with unexpected situations. Another limitation is the effect on the driver of being observed and being on his or her best behaviour, a behaviour that does not reflect the ordinary driving style. This constitutes an argument against driving tests for people with types of dementia that impact impulse control and judgement. Conversely, some drivers perform much worse during a driving test due to nervousness. It might be also argued that some aspects of the driving test (driving in an unfamiliar vehicle with dual controls, in an unfamiliar and sometimes more complex environment and perhaps during a longer time) are too challenging for a driver who has already reduced his or her driving to short local trips.

Finally, financial considerations should be taken into account. Costs related to driving tests, mainly the use of a dual-control car and the participation of a driving instructor, are usually not covered by health insurance or included in national healthcare systems. If the individual patient must pay the corresponding fee (amounting to about 100 euros in our centre), this might deter those with insufficient means from taking the test and appear discriminatory.

When taking a final decision on driving after clinical examinations and an on-road test, it is important to consider all relevant aspects of the clinical picture, such as comorbidities (e.g. sleep disorders, cardiac diseases or physical limitations), use of medication with the potential to affect attention and vision. If the outcome of the on-road test is uncertain, the conclusion might be that the patient cannot show in a convincing way that he or she can compensate for the effects of the dementing disease by showing driving skill and safe behaviour in traffic.

6 Driving Cessation

The issue of driving should be raised early in the disease process, when there is still a good chance the patient will cleared for driving. As many types of dementia are progressive, although rates can differ between individuals, reassessments of the patient must be performed periodically. A suggested interval is one year or more frequently if warranted by the rate of progression. Much can be gained if patient and family at an early stage become aware that the patient must one day give up driving and that the question is not *whether* but *when* this will happen. In this way, they may be able to take timely measures to become less dependent on the patient's driving – for example, by finding alternative modes of transportation or moving to a location closer to public transportation.

There is considerable variation in the number of remaining driver years after a diagnosis of dementia. Many patients have already given up driving at the time of diagnosis, even when the dementia is of the early-onset type [32]. Other patients reduce their driving gradually until they stop altogether. Still others continue driving to the same extent as before diagnosis. A three-year follow-up study of AD patients showed the median time until the patients stopped driving was 605 days for patients with very mild dementia at baseline and 324 days for patients with mild dementia.

Reasons to stop driving were failing an on-road test, an at-fault MVC or dementia progression [11]. In another study over a three-year period, the reported mean time to driving cessation was similar: one year from baseline [1]. In our clinical experience, however, many patients with dementia can continue driving considerably longer. This might reflect that diagnosis is made earlier in the disease process in some national or clinical contexts.

Predictors of driving cessation are more severe dementia with lower cognitive and functional abilities as well as demographic variables (age and sex). Interestingly, there is some evidence that the degree of cognitive impairment and the presence of AD biomarkers predict a shorter time to driving cessation in a study population of older drivers, including a subgroup of individuals with preclinical AD [33]. Women have been shown to have twice the risk of stopping driving compared to men [1]. Social norms and conceptions of gender roles (driving being more strongly linked to the perception of masculinity) thus play a part in decisions about continued driving. A negative bias in the healthcare system is probably not the main cause; rather the cause is the patients' own views, possibly economic factors (as a group, retired women have lower pensions than do men) and the influence of their social network. In fact, as shown in a Swedish registry study [34], male dementia patients were more likely than females to be reported as unfit by physicians.

In the general older population, there is a relationship between driving cessation and adverse outcomes such as depressive symptoms, a compromised relationship between the doctor and the patient [35] and decreased out-of-home activities. People with dementia and their carers describe a shrinking social world following the onset of the disease and restricted opportunities for social participation [5], and services such as volunteer chauffeurs in the community or subsidized taxi trips seldom fully compensate for the loss of autonomous mobility. It is therefore understandable that many patients with dementia react strongly when informed they can no longer drive.

It is clear mobility issues, although important, are not always the main concern. Often driving represents not only a means of transportation but also relaxation, an experience of mastery and a source of self-esteem. The perspective of being able to pursue this valued activity may be the chief motive for going through a stressful and time-consuming fitness-to-drive examination. In our centre, patients may express that life is no longer worth living and that they contemplate suicide. The loss of a licence is definitive and changes the status of the patient from an individual with autonomous mobility to the potentially stigmatizing one of a person in more need of help to get around.

It is also important to note people with dementia are more likely to be socially disadvantaged from the outset because risk factors associated with dementia (e.g. lower levels of education, cardiovascular disease, obesity, lack of physical activity and lower levels of social participation) cluster in lower socio-economic groups [5]. Therefore, there might be a cumulative effect of social class and dementia, leading to a higher risk of social exclusion.

Common reactions are anger, frustration, sadness and lack of initiative, although it is difficult to disentangle them from the broader decline associated with the illness [36]. When the spouse of the patient has initiated the memory assessment, the patient may accuse him or, more often, her of this negative consequence. Indeed, in the period following the licence revocation, the situation of the family may become very challenging, with aggression on the part of the person with dementia and difficulties in preventing him or her from using the car. It is therefore not uncommon that medical professionals advise the caregiver to disable the car (usually by removing or loosening some component) in order to avoid conflict.

Moreover, if the spouse is a less experienced driver, having the partner with dementia as a passenger in the car may represent a source of distraction and a potential risk in traffic. In our experience, the strongest reactions are often seen among patients with the most pronounced cognitive impairments, who are sensitive to this perceived threat to their identity. Moreover, the grief of the patient may concern the anticipated loss related to the foreseeable trajectory of the disease. The loss of the licence thus becomes a symbol of a more general deterioration [36].

When planning a meeting to inform a patient of a negative result after a driving evaluation, the patient should be encouraged to bring a family member or a friend to the clinic. The responsible healthcare provider should devote enough time to explain and discuss the reasons for the decision and to give the patient the opportunity to express feelings and to ask questions. Alternative modes of transportation should be discussed, involving family members if appropriate, in order to allow the patient to pursue valued practical and social activities. It is important from a quality-of-life perspective to enable the person with dementia to take social and recreational trips and not limit transportation to essential purposes such as shopping or healthcare appointments. Frequently, people with dementia who have always driven themselves may be too limited by impairments of memory, orientation and attention to be able to use public transportation and this may lead to an increased burden on family members. To ensure the patient's continued well-being, follow-up meetings can be scheduled or the patient can be referred to other healthcare providers.

7 Future Perspectives

Technological development in automobile design has led to great advances and many features are now part of standard equipment in new cars. A patient who is aware of his or her memory impairment may feel less of a cognitive load when using the adaptive cruise control or the lane assistance devices, because he or she no longer needs to constantly monitor the speed or position of the car and is less worried about inadvertent speeding.

However, given the effect of dementia on the ability to process information and learn new skills, it is far from evident that drivers with dementia will be able to fully benefit from all devices. The GPS system, for example, could be a great help to compensate for the orientation difficulties that are a prominent symptom in Alzheimer's disease, but entering the correct destination might often prove too difficult and using it could be too distracting.

Autonomous cars have the potential to enable people with physical or cognitive limitations or both to travel independently. However, development is still ongoing. There is yet no car that is sufficiently autonomous to never require action on the part of the driver in certain situations. Furthermore, it is likely that the introduction of 'driverless' cars on the roads will take place gradually, and that traffic will be made up of a mix of more or less autonomous and conventional cars for many years. This could be particularly challenging for drivers with dementia, since it might be especially difficult for them to tell the difference and adapt their own driving behaviour accordingly.

8 Concluding Remarks

The issue of driving in people with questionable medical fitness can be viewed from several perspectives. Among these the ethical and political perspectives are particularly important. Medical practitioners confronted with decisions about their driving patients are generally sensitive to the conflicting interests of the individual and society at large. They feel a duty not to unduly limit the autonomy of the patients, and this may be particularly important in cases of dementia, since untimely limitations can contribute to a swifter progression of symptoms. On the other hand, they have an awareness of the obvious interests of the public not to be harmed by unfit drivers. In this respect, the issue is not unlike that of weapons possession, although on a different scale.

Many factors hinder a dispassionate discussion. Patient representatives may legitimately invoke the fact that the increased risk in traffic posed by drivers with dementia is hard to quantify in a precise way (and, in any case, is probably lower than that of drivers under the influence of alcohol or street drugs or that caused by reckless driving). The level of increased risk (whether twofold, higher or lower) that can be accepted is a political or public policy decision, not a scientific or ethical one. As for the question of fitness to possess and use weapons, societies that value personal freedom and a minimal level of state interference in private lives will be more tolerant and less controlling than societies that are more oriented towards public safety.

As in many other areas, in the absence of definite answers (based on scientific evidence) to the question of who may be allowed to drive, societal or political discussions are heavily influenced by events colourfully relayed by media – for example, of instances where a cyclist or pedestrian has been hit by a driver suspected of having a cognitive illness. This leads to a polarization of the debate and simplified arguments on the part of both parties who call for less or more control measures. There may also sometimes be an element of opportunism in the choice of political decision makers to either adopt such measures or to reject or postpone them.

In discussions on the individual level, arguments can also be variously rational. Understandably, a person with dementia may be unwilling to face the certainty of driving cessation, with all its practical and psychological consequences, to avoid a crash that remains a mere possibility. Indeed, our calculations, based on Swedish data from 1992 to 1995, show people between 65 and 74 years of age in the general older driving population have an estimated risk of being killed or injured in a crash of about 0.26 per million person-kilometres. For the age group of 75 to 84 years, the corresponding figure is 0.48. If a driver with cognitive impairment has a twofold increased risk, this means the corresponding estimates would be 0.53 and 0.97 per million person-kilometres, respectively. An at-risk driver 65 to 74 years of age would need to drive about 1,900,000 kilometres and a driver between 75 and 84 years 1,030,000 kilometres to have one single severe or fatal crash.

This is obviously a distance that by far exceeds the projected distance driven during the remainder of the person's driving career. These calculations do not refer to crashes caused by older drivers who are not themselves injured or killed, but it is reasonable to assume results would be similar since crashes are infrequent events in countries with good infrastructure and vehicles in good condition.

Given the frailty associated with ageing, with weaker bones and muscle mass, and less resistance to trauma of large blood vessels, the risk of being severely injured or killed in a crash is far higher for older than for younger road users. This is an important consideration for medical professionals because of their responsibility to protect their patients' health.

It is also important to note that, although the debate about (cognitively impaired) older drivers often focusses on their risk to other road users, it is not unlikely that they themselves are at a higher risk of becoming the victims of other drivers. Limitations in attention and anticipation make it more difficult for an older driver with cognitive impairment or dementia to foresee that other road users will engage in rule-breaking behaviour (e.g. speeding or not respecting right of way). In turn, this lack of anticipation will prevent the older driver to take appropriate defensive measures. However, if the older driver were asked if he or she is willing to give up driving in order not to be injured by another car, the answer would probably be that this is far too high a price to pay to avoid a very unlikely event.

When family members seek to convince an older at-risk driver to give up driving, they often appeal to their sense of responsibility and to their imagination, depicting the terrible consequences of killing a child in the neighbourhood. Other arguments can be financial, weighing the cost of using a car against the equivalent in taxi trips or other alternative transportation. In our experience, the efficacy of such arguments partly depends on the personality of the older driver and on family dynamics.

However, this type of reasoning is not likely to resonate with even older drivers in general, because a majority perceives driving as a '"right" which we all deserve' and older frequent drivers, more than younger, state they are reluctant to give up driving because of the loss of something they enjoy [37]. It is reasonable to assume cognitively impaired drivers will express the same views, but perhaps more forcefully. A continued cognitive deterioration makes it more difficult to notice and remember signs of diminished capacity as a driver and the person will dwell on past experience and expertise rather than trying to compensate for more recent cognitive challenges.

In conclusion, the long-standing issue of driving in dementia remains controversial, with strong opinions, not always supported by scientific evidence, both on the part of more liberally inclined stakeholders and those supporting increased restrictions. The debate is likely to continue for many years to come, despite technical development of vehicles and improvements in the traffic environment. Harmonization of regulations and legislation between different countries is a desirable aim.

Furthermore, it is important to further a general awareness of the fact that dementia is not a uniform and static condition, but one with different and sometimes individual manifestations that evolve over time. This has implications for driving because a person with cognitive impairment (pre-dementia) or mild dementia cannot be considered in the same way as a person with moderate or severe dementia.

The following case description illustrates a situation where an older driver is apprehended because of aberrant behaviour in traffic. The person might have been identified by the healthcare system and social services as needing support because of health problems and failing cognition, but the question of driving has not been raised. It also shows the older driver has difficulties in understanding and accepting the verdict that driving is no longer permissible and that several conversations are sometimes necessary before reaching closure.

The patient's story

Mr B is a 90-year old man who lives alone. He has a university degree and retired at 62 after a distinguished career as an engineer. His wife died 10 years ago and he misses her very much. They had no children, but a nephew helps him with some practical matters and has arranged for bills to be paid automatically by the bank. Meals are delivered to his home; a care assistant comes twice a day and the district nurse visits him once a week to help him with medication.

Mr B says he feels his age and is aware he is not in as good shape as he used to be. Since a stroke, he has difficulties moving about and is afraid of falling. He has always enjoyed driving and takes pride in his car, a vintage Italian model. He feels completely safe and in charge when driving and likes going for recreational trips in the countryside one to two hours from home.

One late November afternoon, he takes a taxi to fetch his car from the garage where it had been serviced. On his way home, he notices a police car behind him. Its rooftop lights are flashing, and Mr B thinks it is chasing a criminal, so he veers to the right and slows down to let the car pass. He does not understand why the police car makes him stop. Two policemen, who Mr B thinks are ridiculously young, explain they have been alerted by other drivers and they need to check if he is drunk. Mr B says he drinks very little and he would never dream of driving after having had a drink. He nevertheless submits to the breathalyser test and is satisfied when it is negative. He is persuaded the matter is closed and is flabbergasted when one of the policemen takes his licence and declares he is going to drive him home in his own car.

After a week Mr B receives a registered letter informing him his licence has been permanently revoked. Mr B is first taken by surprise, then indignant. He immediately applies for a new licence and receives notification from the licencing authority that he needs a medical certificate to show he fulfils medical requirements. To obtain this, he visits his family physician.

Mr B reluctantly comes to the Traffic Medicine Centre, situated inconveniently far from his home. The staff is agreeable enough, but he is surprised by having to take a test in front of three computer screens that involves steering and pushing buttons according to instructions from a nurse. Mr B is a bit confused and is reminded of the games his nephew's children have shown him. He tells the nurse this is nothing like driving a car. He then meets the doctor, who not only performs the usual medical examination but also asks him to draw a clock and a cube and repeat some words. Mr B waits for a chance to go outside with someone from the staff to show his practical driving ability, but this does not seem to be part of the procedure. Mr B tries to make the doctor understand what happened with the policemen was a misunderstanding, but the doctor is completely unsympathetic.

At the end of the examination, Mr B is completely surprised when the physician informs him he will not be receiving the certificate he needs to apply for a new licence. He is asked if he accepts a referral to his family doctor for a memory assessment. Mr B, believing this might increase his chances of obtaining the certificate, accepts.

The outsider's view

The patient is known to his family doctor. His medical history includes a variety of conditions such as a previous myocardial infarction, prostate cancer and a cerebral infarction seven years ago. He needs daily assistance and all caregivers have noticed he has become increasingly forgetful, but he still seems to manage quite well at home.

The police are patrolling a suburban expressway on a late November afternoon. The light and weather conditions are not very good. The police are alerted that a car has been observed swaying from side to side on the road. The police car soon identifies the car and follows it. The police notice the speed of the car is very variable and that its lane keeping is bad. They have difficulty in stopping the car but succeed by braking in front of it. The driver of the car turns out to be an elderly man, who seems shocked. He has difficulties finding his driver's licence and following instructions for the breathalyser test. The policemen quickly conclude the driver might have medical conditions that make him unfit for driving and one of them drives him home. His licence is provisionally confiscated and he is reported to the driving licence authority. The authority decides that, in view of his traffic behaviour, the driver no longer fulfils medical requirements for holding a licence.

The family doctor is surprised when the patient, who is usually very calm, insists he needs a certificate of medical fitness to drive. The patient does not explain why he needs this certificate and the doctor is at a loss, feeling very uncertain regarding the patient's physical and mental fitness. They agree a referral to a specialized medical unit is the best solution.

The medical driving evaluation includes a simple test of simulated driving (essentially testing psychomotor coordination, reaction speed and divided attention). Here the patient remains quite passive and seems to have great difficulties in understanding the task and remembering what to do. His steering is sometimes very unstable and his reaction times are close to twice the normal levels when he is required to divide his attention between two simultaneous tasks. The patient fails to react to many signals (missed signals are deemed unacceptable) and presses the wrong button on more than half of the trials.

The examining physician notes the patient moves slowly and uses a walking aid but is very unsteady and close to falling several times. He speaks slowly, is calm and amenable and follows instructions but gives a clear impression of cognitive impairment. His insight appears to be limited and he constantly returns to his preoccupation that the authorities are persecuting him and that his licence has been wrongly revoked.

The doctor performs some cursory tests of memory and visuospatial ability. The patient has impaired memory and cannot copy a three-dimensional cube. He cannot write today's date correctly and is unable to draw a clock face and set the hands to show the correct time. Even with his own glasses, his visual acuity is barely above the minimum limit.

The conclusion is that the patient does not fulfil cognitive requirements for licensure. Due to signs of cognitive impairment, a referral is made (with the patient's consent) for a memory assessment in a primary care setting. A medical certificate is sent to the licencing authority (with a copy to the patient), stating the medical requirements for licence holding are *not* fulfilled.

The patient calls the physician four days later, telling him the police report that led to his licence revocation contained outright lies and has questions about how the medical assessment was performed. The physician explains the conclusion of unfitness was based on the results of the clinical tests, not on the observations of the police.

(cont.)

When Mr B receives the copy of the medical certificate, he feels the contents are cold and uncaring. He cannot understand why no one is interested in his true driving ability and the fact that there is not a single misdemeanour on his driving record. He strongly believes things would have gone differently if he had not been stressed by the police car that chased him. He calls the physician a few days later to explain his point of view. Since the physician is not convinced by Mr B's arguments, Mr B writes to the licencing authority stating he has driven without problems for most of his life and he needs his car because of his difficulties to walk. He quickly receives a bureaucratic response informing him the decision will not be changed.

Mr B feels he should have a better chance with the tests at the Traffic Medicine Centre now that they are not unfamiliar to him. After all, people who want a first-time driving licence are allowed to take the tests as many times as they need if they do not succeed the first time. He therefore calls the physician again and asks for a new assessment. Mr B. cannot understand why he cannot obtain a new assessment and feels very frustrated.

Mr B's condition deteriorates. He does not think about his car all the time, but he feels unhappy and frustrated when he does. He dies less than six months later.

The patient calls the physician yet again, repeating his arguments and insisting on a new assessment so he can obtain better results and regain his licence. The physician explains the results are not likely to improve to the extent that he would be considered fit to drive. The physician also notes the patient immediately seems to forget what is said, despite great effort on the part of doctor to express himself clearly.

References

1. Connors MH, Ames D, Woodward M, Brodaty H. Predictors of driving cessation in dementia: Baseline characteristics and trajectories of disease progression. *Alzheimer Dis Assoc Disord*. 2018; **32** (1): 57–61.

2. OECD. Traffic safety of elderly road users. Paris: Organisation for Economic Cooperation and Development; 1985.

3. Martin A, Balding L, O'Neill D. Are the media running elderly drivers off the road? *Br Med J*. 2005; **330**: 68.

4. Heikkinen S. *Att köra eller inte köra. Hur de äldre, åldrande och bilkörning har diskuterats i svensk transportpolitik*. Uppsala, University of Uppsala, 2008.

5. Biggs S, Carr A, Haapala I. Dementia as a source of social disadvantage and exclusion. *Australas J Ageing* 2019; **38** Suppl 2: 26–33.

6. Chee JN, Rapoport MJ, Molnar F, Herrmann N, O'Neill D, Marottoli R, et al. Update on the risk of motor vehicle collision or driving impairment with dementia: A collaborative international systematic review and meta-analysis. *Am J Geriatr Psychiatry* 2017; **25**(12): 1376–90.

7. Adler G, Rottunda S, Dysken M. The older driver with dementia: An updated literature review. *Journal of Safety Research* 2005; **36**: 399–407.

8. Liljegren M, Naasan G, Temlett J, Perry DC, Rankin KP, Merrilees J, et al. Criminal behavior in frontotemporal dementia and Alzheimer disease. *JAMA Neurology* 2015; **72** (3): 295–300.

9. Fujito R, Kamimura N, Ikeda M, Koyama A, Shimodera S, Morinobu S, et al. Comparing the driving behaviours of individuals with frontotemporal lobar degeneration and those with Alzheimer's disease. *Psychogeriatrics: The Official Journal of the Japanese Psychogeriatric Society* 2016; **16**(1): 27–33.

10. Charlton JLKS, O'Hare M, Andrea D, Smith G, Khodr B, Langford, J, et al. Influence of chronic illness on crash involvement of motor vehicle drivers. Monash University Accident Research Centre; 2004 March, 2004. Contract No.: Report No. 213.

11. Ott BR, Heindel WC, Papandonatos GD, Festa EK, Davis JD, Daiello LA, et al. A longitudinal study of drivers with Alzheimer disease. *Neurology* 2008; **70** (14): 1171–8.

12. Meuleners LB, Ng J, Chow K, Stevenson M. Motor vehicle crashes and dementia: A population-based study. *J Am Geriatr Soc*. 2016; **64**(5): 1039–45.

13. Ball KK, Roenker DL, Wadley VG, Edwards JD, Roth DL, McGwin G Jr, et al. Can high-risk older drivers be identified through performance-based

measures in a Department of Motor Vehicles setting? *J Am Geriatr Soc.* 2006; **54**(1): 77–84.

14. Masters MC, Morris JC, Roe CM. 'Noncognitive' symptoms of early Alzheimer disease: A longitudinal analysis. *Neurology* 2015; **84**(6): 617–22.

15. Babulal GM, Stout SH, Head D, Holtzman DM, Fagan AM, Morris JC, et al. Neuropsychiatric symptoms and Alzheimer's disease biomarkers predict driving decline: Brief report. *J Alzheimers Dis.* 2017; **58**(3): 675–80.

16. Johansson K, Bogdanovic N, Kalimo H, Winblad B, Viitanen M. Alzheimer's disease and apolipoprotein E epsilon 4 allele in older drivers who died in automobile accidents. *Lancet* 1997; **349**(9059): 1143–4.

17. Kim YJ, An H, Kim B, Park YS, Kim KW. An international comparative study on driving regulations on people with dementia. *Journal of Alzheimer's Disease* 2017; **56**(3): 1007–14.

18. Siren A, Meng A. Cognitive screening of older drivers does not produce safety benefits. *Accid Anal Prev.* 2012; **45**: 634–8.

19. Martin AJ, Marottoli R, O'Neill D. Driving assessment for maintaining mobility and safety in drivers with dementia. *Cochrane Database Syst Rev.* 2013; (1): CD006222.

20. Tyrrell M, Religa D, Fossum B, Hedman R, Skovdahl K, Hilleras P. Embarking on a memory assessment: Voices of older persons living with memory impairment. *Dementia* (London) 2020: 1471301220910637.

21. Guss R, La Fontaine J, Buckell A, Knibbs T, Palfrey M. *Clinical Psychology in the Early Stage Dementia Care Pathway.* Leicester, British Psychological Society, 2014.

22. Carr D, Stowe JD, Morris JC. Driving in the elderly in health and disease. *Handbook of Clinical Neurology.* 2019; **167**: 563–73.

23. Manning KJ, Davis JD, Papandonatos GD, Ott BR. Clock drawing as a screen for impaired driving in aging and dementia: Is it worth the time? *Arch Clin Neuropsychol.* 2014; **29**(1): 1–6.

24. Lundberg C, Johansson K, Ball K, Bjerre B, Blomqvist C, Braekhus A, et al. Dementia and driving: An attempt at consensus. *Alzheimer Dis Assoc Disord.* 1997; **11**(1): 28–37.

25. Reger MA, Welsh RK, Watson GS, Cholerton B, Baker LD, Craft S. The relationship between neuropsychological functioning and driving ability in dementia: A meta-analysis. *Neuropsychology* 2004; 18(1): 85–93.

26. Bennett JM, Chekaluk E, Batchelor J. Cognitive tests and determining fitness to drive in dementia: A systematic review. *J Am Geriatr Soc.* 2016; **64**(9): 1904–17.

27. Hird MA, Egeto P, Fischer CE, Naglie G, Schweizer TA. A systematic review and meta-analysis of on-road simulator and cognitive driving assessment in Alzheimer's disease and mild cognitive impairment. *J Alzheimer Dis.* 2016; **53**(2): 713–29.

28. Edwards JD, Ross LA, Wadley VG, Clay OJ, Crowe M, Roenker DL, et al. The Useful Field of View Test: Normative data for older adults. *Arch Clin Neuropsychol.* 2006; **21**(4): 275–86.

29. Radford KA, Lincoln NB, Murray-Leslie C. Validation of the Stroke Drivers Screening Assessment for people with traumatic brain injury. *Brain Inj.* 2004; **18**(8): 775–86.

30. Winblad B, Amouyel P, Andrieu S, Ballard C, Brayne C, Brodaty H, et al. Defeating Alzheimer's disease and other dementias: A priority for European science and society. *Lancet Neurology* 2016; **15**(5): 455–532.

31. Piersma D, Fuermaier ABM, de Waard D, Davidse RJ, de Groot J, Doumen MJA, et al. Prediction of fitness to drive in patients with Alzheimer's dementia. *PloS One* 2016; **11**(2): 1–29.

32. Velayudhan L, Baillon S, Urbaskova G, McCulloch L, Tromans S, Storey M, et al. Driving cessation in patients attending a young-onset dementia clinic: A retrospective cohort study. *Dement Geriatr Cogn Dis Extra* 2018; **8**(1): 190–8.

33. Stout SH, Babulal GM, Ma C, Carr DB, Head DM, Grant EA, et al. Driving cessation over a 24-year period: Dementia severity and cerebrospinal fluid biomarkers. *Alzheimer Dement: J Alzheimer Assoc.* 2018; **14**(5): 610–16.

34. Lovas J, Fereshtehnejad SM, Cermakova P, Lundberg C, Johansson B, Johansson K, et al. Assessment and reporting of driving fitness in patients with dementia in clinical practice: Data from SveDem, the Swedish Dementia Registry. *J Alzheimer Dis.* 2016; **53**(2): 631–8.

35. Redelmeier DA, Yarnell CJ, Thiruchelvam D, Tibshirani RJ. Physicians' warnings for unfit drivers and the risk of trauma from road crashes. *N Engl J Med.* 2012; **367**(13): 1228–36.

36. Sanford S, Rapoport MJ, Tuokko H, Crizzle A, Hatzifilalithis S, Laberge S, et al. Independence, loss, and social identity: Perspectives on driving cessation and dementia. *Dementia* (London) 2019; **18**(7–8): 2906–24.

37. Arai A, Mizuno Y, Arai Y. Differences in perceptions regarding driving between young and old drivers and non-drivers in Japan. *Int J Geriatr Psychiatry*. 2010; **25**(12): 1239–45.

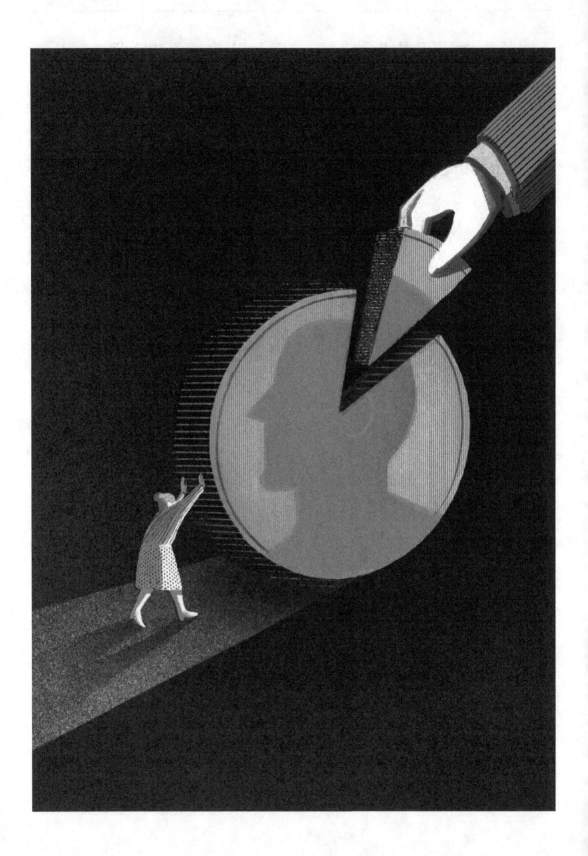

Social and Private Costs of Dementia

Patrick Cloos, Martin Knapp, Jeroen Luyten, Erik Schokkaert and Cheng Shi

1 Introduction

The main focus of this book is on the quality of life and social integration of persons with dementia. Good-quality dementia care can be effective in slowing down and alleviating the symptoms associated with dementia and providing support to families. Yet dementia also has large social and economic impacts because many resources are invested in caring for patients (including money, time, labour and social capital). This economic impact or cost can be translated into well-being terms: resources have to be used for care rather than for other purposes such as private consumption, environmental policy or social housing.

In this chapter, we provide an overview of these economic aspects. We discuss actual expenses incurred (e.g. for treatment) and costs that are incurred but hard to quantify (e.g. associated with caregiving), but we also look at the costs of the efforts invested to counter or mitigate the health consequences of the disease (e.g. through research and development (R&D) to find a cure for dementia or to improve care services) or to protect ourselves against the financial impact of dementia (through insurance).

In Section 2, we give an overview of the overall economic burden of dementia and how that is usually estimated in cost-of-illness studies. Special attention is devoted to the importance of unpaid (sometimes called informal) care and to difficulties in quantifying its value. Moreover, we argue traditional cost measures are culture-dependent and reflect the choices made in different societies.

Given the huge and increasing loss of well-being as a consequence of dementia, it would be great if we could find a medical (pharmacological) cure or identify actions that could be taken earlier in life to prevent it. A private firm that would be the first to discover a really effective product would certainly expect to make large profits. Yet, despite this strong incentive, it turns out to be very difficult to find such a cure. The roots of this difficulty are discussed in Section 3. It is very likely that government support is needed in the search for a treatment, but such support is less evident in a period of high and increasing pressure on government budgets.

Without cure, care becomes even more important for the quality of life of persons with dementia. Yet care is costly, including for the individuals involved. Moreover, more attention should also go to prevention – that is, to changing the modifiable risk for dementia. As shown in Section 4, there is a social gradient in the prevalence of dementia and in the use of care. Therefore, distributional issues cannot be neglected when we move from the analysis of the overall impact from and on society to the analysis of the challenges for individuals living with dementia.

In Section 5, we look at the private costs of dementia for a household which includes someone with dementia. Again, these 'economic' costs should be interpreted in the right way: if households have to bear a large financial burden, this has immediate implications for their health and well-being.

If personal costs can be huge and they are distributed unequally, the question arises as to how to protect households with a person with dementia, with special attention to poorer population subgroups. Private insurance markets for dementia care are largely missing and, even if they existed, they would be inadequate for lower-income groups. There is a need for government intervention, from both efficiency and equity points of view. Yet, at the moment, government financing is also insufficient to fully protect people with dementia and their households. This is discussed in Section 6.

Government intervention should not be restricted to financial support. There is also a need for a strong public healthcare system that focusses not only on curative care and hospitals but also on disease prevention and health promotion and on programmes like home care and social support. These issues are discussed in great detail in other chapters of this book.

2 The Global Economic Cost of Dementia

2.1 Cost-of-Illness Estimates

The demand for medical and social care by individuals with dementia has specific features caused by the combination of high levels of dependence, complex care needs and increasing morbidity as the disease progresses. Therefore, in addition to the potential social suffering associated with dementia, the impact on the economy is substantial. On a worldwide scale, the cost of dementia was estimated at about US $1 trillion in 2018, a number expected to double by 2030 [1]. Yearly costs per person have been estimated at about £30,000 in the United Kingdom and $50,000 in the United States [2].

Cost-of-illness studies typically categorize dementia costs into three groups: medical costs, social care costs and unpaid care costs. *Medical costs* are all healthcare costs directly related to diagnosing and treating dementia, including neuroimaging, diagnostic tests, anti-dementia drugs, cognitive stimulation therapy, hospital stays and doctor visits. In terms of medical costs, dementia generates less than 1% of total healthcare expenditure [3]. For healthcare payers, dementia is therefore, considering its high prevalence, a relatively 'affordable' disease.

For comparison, in the European Union, the direct medical costs of cancer care are estimated at 6% of total healthcare expenditure [4]. However, on top of these medical expenditures, dementia mobilizes other resources such as professional *home care* or *residential and nursing home care*, costs often borne by other budgets such as social care agencies, or by individuals and families themselves.

Both medical and social care costs are real expenditures. But costs can also be incurred without actual expenditure. A third and often high cost is associated with *unpaid or informal caregiving* by family members or friends (so-called carers or caregivers). These costs are not real monetary expenditures (in the sense that nobody has to pay for these services). They are nonetheless costs to be attributed to dementia. Caregiving is a usually unpaid, time-costly activity that can often imply a substantial well-being burden on people.

From an economic perspective, it is therefore important to count these as costs and it may be useful to (try to) put a monetary value on these time losses. Two main methods are used to do this. The first one is to value hours of informal care by the (average) wage lost because of being less available for the labour market (the *forgone wage approach*). The second method is to impute the cost of hiring a professional (the *replacement cost approach*). A third method has been used much less often, which is the *well-being approach* that asks carers directly about their willingness to provide care, and then estimates the income necessary to maintain the same level of well-being for the carer. On a global level, unpaid informal care costs are estimated at between 60% and 80% of total dementia costs [5]. We come back to the costs of unpaid care later in the chapter.

Obviously, the scale of care costs is highly context-dependent. The higher the average income across countries, the larger the share of the social care component in the total cost estimate will be. In high-income countries, the share of medical costs therefore tends to be lower, whereas care costs tend to be higher. An interesting evolution is that an increasing number of people with dementia are accommodated in care homes in middle-income countries, often because families no longer can afford the (opportunity) costs of support in community settings. Some of these countries, such as Thailand, are promoting themselves as international hubs for dementia care.

2.2 Caveats

Cost-of-illness estimates clearly demonstrate dementia has a large economic impact on our societies. However, for at least three reasons it is not always clear what these cost estimates imply exactly, or how they need to be interpreted by policymakers or others in charge of resource allocation decisions.

First, costing is not an exact science and any estimates are dependent upon the resources that are considered relevant and the methods used to value them. This caveat is most relevant regarding the value of unpaid care costs and whether (and how) to include them. In one study, the cost per person with dementia was 35% higher when unpaid care costs were estimated through a 'replacement cost' method instead of a 'forgone wage' approach [2].

Also as unpaid care costs are not 'real' expenses, these total cost estimates cannot easily be compared to other costs that do not include similar 'indirect' costs. For instance, the total global cost of dementia ($1 trillion per year) is sometimes compared to the GDP of a country like the Netherlands or Indonesia, or the combined market value of companies like Apple or Google, mainly to highlight the magnitude of the dementia challenge. However, such comparisons do not compare like with like, as time costs are not included in GDP calculations or business valuations. As such, cost-of-illness estimates might produce artificially high estimates of the economic impact of dementia, at least when compared to metrics of economic impact of other social issues.

Second, some important social cost categories are excluded in cost-of-illness studies. One cost that is ignored is the broader set of spillover and interaction effects dementia can have on the economy. As larger shares of the labour force become affected by dementia (through developing the condition or through the need to provide care for others), it will begin to have structural macroeconomic effects that go beyond what is quantified in a micro-costing study. Unpaid care implies lower participation in the labour market, earlier retirement or participation of lower quality/intensity, with lower family income as a result, but also lower tax contributions and reduced production of economic goods and services. Studies tentatively show the scale of these indirect costs can be large enough to create significant macroeconomic effects [6].

Another ignored 'cost' is the 'intangible cost' of the health impact of dementia itself as a value lost to society (in addition to all of the resources used to mitigate the impact of this loss). A prime example is the cost of lost 'human capital' due to the cognitive decline of dementia. Elsewhere a measure of 'cognitive footprint' has been suggested, aiming to capture the impact a disease such as dementia (but also other exposures such as air pollution or alcohol) has on cognitive functioning of individuals and the value that is therefore lost to society [7].

A third caveat in interpreting cost estimates of dementia is that these figures are not only less precise than is being suggested, but that it is not clear what exactly policymakers should learn from them. The total costs incurred merely reflect our default ways of responding to the dementia challenge, but from such estimates we cannot infer whether this way of responding is appropriate, particularly whether incurred levels of costs are warranted by provision of adequate, cost-effective care. In this sense, costs incurred reflect how much priority society *is willing to allocate* to address dementia: how quickly it is being diagnosed, how families respond to a diagnosis, what types and levels of care are provided by healthcare systems and so on.

For instance, when stigma is involved and people tend to postpone seeking a dementia diagnosis, then cost-of-illness studies reflect these attitudes, but it is likely that there would be a different pattern of care in a scenario where societal attitudes were less discriminatory. This does not mean costs would be lower (they might even be higher), but the care received for the money (and its translation to quality of life) might be higher. It therefore makes sense to distinguish between 'good' costs and 'bad' costs. The former stem from appropriate use of resources in a way that maximizes benefits to patients and society, while the latter stem from inappropriate care or overly late diagnoses that necessitate more expensive and less effective care.

Cost estimates also hide what might be wide regional differences in the cost of dementia. On a global level, cost differences between countries are closely associated with differences in GDP per capita. The relative contribution of unpaid care is greatest in the African regions and lowest in North America, Western Europe and some South American regions, while the reverse is true for social-sector costs [1].

2.3 Future Cost Projections

What can be expected for the future in terms of dementia costs? Global costs are likely to grow because life expectancy will rise due to reductions in mortality from other causes and, as age is the main risk factor for developing dementia, global incidence and prevalence of dementia may increase – although this latter point is disputed (see Chapter 8). Also, the cost of any given service or item of care (usually) inflates over time. As developing economies grow, the cost of care might increase more rapidly than the average price level. So the cost of dementia care, due to its high dependence on labour, might rise faster than inflation in these regions, even without any increase in prevalence.

It is possible that economic growth may also result in increased awareness, help-seeking and medical diagnosis (leading to increases in direct medical care costs) and a shift from unpaid informal care to direct costs from the social-care sector. Some studies suggest the proportion of people with dementia living in residential care has begun to decline in high-income countries, consistent with policy initiatives to provide care at home where possible. However, such a strategy may not be associated with reduced costs when all of the costs of home care, including unpaid care, are properly accounted for.

A UK study mapped out the economic consequences of dementia under different scenarios about the availability of evidence-based treatment and care [8]. The estimated total cost of dementia at the time of that study was £21 billion a year, or about £30,000 per patient. A first scenario examined the situation in which no dementia diagnoses were made at all and the disease was left to take its natural course in the entire population. It was therefore assumed no use was made whatsoever of the currently available insights regarding effective symptom-alleviating medication or adapted, adequate care. This would lead to an additional cost of £350 million due to extra care, in addition to the obvious loss of quality of life for people with dementia. Carrying out a diagnosis, without subsequently offering appropriate care, would add up to £500 million annually.

A second scenario consisted of making better use of the available scientific insights – that is, providing more adequate care to patients in accordance with the current state of knowledge of what works and what does not: effective medication that reduces symptoms, cognitive stimulation therapy, case management and a coping intervention for family carers. The most important effects are in the area of the substantial

improvement of the quality of life of people with dementia.

In terms of cost impact, these scenarios of 'improved care' have their own costs and sometimes have a cost-reducing and sometimes a cost-increasing effect. Even in the latter case, when a sufficiently broad horizon is considered in which all relevant effects are included, the additional costs come with health improvements and quality of life gains that make the whole scenario cost-effective according to conventional standards.

The conclusion of this study is that even in the most positive (but realistic) scenarios, dementia will continue to represent a large, non-negligible social cost. However, great gains can be made in the area of quality of life of people with the condition and their carers, through effective prevention and adequate organization of social support programmes.

This UK study also investigated a number of hypothetical scenarios in which an effective treatment for dementia was discovered. What emerged from this study is that a treatment is not a 'magic bullet', as the economic benefits will largely depend on when during the course of dementia this hypothetical treatment would influence disease progression (degree of delay of disease onset) and how the process would be affected (delay of disease progression and/or prolongation of life expectancy).

A more recent exercise by the same team explored their economic effects in a situation where a likely maximum price for a hypothetical new treatment would be set in order for it to satisfy the cost-effectiveness requirements associated with the National Institute of Health and Care Excellence (NICE). There could be major economic as well as quality of life benefits from deferring the onset of Alzheimer's disease, reducing the transition rate from prodromal to full dementia or reducing the transition rate to more severe stages of the condition [9, 10].

In this respect it is important to see there is also a strong economic case for prevention, as is shown in the cost-effectiveness analysis by Mukadam et al. of four midlife interventions to reduce the later-life risk of dementia [68]. In this chapter, we do not go deeper into the costs and benefits of prevention. More about this can be found in Chapter 8.

Although a treatment is not a 'magic bullet' from the economic point of view, there certainly is a large consensus in society that the optimal way to tackle the dementia challenge would be to find an effective cure. One would therefore expect that the prospect of such a large market attracts many pharmaceutical companies to invest into R&D for a dementia treatment, as such a treatment should surely be a 'blockbuster'. However, the reality is that investment in dementia research is low compared to other diseases, and some companies are even pulling out of dementia research. In the next section, we first look at the possible explanations for this seeming paradox. From Section 4 onwards, we focus on the costs of care.

3 The Social Costs of 'Cure': Research on Medicines for Dementia

In January 2018, Pfizer, the world's biggest pharmaceutical company in terms of yearly revenue, announced it would stop conducting Alzheimer's research. Other big pharma companies such as Novartis, Janssen, Biogen and Eli Lilly pledged to keep active in research, and large public or non-governmental organization (NGO) funders such as England's National Institute for Health Research (NIHR) and Alzheimer's Research UK and the National Institutes of Health (NIH) in the United States also keep funding research. But it is widely acknowledged that dementia is a difficult market for the private sector. Why? If expected profits of an effective medicine are huge and quasi-certain, the only explanation can be that R&D must be too costly and that, in the end, return on investment is not as attractive as it is for other diseases.

Although the pharmaceutical industry is a highly profitable sector, drug development in general is expensive and risky. Studies that have investigated how much it costs to discover and develop a safe and effective medicine have produced estimates of up to $2.6 billion [11], although that number remains controversial. A more recent estimate based on publicly available data estimates the average cost rather at $1.3 billion [12]. However, experts estimate the costs of an Alzheimer's disease drug development programme at $5.6 billion (CI: 3.7–9.3 billion) [13].

Research and development costs have four components, each contributing to making dementia R&D more expensive. There are the direct research costs: (1) costs of basic and pre-clinical research leading to an 'investigational new drug' (IND) and (2) costs of executing phase 1–3 trials of an IND, testing safety, efficacy and effectiveness. On top of these costs we have to add (3) a 'cost of failure'. For every drug that is successful, many other drug candidates are not. On average, across therapeutic areas, about 1 in 10 INDs ends up receiving market approval by bodies such as the Food and Drug Administration (FDA) in the United States, but there are differences between therapeutic areas. These costs have to be recouped by those products that become successful.

Finally, there is (4) the cost of capital: the compensation investors need to be paid in order to be willing to invest financial resources into drug development. This consists of compensation for the opportunity cost (if money were invested elsewhere e.g. government bonds, profits would be received for certain) and a risk premium (there is a chance the project fails). A standardized way to express this cost is by means of the 'weighted average cost of capital' (WACC): a combination of private funding, loans, equity and so forth, and how much that costs on average. In the drug industry, the WACC can go up to 11% per year of resources invested.

Why are these costs of drug R&D higher for dementia? First, our basic biomedical knowledge about dementia as a disease is limited compared to our knowledge of other diseases such as cancer. For decades, the cause of Alzheimer's, the most common form of dementia, was thought to be located in the build-up of abnormal proteins called amyloid and Tau in the brain. But the causal effects of this mechanism are still unproven. Today, there are also alternative theories rooting dementia in completely different biological mechanisms such as inflammation, metabolic disorders and numerous environmental toxins, or viral, bacterial and fungal infections.

Even beyond our understanding of the disease process itself, there is a lack of accurate diagnostic tools to indicate who has dementia. A key requirement for the development of therapies is an accurate diagnostic to identify who has and does not have the disease. The heterogeneous nature of dementia makes diagnosis difficult. In living patients, diseases like vascular dementia and Lewy body dementia can be indistinguishable from Alzheimer's. Similar dementia symptoms may have completely different underlying disease mechanisms and may in fact point at entirely different diseases (with similar symptoms).

A significant fraction of dementia has multiple causes and some cases cannot be clearly categorized even in an autopsy. This indicates that the preclinical research phase, in which potentially effective drug pathways are explored based on the state of the art in basic science and understanding of dementia, is more difficult, less developed and therefore more costly than is the case in other diseases.

On top of that, finding promising drug candidates to treat dementia is especially difficult because the brain is more inaccessible and harder to test and deliver compounds to compared to other human organs. For instance, the brain is protected behind the 'blood-brain barrier', which regulates the interaction between blood vessels and brain tissue, and which provides a defence against disease-causing pathogens and toxins that may be present in our blood. Even if one has a potentially effective compound, it may not reach its target.

Second, as a consequence, the risk of failure is higher in dementia drug R&D. A study that looked at the Alzheimer's disease drug development pipeline between 2002 and 2012 identified 413 trials investigating 244 different compounds [14]. Only one of these investigated compounds (memantine, a symptomatic cognitive enhancer) eventually received FDA approval for marketing. The researchers report that this gives Alzheimer's disease drug candidates one of the lowest success rates of any disease area: 0.4%.

Third, when a promising drug candidate emerges from preclinical research, phase 1–3 trials are needed. These are more expensive for dementia because they take longer and require more participants than average. It is important that interventions occur early in the dementia disease process. However, a disease-modifying treatment would need to show slowing in the rate of cognitive decline and there is often a long time interval between disease onset and emergence of symptoms.

In patients with early stages of dementia this requires a very long follow-up period. In patients with advanced dementia, follow-up periods would be shorter, but treatments may be less effective as the disease has progressed further and there are fewer opportunities for drugs to become disease-modifying. It may even be required for disease-modifying medicines that they are tested in patients before *any* symptoms occur. Symptoms

occur a decade later, however, so trials take a very long time and are therefore relatively expensive.

Moreover, trials are not only longer but also need larger numbers of participants. As there are many possible underlying dementia mechanisms, participants recruited into a trial may have widely diverging forms of dementia. This heterogeneity is important to understand in order to judge whether drugs are effective (and, if so, for which types of dementia patients in particular). It is important that trials have large numbers of participants so subgroup analysis, in which a particular drug may have greater effect, can be distinguished at statistically significant levels.

Fourth, and partly as a consequence of the previous three points, the cost of capital of drug R&D in the field of dementia is likely to be higher than elsewhere. Given the longer trial duration, the costs of capital, which can be up to 11% per year, increase exponentially. Moreover, given the risky nature of dementia trials, even higher capital costs can be expected for companies investing in dementia research compared to similar companies investing in other drug R&D. In fact, the extremely low chance of success of a dementia trial changes the very nature of the risks involved.

Economists sometimes distinguish between 'risk' for which the probability of success is known and where the risks can to some extent be hedged through mechanisms of risk diversification, and more radical (or 'Knightian') 'uncertainty', where probabilities of success are unknown and where compensation strategies are absent. Making such an investment comes closer to taking a 'gamble' than to taking a 'calculated risk'.

On top of these extra expensive R&D costs, additional problems may hinder the market development of dementia drugs. For instance, there is a risk of inadequate patent protection. To receive market approval, a drug needs to show efficacy in concrete outcomes such as cognition or activities of daily living (ADL). These end points are not quick to measure in the case of dementia. A patent on a molecule can expire before trials have sufficiently demonstrated its safety and effectiveness.

Without adequate patent protection, R&D investment, just as any other form of publicly accessible knowledge, suffers from the 'free-rider problem'. Knowledge is a public good and without government protection those who have invested in creating it will not be able to exclude others from using it for their own advantage. In a competitive market other companies would have a large incentive to 'free-ride' on the efforts of the originator firm.

In terms of budget sizes, there is a mismatch between the immense social costs of dementia and the resources society dedicates to research on it. For instance, costs for the United States have been estimated at more than $216 billion annually, whereas the main funding body, the NIH, has a budget of $1.8 billion [15]. It will be necessary to increase the scale of funding in order to make the dementia R&D pipeline productive, especially regarding the development of new compounds in the preclinical research stage.

A major concerted effort is needed from a wide variety of sources: pharmaceutical companies, national science funders, advocacy organizations, philanthropy and others. Currently, more than 70% of all trials for dementia are funded by the pharmaceutical industry [16], but there are many public institutions funding dementia research, including the NIH, the Veterans Affairs and the Centers for Medicare and Medicaid Services in the United States and the Medical Research Council and the NIHR in the UK.

Besides increased funding, there is also a need for a different research infrastructure. A complex financial ecosystem is needed to pool the necessary resources for dementia drug development, including public-private partnerships, so economies of scope can be maximized and individual research teams can be encouraged to build on the work of others rather than lose continuity or, worse, redo the same studies.

Trial platforms must be established that can investigate biomarker and drug combinations across companies. One major leap of progress would be development of (surrogate) biomarkers with sufficient sensitivity and specificity. Being able to identify patients with specific types of dementia (diagnostics) and being able to indicate in the short run what will happen to patients in the long run (through surrogate biomarkers) could enable large cost savings in the R&D process. It would be a major contribution to selecting the right patients in trials but also towards providing an early indication that a drug is having an effect that will ultimately lead to improvements in cognition. Without such information, ineffective drug candidates (that are nonetheless promising and safe) can advance to phase 3 trials (provided they are safe and tolerable), which is the longest and most expensive trial phase.

Additional government financing is important if the search for a cure for dementia is to be sped up. This puts additional pressure on government budgets and hence further increases competition for scarce government resources. This raises the issue of whether research funds should primarily go to the search for a cure or to the investigation of the effectiveness of different forms of care. We do not discuss this issue in depth, but we strongly feel the two should not be seen as competitors and a two-pronged research effort to improving the well-being of persons with dementia is needed (see [67]).

In any case, since an effective cure is not within reach in the short term, the financing of high-quality care for persons with dementia becomes a crucial challenge. We discuss the challenge of the public financing of such care in Section 6. Before turning to that question, we argue that distributional issues are an essential part of the overall picture (Section 4) and describe the importance of the personal costs for persons with dementia and their households (Section 5).

4 The Socio-economic Gradient of Dementia

In Section 2, the cost of dementia was described at the global level. We now turn to the costs for the persons with dementia themselves. To get a clear perspective on the distribution of that burden over society, one has to take into account the existence of a social gradient in dementia. This section explores issues of inequalities related to ageing, dementia and dementia care. We start from a general picture of the social determinants of health and illness and then go into the specific case of dementia.

4.1 The Social Determinants of Health and Illnesses

It is well known that social factors are powerful determinants of health and that groups and individuals with lower socio-economic status have worse health than those with better socio-economic status. The circumstances in which people grow, live, work and age are shaped by political, economic and social forces, and these factors are 'at the root of much of health inequalities' [17].

Structural factors (social protection–related policies and social position – socio-economic status, gender, racism, migration status), social capital (social support, social network), working and living conditions, healthcare organization, cultural and psychosocial factors (e.g. control over life) interact with each other and with genetic components to determine biological and physiological processes that shape morbidity, mortality and quality of life.

Social inequalities in health persist across the life course and in older ages. A substantial part of these years is lived with disabilities, and both life expectancy and disability-free life expectancy relate to socio-economic status [18]. Education level is a strong determinant of life expectancy: people with the highest education level can expect to live longer than persons with the lowest level. Lower educational level is associated with poorer health, chronic diseases and disability among older persons.

Inequalities in health in old age are the result of accumulated disadvantage related to gender and socio-economic status, ageism and inadequate laws and policies [18]. Elderly persons from ethnic minorities experience even more strongly multiple disadvantages (ageism, racism, gender disparities, class issues, lack of access to health and welfare resources) that have potential negative health impacts [19]. Ageism is of special concern as it has deleterious consequences for the health and well-being of older people: stereotypes refer to elders and disabled people as high in warmth and low in competence [20]. As discussed in detail in Chapter 2, stereotyping is particularly strong and damaging in the case of dementia.

4.2 Dementia: The Interaction between Environmental, Biological and Medical Factors

The general picture of a socio-economic gradient in health also applies to the specific case of dementia. Socio-economic status (education level and wealth) has been shown to have influence on dementia risk and on the decline in cognitive function with age. Different risk factors for dementia have been described in detail in Chapter 8, and many of them are directly related to socio-economic status.

Vascular risk factors are particularly important. As argued elsewhere in this book, the most common types of dementia described in the literature are Alzheimer's disease and vascular dementia (see Chapter 1). Their frequency increases with age in the presence of vascular risk factors [21]. Vascular risk factors (e.g. hypertension, smoking, diabetes, general atherosclerosis, physical inactivity and obesity) are common to cardiovascular (coronary heart disease, angina or heart attack) and cerebrovascular disease (e.g. stroke), both diseases being viewed as mutual risk factors and as risk factors for dementia. Some authors are specifying that midlife vascular risk factors (hypertension and obesity) accelerate cognitive decline later in life [22] and increase the likelihood of both Alzheimer's disease and vascular dementia [23]. The link with socio-economic background is clear, as socio-economic disadvantage increases the likelihood of cerebrovascular and cardiovascular disease.

The evidence of a link between socio-economic status and dementia depends on the level of analysis (individual, neighbourhood). Dementia incidence increases with lower individual wealth (e.g. property, possessions, housing, investments), deprivation and social isolation [23]. The effect of area deprivation on dementia is less clear. Cadar et al. [24] suggest the individual socio-economic characteristics rather than the features of the area explain the deleterious effect of deprivation on cognitive decline. According to these authors, possible explanations could be that wealth improves cognitive reserve and the possibility for individuals to be involved in digital literacy, social networks and cultural activities. Indeed, less social interaction is associated with the development of dementia and greater social relations seem to increase the cognitive reserve and, subsequently, be a protective factor against dementia. High social engagement is associated with a lower risk of dementia. Possible explanations could be that a stimulating environment and social relations could contribute to reducing stress, which in turn could reduce the risk of dementia [25].

Some studies suggest a relation between air pollution exposure and dementia. Causal pathways are unclear, but air pollutants are known to increase cardio and cerebrovascular diseases that are in turn known to be associated with an increased risk of dementia [26]. Air pollution exposure on its turn also shows a social gradient.

4.3 Social and Cultural Context of Ageing and Dementia Care

Not only is there a social gradient in the prevalence of dementia, there is also a social gradient in the implementation of services, treatments and care for people with dementia and their carers. The social and cultural context (policies, norms, socio-economic group, social capital) shape experience of and attitudes towards dementia and access to diagnosis, care and treatment. The lack of social network (a family or friend carer) represents a barrier for people with dementia to access care [27].

Poor neighbourhoods provide limited resources to assist older people with disabilities [18]. Limited mobility, poor transportation and long distances to healthcare centres can prevent access to healthcare. Ageism and stigmatization are other factors that impede access to quality care for older people and those with dementia, and can also be a source of mistreatment within long-term care institutions [28].

People with dementia, especially women living alone without a carer, receive less primary and preventive healthcare compared to people without dementia [27]. Migrant populations represent a social category with particular difficulties. Some authors are suggesting ethnic disparities in dementia due to various social, economic and cultural factors [29, 30]. Ageing migrants are often overlooked by authorities, social care services and society. It has been suggested there are biases among studies on dementia involving minority groups in countries like the UK (lack of valid diagnostic and screening instruments, amalgamation of ethnicities, miscommunication). Difficulties for minority groups may relate to diagnostics (racism and prejudice of clinicians, stigma of mental illnesses and lack of awareness in certain communities), to pathways to dementia care (lack of awareness of services, inadequate or inaccessible services) or to more difficult access to primary and secondary healthcare (that can influence the diagnosis and management of dementia) [19].

All these findings lead to the strong conclusion that social inequalities should not be neglected when thinking about the personal and social costs of dementia. The financial cost of care will weigh more heavily on households with a lower income. This implies they will have to spend less on consumption goods or refrain from spending on care. A concern for access and affordability for all should influence the design of protective government measures. We discuss in more detail in Section 6 how the amount and the structure of public funding – for example the availability of financial support of informal carers or the supply of subsidized formal care – can counteract (or not) socio-economic inequalities in the care for persons with dementia. The large variation in the degree of public financing between different countries will therefore be reflected directly in international variation in the distribution of the financial burden of care over different social groups. We now give a general overview of the private costs of dementia.

5 The Private Costs of Dementia for Households

Dementia has potentially considerable financial (and hence well-being) impacts on people living with the condition and their households, families and communities. Those impacts will vary between individuals and some are patterned by, for example, severity of dementia symptoms, the presence of other health problems, socio-economic group and personal preference. In turn, those factors are influenced by the context set by availability of, and access to healthcare and social care provision, how funding arrangements balance collective and individual responsibilities and societal attitudes to dementia.

5.1 Out-of-Pocket Payments

Private costs vary: some are more direct than others and some are more tangible than others. Most obviously, they include out-of-pocket payments (or self-funding) for services that are not funded by 'collective' risk-pooled healthcare and social care systems – that is, not covered by universal healthcare, social or private insurance. (These different modes of funding are discussed in the next section.) There are, for example, various forms of co-payment in insurance-based systems (e.g. where the service user pays the first €500 or 10% of total cost) and user fees for public services that operate means-testing regimes (e.g. where fees are payable by people with wealth holdings above a specified threshold).

There might also be payments for supplementary services such as low-level or more intensive psychological therapies or complementary and alternative therapies not available through 'mainstream' healthcare and social care structures. Individuals or their families might purchase assistive technologies (handrails, bathing adaptations and so on). Increasingly, if slowly, families are purchasing *technology-based* devices: safety interventions such as smoke detectors and panic buttons, interventions to enhance memory such as global positioning system devices and voice prompts and technology-aided reminiscence or therapeutic care for people with dementia and their carers [31]. Individuals may also hire help with 'everyday' functions they struggle to do because of increasing frailty, such as domestic cleaning, gardening and dog walking. Other private expenditures linked to dementia could include travel costs to attend hospital appointments or day care.

Even in countries with high coverage of collective healthcare and care services, out-of-pocket expenses on medical and non-medical services can impose quite significant burdens on households, with these economic impacts often largely invisible from administrative or other data systems. These payments may also arise because individuals with dementia or their families want to shorten the waiting time for services that *are* covered collectively, or to pay for services that are more personalized or of higher quality than those offered within the public system.

Private costs for people living with dementia and their families arise in many countries because the condition is not covered financially in the same way as most other health issues. This is partly because of the separation of long-term care from healthcare services, with the former often not included within healthcare financing arrangements. For example, in the United States, out-of-pocket expenditures for people living with dementia (including nursing home services, medications and other care) were estimated to be three times greater than for people with 'intact cognition' [32].

Another study looked back five years from time of death, finding that average cost per decedent with dementia was significantly greater than for people who died of heart disease, cancer or other causes; average out-of-pocket spending was 81% higher than for non-dementia patients [33].

A third US study gives some indication of both the scale of private costs in a private insurance system and of some marked variations: 'Dementia is associated with a loss of 97% of wealth among black Americans, compared with 42% among nonblack Americans, while wealth loss among black and non-black Americans without dementia did not differ substantially (15% versus 19%)' [34].

In England, many of the costs of supporting someone with dementia are considered social care rather than healthcare. Under current financing arrangements, these services are means-tested, so individuals with wealth holdings above a relatively modest amount have to pay for at least part of their care: currently about half of all people receiving adult social care make such a contribution [35]. For many older people, this means selling their home to pay for their care. To make matters worse, prices of social care are usually negotiated individually by self-funders and tend to be higher than prices paid by local authorities (which have the purchasing power to negotiate prices down): self-funders are generally cross-subsidizing publicly funded service users [36].

In Hong Kong, there are almost no user fees for publicly funded social care if an individual is eligible on the grounds of need for support, but waiting times are long for both community and residential care, so many people use private services or hire live-in foreign domestic helpers [37]. In contrast, in Germany, the compulsory long-term care insurance system fully covers cognitive and psychological impairments as well as physical care needs.

Out-of-pocket costs can impose large financial burdens on families that have to pay them. There is another, equally worrying side to the medal: out-of-pocket costs can also threaten access to care if families avoid them by reducing the use of healthcare facilities. In fact, this raises the issue of whether family members are willing to bear the costs of care for a person with dementia. They may weigh the care cost against their future inheritance. Also for people with dementia themselves, spending their money for care rather than passing their savings to their children can cause psychological distress. Therefore, a complete picture should include, in addition to a measure of out-of-pocket costs, an indicator of 'unmet need'.

5.2 Unpaid Care

As we noted earlier, there is considerable reliance on unpaid care inputs from spouses and family members of people with dementia across the world. Unpaid or informal care was defined by the World Health Organization (WHO) in 2015 as support by individuals who have low or no 'diverse training, expertise, status and remuneration level' [38]. For people with dementia, such care is often intensive and typically provided at home. Carers (or 'caregivers') are spouses, partners, family members, friends or neighbours of recipients providing care and support; the majority are women. Without their inputs, support would have to be provided and/or paid for by the state, third-sector organizations or care recipients themselves.

Some family members and friends spend considerable amounts of time taking responsibility for daily care and supervision. This is usually unpaid, as suggested by the label we are using, but some carers might be remunerated in cash or kind (and personal budgets complicate the picture somewhat: see later in this chapter). It is important to re-emphasize, however, that unpaid care does not mean *free* care: time devoted to care could be spent in other ways, such as paid employment and leisure activities, and so represents an opportunity cost over and above any out-of-pocket expenditure on services.

There can also be impacts upon the health and well-being of carers themselves. This is why policymakers should not neglect the well-being and costs of caring or they may make over-optimistic assumptions about the longer-term availability of family and other unpaid support. If the costs borne by carers (directly or indirectly, out of pocket or in kind) are sufficiently high to compromise their ability or willingness to continue to provide care, then dementia support structures would be severely stretched.

Putting a monetary value on the cost of unpaid care is not straightforward. One reason is that it is hard to define exactly what constitutes such care and so to quantify the number of hours provided. For example, are cooking, cleaning and shopping by a spouse or other co-resident family member simply regular household tasks or do they constitute 'care'? What counts as 'supervision' rather than just sharing the same home, particularly

where joint activities such as watching television are concerned?

Second, and as we noted earlier in the chapter, there is more than one way to then attach a unit cost to each hour of unpaid care: the *opportunity cost method* values the wages forgone and other time lost by being a carer, the *replacement method* calculates what it would cost to bring in substitute paid support (such as a home care worker or community nurse) and the *well-being method* tries to estimate what income compensation a carer would need to continue to provide care.

Replacement cost methods are most frequently used, and well-being methods are rarely used. Some studies use more than one method, either to check how sensitive the overall study conclusions are to the different approaches, or to attach different monetary values to different care tasks. For example, in a recent English study, carer time spent on supporting ADL tasks was valued as the cost of replacement of home care, while time supporting instrumental activities of daily living (IADL) tasks and supervision was valued using two different opportunity cost assumptions for carers who had or had not formally retired from paid employment [39].

Not surprisingly, different methods will generate different total and component costs. Differences are also generated by context: the Right Time Place Care study investigated patterns of transition from home care to institutional dementia care for people with dementia in eight European countries (Estonia, Finland, France, Germany, Netherlands, Spain, Sweden, UK). Using identical methods across countries, unpaid care (supporting ADLs, IADLs and supervision) was found to contribute an average of 52% of total cost, but varied from 28% in the Netherlands to 75% in Estonia [40].

The well-being method could, in principle, capture the non-pecuniary impacts of being a dementia carer. Not only are carers giving up the opportunity to enjoy their lives as they choose (leisure, enough sleep and so on) but they are also risking burnout, leading to worse health, particularly mental health. Some co-resident dementia carers might see their responsibilities as extending to 24 hours per day:

> It should be noted that being a carer for someone with dementia may affect the carer's physical and mental health and well-being and social relationships. Health systems must consider both the

substantial need of people with dementia for help from others and its significant impact on carers and families, including economic impact. Carers should have access to support and services tailored to their needs in order effectively to respond to and manage the physical, mental and social demands of their caring role.

(World Health Organization 2017, [41])

In response, governments often introduce policies to encourage and support family and other carers (see Chapter 7). Effective support mechanisms include partial 'replacement' care (i.e. 'paid' community health and social care services), flexible working conditions for those carers still in employment, support groups and interventions based on psychological therapy, training and raising awareness.

In the latter category, one of the most successful approaches in the UK is the multifaceted START (STrAtegies for RelaTives) intervention: it provided family carers of people with dementia with information on where to get emotional support and taught personalized techniques to understand and manage behaviours, change unhelpful thoughts, promote acceptance, improve communication, plan for the future and relax and engage in meaningful enjoyable activities. START significantly improved the mental health and wellbeing of family carers and was cost-effective both in the short-term and even after six years [42].

5.3 Other Private Costs

A further private cost of dementia is the value of *productivity loss* of people living with dementia, whether from disruption to labour market participation, social activities or family roles and responsibilities. Worsening symptoms will eventually make it impossible for people with dementia to continue to work, contribute to their communities, act as grandparents, help with household tasks and so on. It is not uncommon for an older person who is a carer for their spouse to develop dementia and themselves become the cared-for person: the opportunity costs are complex and potentially large.

Some services are delivered by *volunteers* – that is, unpaid workers who have not necessarily had previous connections to the people they support – whereas carers will generally have had such links through kinship or friendship. The help volunteers provide can be variable, and the personal, complex

and developmental nature of some of the symptoms and needs associated with dementia might mean family carers or paid care workers are more suitable. For an individual whose cognition is deteriorating, leaving them confused, an unfamiliar volunteer might be less suitable [43].

The costs associated with volunteering are, in some respects, similar to the costs associated with unpaid care. Volunteers may not be paid a wage, but they are generally not necessarily 'free' because of the opportunities forgone by volunteering. In attaching costs in evaluative studies, similar methods have been used as when costing unpaid care. A difference between the two groups, however, is that some volunteers are undertaking these activities as a stepping stone into (or back into) paid employment, and so volunteering may, in some respects, also represent a personal investment in human capital.

There might also be costs associated with *stigma and public attitudes* towards dementia (see Chapter 7). Attitudes vary considerably across the world, but are generally negative. Often these attitudes are shaped by the view that dementia is just a 'normal' part of ageing rather than a condition that can to some extent be prevented and certainly for which some symptoms can be delayed or ameliorated, even if progression of the underlying disease cannot be halted. Research in the wider mental health field has shown sizeable economic impacts flowing from stigma [44].

One consequence is that access to services may be more difficult for people living with dementia and their family carers, with cognitive needs given lower priority than physical health needs or disabilities. The built environment may be unsympathetically designed for people experiencing visual hallucinations or other impairments as a result of their cognitive decline (more details in Chapter 8). Carers may feel ostracized because of a lack of understanding about what dementia is and the stresses it can generate for them. People with dementia and their carers may choose to avoid interpersonal contact because of self-stigma. The effect will almost certainly be diminished quality of life. Anti-stigma initiatives have been shown to work in relation to some mental health problems, but dementia-focussed efforts remain relatively unexplored. Reducing dementia stigma is a key aim in WHO's recommendations [45].

5.4 Personal Budgets

A final form of private cost, growing in importance, even though relatively modest as yet, is self-directed support. Governments in some high-income countries have introduced mechanisms to devolve some control of public funds to individuals with long-term care needs. In England, these are called direct payments and personal budgets. These transfers therefore represent public or collective expenditure (funded from taxes or social insurance contributions) controlled by private individuals or households. In some countries, these devolved funds can be used to pay family or other carers for the support they provide. These self-directed budgets are usually subject to some degree of oversight by social workers or other authorized persons. By enhancing control over care, these approaches expand the choice options for individuals with long-term care needs (including people with dementia).

Evidence from evaluations suggests quality of life is improved as a result of these transfers of financial responsibility. For younger adults, the evidence also suggests there is access to more appropriate support, improved mental health and well-being, social participation and relationships and confidence and skills [46]. Although this form of self-directed support is perhaps less popular with older persons than with younger adults with disabilities [47], the flexibility and opportunities offered by direct payments or similar mechanisms open up new models of care, increase well-being and improve health and care system efficiency.

5.5 Inequalities

Of course, as discussed in Section 4, there are marked variations across the population in many respects, with lower socio-economic categories at higher risk of dementia [48], linked in part to higher exposure to risk factors such as lower education [49]. There is then the double jeopardy that population subgroups facing higher risks of dementia are also less able to afford treatment and care, or (in universal healthcare systems) less able to pay for supplementary services.

There are other variations, linked to place of residence, whether someone with dementia has a carer (given that some countries give more support to individuals without carers), quantity and quality of participation in local communities and so on. One of the purposes of risk-pooled healthcare and social care financing systems is to redistribute benefits (well-being) from the less sick to the more sick; many of those systems are also redistributive in relation to socio-economic status. We now consider the public financing of dementia care.

6 The Social Cost of Care: Willingness-to-Pay and the Financing of Dementia Care

We have seen in Section 3 that, at present, there is no effective disease-modifying pharmacological treatment of dementia, and that it does not look as if one will become available in the near future. There is strong evidence that donepezil, galantamine and rivastigmine (which are all cholinesterase-inhibitor medications) and memantine (which has a different mechanism of action) are cost-effective in the treatment of people with mild-to-moderate Alzheimer's disease [50]. Indeed, these medications are now off-patent in many countries, and so their prices will have dropped through competition, making the economic case even stronger today.

For people with moderate-to-severe Alzheimer's disease, the best evidence comes from the DOMINO trial which found that donepezil was both effective and cost-effective compared to placebo over a one-year period [51], and also appeared to reduce the risk of nursing home placement over a four-year period [52].[1] This would support the case for these medications being reimbursed through health insurance or taken up in the coverage of healthcare systems – as, for example, they are in England – but certainly care for persons with dementia will remain necessary in the future.

In the present state of affairs, the care of people with dementia already has a huge impact on society, as we outlined earlier in this chapter. Moreover, in many chapters of this book, proposals are made to improve care for people with dementia or provide better support for family and other unpaid carers. Implementing these proposals is likely to increase further the economic costs of care. As documented in the previous section, this may also lead to substantial personal costs for the households involved. In this section, we discuss how collective

---

[1] More information on the DOMINO trial can be found in Chapter 5.

government-organized systems can protect people with dementia and their households against these huge private costs. What could be the role of government in alleviating this financial burden? In answering this question, special attention should go to weaker socio-economic groups.

We focus on the distribution of the burden and not on its size. We also consider that distribution from a broader welfare point of view. Let us illustrate these two points by means of the example of unpaid care. As we have seen in the previous sections and in other chapters of this book, the cost of unpaid care can be large, both in economic terms (income losses) and in well-being terms (the health effects on carers). This raises two questions. First, is the overall cost of unpaid care larger or smaller than the cost of congregate care? This question about the size of the care burden for society is highly relevant but is not tackled in this section. Second, who has to bear that burden? Unpaid care costs are not borne by the government (at least not directly) and, if formal or congregate care is financed by the government, a shift from formal to informal (unpaid) care softens the pressure on government budgets. Yet the 'government' is not 'society'.

From the point of view of society, unpaid care costs are true economic costs also when they are borne by the individuals themselves. A shift to unpaid care can then increase or decrease the total burden (that is the first question), but it is in the first place a shift of the burden from society (the average taxpayer) to people with dementia and their social environment. It is this distributional perspective that we take in this section.

The optimal way to protect individuals against the financial burden of any disease (including dementia) is a system of insurance. Saving can never be optimal in a situation of uncertainty, when future costs are unknown, because individuals will save too much (if they are lucky) or too little (if they are hit severely). Pooling of risks through insurance is the best solution to this problem and purchasing insurance against care costs is the optimal solution for rational individuals. It is then somewhat surprising that private care insurance markets are missing or underdeveloped, even in high-income countries. Economists have even coined the term the 'care insurance puzzle' to refer to this issue that private insurance markets for long-term care are missing

[53, 54]. We first summarize briefly the potential explanations for this puzzle and show they also help to explain the specific challenges of government financing of dementia care. We then discuss willingness-to-pay for dementia care in society and conclude with some prospects for the future.

6.1 Why Are Private Insurance Markets Underdeveloped?

The fact that private long-term care insurance markets are underdeveloped is a general issue, but most of the explanations put forward for it are also highly relevant in the specific case of dementia care. Note first that private insurance in principle is meant to cover formal care in congregate settings or otherwise. To some extent it can be seen as a substitute for unpaid care. This has effects that may play in two directions

On one hand, if one strongly prefers to be cared for by one's partner or children, this will have a negative effect on the willingness to take private insurance, as this would strongly lower the threshold to be relegated to formal care. On the other hand, if parents are altruistic, they may opt to take private insurance just to avoid putting too large a burden on their children (in terms of direct costs or lost inheritance). Empirical evidence for the latter effect is found in SHARE data for France [55]. The two effects go in opposite directions and the net effect is unknown: it depends on culture and on family norms in a given society.

There are technical explanations for the lack of private care insurance markets. Long-term care in general and dementia care in particular are to some extent collective risks. Costs have been strongly increasing over time, both because the prevalence of dementia has been increasing and because the potential for unpaid care is decreasing because of smaller family sizes and increasing labour force participation by women, who have historically been the main providers of family care.

On a private market, where there is no compulsory contribution at a younger age, people will (rationally) wait as long as possible before they start contributing to the insurance. This makes it very difficult to diversify the risk of care over the population. Private insurers, who cannot organize intergenerational redistribution, have difficulties insuring such collective risks and, in any case, will have to raise high premiums. Moreover, private markets have difficulties coping with adverse selection – that is, the fact that insurance is more attractive for people with a higher risk, and that individuals themselves can form a better estimate of their risk than the insurers (see e.g. [56]).

This leads to the phenomenon that the pool of patients is 'selected' and consists mainly of 'expensive' persons. In turn, this leads to an increase in private market premiums, so that the resulting policies are no longer attractive for the better risks (or the population at large). All of these factors together could lead to premiums that are too high even for high-income households and that certainly are prohibitive for low-income households.

Even more important for long-term care is the issue of moral hazard – that is, the phenomenon that insured people will change their behaviour when they do not have to bear the costs. In the case of dementia, one should not think in the first place that this would encourage people to lessen their prevention efforts, as it seems unrealistic to assume people will become less concerned about developing dementia when they are insured.

However, moral hazard may play a role when circumscribing the need for care when one has dementia. It is, for example, likely that people with dementia (or their families) would opt for more expensive nursing home care or expensive formal home care if they were fully insured for the costs. It is even more difficult to define the 'need' for unpaid care. For private insurers it is necessary to control these forms of moral hazard, but this is difficult as the definition of needs in this setting has a strong subjective component. As a consequence, policies offered by private insurance companies often contain caps on the amount that can be reimbursed, or offer only fixed (and rather low) lump sum benefits. Caps and lump sum benefits restrict the possibility of moral hazard, but also make insurance policies much less attractive for the clients.

In addition to these technical factors, recent fascinating insights from behavioural economics contribute to the explanation from the demand side. Many individuals underestimate the probability they will need care in the future. As an example, Finkelstein and McGarry [56] report that more than 50% of older people in the United States (the average age of the sample is 79) estimate they have a 0% chance of being admitted to a nursing home in the coming five years.

This biased evaluation of personal risk can be due to two factors. It may be linked to a lack of information. In that case, it may seem rather easy to solve the problem: just try to inform individuals better about their true risk. More difficult, however, is to tackle the psychological phenomenon that people want to deny the fact that they will become dependent: they know, but they refuse to accept, because they cannot live with the prospect of ending up in a nursing home. Even large information campaigns will not solve that problem. Given the widespread negative perception of dementia in society, it is likely that this phenomenon of denial plays an important role in the present context.

The same is true for another behavioural phenomenon. An insurance contract implies one pays a premium when healthy in order to be compensated when sick. In a certain sense it boils down to a 'transfer' from healthy to sick states which is welfare-improving if needs are larger when sick. However, if there is a widespread feeling in society that one will no longer be conscious or aware of one's circumstances when experiencing dementia, or that one will anyway not be capable of really enjoying the care one gets, such a transfer might be seen as just a waste of money. Why pay a premium (and lower present consumption) when healthy, if having a larger income in the state of dementia is perceived not to add to quality of life in that state?

Finally, the lack of private insurance markets can also be explained by the fact that there is some public care provision. This argument is mainly put forward for the United States, where the availability of means-tested Medicaid as a support of last resort is assumed to crowd out the motivation to take private insurance [54].

6.2 The Challenge of Public Financing of Dementia Care

Confronted with underdeveloped private insurance markets, the only way to help people with dementia and their families is to install public insurance. Without insurance, they would have to pay the full cost of care out of their own pocket, and this would be prohibitive for many. Note that when we talk about public 'insurance', this is not meant to refer only to Bismarckian collective insurance systems but also includes tax-based public care systems. There are obvious and important differences between the two, but for the purposes of this chapter the relevant criterion is that the costs are to some extent borne or the care services are to some extent provided by a collective, non-market system.

It is well known that public insurance can in principle take care of collective risks (because it can set up intergenerational transfers) and of adverse selection (by making premiums compulsory). Like the private market, it will nevertheless also have difficulties with moral hazard, but public authorities usually have more coercive power than private firms. In general, it is less imperative for public insurance to define and accurately predict risks, just because there is always the outlet (the 'safety net') of compulsory taxation.

Not only can public insurance offer an answer to some of the technical issues that hamper the development of private markets, it can go further than private insurers in coping with socio-economic inequalities. The government can make premiums independent of risk and of income. It can also link benefits to individuals' economic situation. This is very important for a situation like dementia where, as we have seen in Section 4, there is a clear social gradient in prevalence. Public insurance is not only efficient, it can also lead to a more equitable distribution of the burden.

Yet, and this is then another puzzle, public long-term care insurance is also underdeveloped, even in rich countries. Indeed, the recent experience of the COVID-19 pandemic has convincingly uncovered many weaknesses in our systems of care for older people, in all countries. Some evidence on the financial consequences of long-term care is summarized in Figures 14.1 and 14.2 [57].

Figure 14.1 shows out-of-pocket costs – that is, what remains to be paid by people with dementia themselves after government intervention, for someone with median income. For home care, a distinction is made between different levels of needs: low, moderate and severe needs correspond respectively to 6.5, 22.5 and 41.25 hours of professional home care per week. The costs are compared to an affordability threshold: for home care this is defined as the maximum threshold of out-of-pocket expenditures, beyond which individuals would end up in poverty.

For congregate care (called 'institutionalized care' in the Organisation for Economic Co-operation and Development (OECD) report, although this would be a misrepresentation of what is usually provided), it is assumed individuals can afford to spend their whole income on care, as living costs are covered by the nursing home. This is a very tough measure, as it implies the person with dementia would not have any income left for other personal expenditures. While there is a lot of international variation, the top panel shows formal home care is in most countries not affordable for people with severe needs. In fact, panel B suggests congregate ('institutional') care can act as a substitute solution for these persons, but with the consequence that they have to spend a large fraction of their income to cover the costs.

Figure 14.1 focusses on people with median income. Figure 14.2 considers the financial situation of people with moderate needs (22.5 hours of care per week) with either a 'low' income (20th percentile of the distribution of disposable income of the population aged 65+) or a 'high' income (80th percentile of that same income distribution). Although most public systems take into account the income position of the individuals concerned (or have strict means-testing), panel A shows that in many countries home care is far from affordable for people with low incomes. Even for those with high incomes, the financial burden is substantial (panel B).

The results in Figure 14.1 and 14.2 should be evaluated by comparison with what would be optimal insurance. It is well known in economic theory that in a hypothetical situation without moral hazard or administrative costs, full insurance is socially optimal – that is, individuals should have the same income whether or not they need care (and have to pay the premium). With moral hazard, full insurance is no longer optimal, but the observed out-of-pocket costs are certainly much too large from an optimal insurance perspective. In fact, Drèze et al. [58] argue an optimal scheme should offer full insurance above a deductible.

If we want to improve the public financing of dementia care, it is important first to understand why it is deficient right now. Why is there apparently insufficient political support for increasing the care budget (and less support than for increasing the health budget)? Of course, government

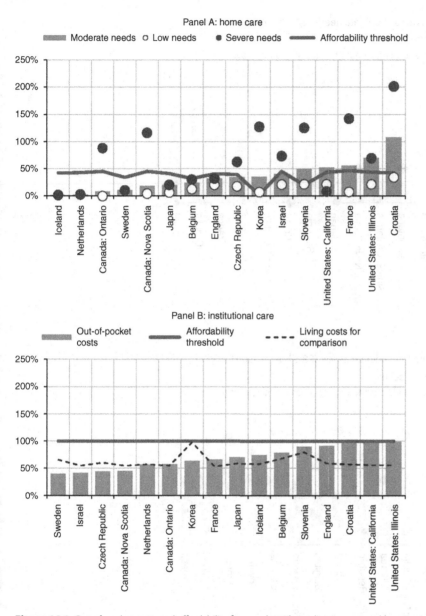

Figure 14.1 Out-of-pocket costs and affordability for people with median income and low assets [57]

budgets have been under pressure everywhere. Many critics do not distinguish between different parts of that budget, and care expenditures then suffer from this general feeling of distrust of government. Indeed, public financing of care is not fully transparent for citizens and is therefore not perceived as an insurance system, which ultimately is welfare-improving for everybody.

At a deeper level, the behavioural economic factors described in the context of private insurance also play a role in the political decision-making

process as they have an impact on the willingness to contribute. Citizens who underestimate the probability that they will need care (either because of a lack of information, or because they do not want to accept the negative message), or who have the feeling that care for persons with dementia is largely useless because they cannot enjoy it anyway, will not be inclined to pay higher contributions for dementia care. If dementia care has to compete with other uses of the money within a fixed budget for health and care, treatments which aim to cure the sick

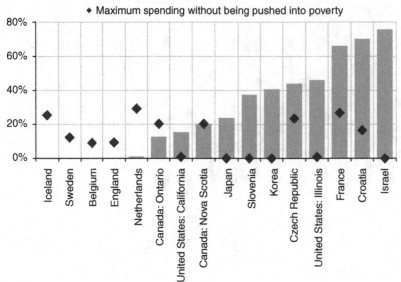

Panel A: home care for moderate needs (22½ hours), low income
- ■ Out-of-pocket costs
- ◆ Maximum spending without being pushed into poverty

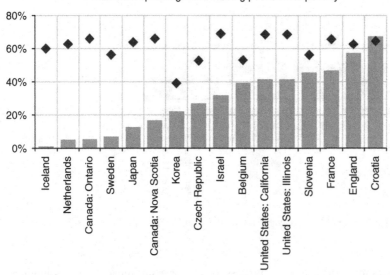

Panel B: home care for moderate needs (22½ hours), high income
- ■ Out-of-pocket costs
- ◆ Maximum spending without being pushed into poverty

Figure 14.2 Out-of-pocket costs by income for someone with low assets and moderate needs [57]

(even if very expensive, e.g. immunotherapy for cancer treatment) will be more popular than care that is perceived to have a negligible effect on quality of life.

To some extent, this may create a kind of vicious circle. Decisions related to the organization of care will, on one hand, reflect the (limited) willingness to contribute, and on the other hand also influence it. If nursing homes are not attractive and citizens have the impression they cannot be made *more* attractive, this will have an impact on their willingness to finance nursing homes. As a result, the lack of financial means makes it difficult to make nursing homes more attractive. If the impression is created that family and other unpaid care is better for people with dementia than nursing home care (this may in some cases be true), and that it is not necessary that carers are financially supported by the government (which is highly debatable), this may be used as an easy excuse not to increase the care budget.

In other chapters of this book it has been argued that the gloomy assumptions underlying this negative attitude are not realistic. Care for people with dementia can improve their quality of life and is in many cases cost-effective. It can therefore be argued that increasing the public care budget would improve welfare. However, increasing the public care budget means increasing the contributions to be paid by citizens. Ultimately this boils down to a choice between private consumption and more and better care. Are individuals willing to give up some private consumption and accept an increase in contributions? How much are they willing to pay for dementia care?

6.3 Willingness-to-Pay for Dementia Care

It is mainly economists who have explicitly studied the 'willingness-to-pay' (WTP) for dementia care. Some take the position that WTP is the best criterion to ethically evaluate government intervention in a democratic society as it is a measure of the preferences of citizens. Critics of this position argue the ethical desirability of care for the weakest in society cannot be determined by this kind of individualistic calculation, and, moreover, individual willingness-to-pay can be based on wrong or incomplete information. We have given examples of such biases in the previous sections. This is not the place to go into this ethical debate, but we do not interpret WTP as offering the basic ethical foundation for the analysis of government policy. We just see it as an approximation of the willingness of citizens to contribute to the system, and hence as a measure of the support in the population for more dementia care. If WTP is low, it is still possible to defend public intervention in dementia care on

ethical grounds, but it will be more difficult to foster sufficient political support for it.

Most studies on the WTP for dementia care use some questionnaire technique, either contingent valuation or discrete choice. The results obtained in different studies and with different techniques are not always consistent, but the broad picture is nevertheless rather robust. We only sketch that broad picture here.

In line with what we hinted at in Section 3, WTP for a cure is high (see e.g. [59]). There certainly is a large potential market here. It also seems individuals attach value to information: in a study with American citizens, more than 70% would take a predictive test, if it were available, even if taking the test does not have any implications for treatment [60]. The mean WTP for such a test is between $400 and $500. This result is less robust, however: 40% of a Swiss sample of the general population did not want to pay for the inclusion of early detection of dementia in public health programmes [61].

The same Swiss sample is willing to pay a substantial amount for more generous support given to family and other unpaid carers [61]. This result is also found in the Netherlands [62], with a strong emphasis on supporting social contact and social activities, and in Spain [63], where day centres are especially valued. Not surprisingly, studies with carers themselves also reveal a large WTP for more and better support ([64] for France; [65] for Switzerland). The latter study shows people providing unpaid care for people with mild-to-moderate dementia symptoms would be willing to give up 23% of their total wealth for a stabilization of the situation of the people they support.

Some studies have tried to measure the WTP to remain living in the community rather than to move into a nursing home. Costa-Font [66] calls this 'institutionalization aversion' and it turns out to be substantial. His Spanish respondents were asked the following question. 'In the event of suffering some form of mild impairment, would you be willing to pay ## monthly to avoid entering a nursing home if you would receive instead equivalent care without being institutionalized?' They were willing to pay on average 16% of their income to avoid the nursing home. Nieboer et al. [62] found similarly strong feelings against being admitted to a nursing home in the Netherlands.

Of course, this small set of results immediately raises the question: if WTP in these hypothetical studies is substantial, why is this not reflected in actual policies and care budgets? An easy, but too easy, answer is that the results in these studies are not reliable. It is indeed true the answers to these hypothetical questions cannot be used immediately to predict behaviour, either on the market or in the voting booth. Yet the answers are certainly not random, and the overall picture is surprisingly coherent. Even if we interpret the numbers cautiously, we still face the question of why this apparent WTP for better care does not get translated into government action.

6.4 Room for Optimism?

One possible explanation for this apparent paradox is that the population is not informed, or is insufficiently aware of the underfinancing of care for older people in general, and for people with dementia in particular. Of course, here also the effect can be due both to a real lack of information or to a denial of what one knows. The recent COVID-19 experience seems to have brought this paradox to the fore. Without generalizing too easily, it can still be stated that in almost all countries there has been evidence of low quality of care, insufficient preparation and an unnecessarily high number of deaths in nursing homes. Home care was also severely hit and not able to respond adequately. A large part of the population was shocked, and many see the COVID crisis as a wake-up call and hope it may lead to increases in government budgets for care in the future.

In a certain sense, the COVID experience shows the way that should be followed to foster political support for the public financing of dementia care. Citizens should be better informed about the real risks associated with dementia. Even more important is to inform them about the possibility to improve quality of life with adequate care, to fight the stigma associated with dementia, to organize dementia-friendly communities. The potential for insurance and public policies to improve the well-being of everybody should be explained, as should be their potential to mitigate socio-economic inequalities.

All of this is related to the other chapters in this book. There are important interactions between ideologies, social policies, quality of care, information about quality of care and the willingness of the population to pay for it. Many of the proposals in this book to improve care can only be realized with better public financing, and support for public financing can only grow if (the perception of) dementia care improves.

7 Conclusion

Dementia leads to huge and increasing economic costs. Informal and unpaid care is an important component of these costs, both from a personal and from a societal point of view. Yet society should keep the ambition to provide affordable and high-quality care to all persons with dementia.

Public intervention is needed to reach an optimal solution. First, although an effective pharmaceutical cure for dementia would undoubtedly be a blockbuster drug for private companies, economic features of the production process of dementia medicines explain the relative underinvestment in private research. Second, there are no well-functioning private insurance markets for long-term care expenditures. Public intervention is needed to stimulate research, to finance care, to reduce inequalities in health and well-being and to address barriers to access to effective treatment and supportive care. This is even more important because of the clear socio-economic gradient in care needs: only public insurance can implement the necessary mechanisms to make care affordable and accessible for the poorer socio-economic groups.

While the need is clear, we see that long-term care in general and dementia care in particular are underfinanced in all countries. This can be at least partly explained by the psychological mechanism through which citizens deny the fact that they are likely to need care when they grow old, and by the dominating conviction among a large share of the population that care for persons with dementia does not yield substantial improvements in their quality of life. One of the main messages of this book is that this conviction is wrong. High-quality care *does* improve the quality of life of persons with dementia and is in many cases cost-effective.

Given that curative possibilities against oldest age and irreversible dementia will remain limited in the coming years, preventive strategies should be the priority, along with improved dementia care and social support. But for this to happen, public health institutions, social policies and practices should be a funding priority. There may be a virtuous circle here: better public financing may lead to fewer social inequalities and better quality care, and support for public financing could grow if better care is indeed provided and perceived as such by the population.

References

1. Patterson C. *World Alzheimer Report 2018: The State of the Art of Dementia Research.* London, Alzheimer's Disease International, 2018.

2. Hurd MD, Martorell P, Delavande A, Mullen KJ, Langa KM. Monetary costs of dementia in the United States. *New England Journal of Medicine* 2013; **368**(14): 1326–34.

3. Prince M, Comas-Herrera A, Knapp M, Guerchet M, Karagiannidou M. *World Alzheimer Report 2016: Improving Healthcare for People Living with Dementia.* London, Alzheimer's Disease International, 2016.

4. Hofmarcher T, Lindgren P, Wilking N, Jönsson B. The cost of cancer in Europe 2018. *European Journal of Cancer* 2020; **129**: 41–9.

5. Schaller S, Mauskopf J, Kriza C, Wahlster P, Kolominsky-Rabas PL. The main cost drivers in dementia: A systematic review. *International Journal of Geriatric Psychiatry* 2015; **30**(2): 111–29.

6. Keogh-Brown M, TarpJensen H, Arrighi M, Smith RD. The impact of Alzheimer's disease on the Chinese economy. *EBioMedicine* 4: 184–90.

7. Rossor M, Knapp M. Can we model a cognitive footprint of interventions and policies to help to meet the global challenge of dementia? *Lancet* 2015; **386**(9997): 1008–10.

8. Knapp M, Comas-Herrera S, Wittenberg R, Hu B, King D, Rehill A, Adelaja B. *Scenarios of Dementia Care: What Are the Impacts on Cost and Quality of Life?* London, PSSRU/CPEC, LSE, 2014.

9. Anderson R, Knapp M, Wittenberg R, Handels R, Schott JM. Economic modelling of disease-modifying therapies in Alzheimer's disease. Care Policy and Evaluation Centre, LSE, 2018.

10. Editorial. Dementia in the UK: Preparing the NHS for new treatments. *Lancet* 2018; **391**: 1237.

11. DiMasi JA, Grabowski HG, Hansen RW. Innovation in the pharmaceutical industry: New estimates of R&D costs. *Journal of Health Economics* 2016; **47**: 20–33.

12. Wouters OJ, McKee M, Luyten J. Estimated research and development investment needed to bring a new medicine to market, 2009–2018. *Journal of the American Medical Association* 2020; **323**(9): 844–53.

13. Scott TJ, O'Connor A, Link AN, Beaulieu TJ. Economic analysis of opportunities to accelerate Alzheimer's disease research and development. *Annals of the New York Academy of Sciences* 2014; **1313**(1): 17–34.

14. Cummings JL, Morstorf T, Zhong K. Alzheimer's disease drug-development pipeline: Few candidates, frequent failures. *Alzheimer's Research & Therapy* 2014; **6**(4): 37.

15. Cummings J, Reiber C, Kumar P. The price of progress: Funding and financing Alzheimer's disease drug development. *Alzheimer's & Dementia* (NY) 2018; **4**: 330–43.

16. Cummings J, Lee G, Mortsdorf T, Ritter A, Zhong K. Alzheimer's disease drug development pipeline: 2017. *Alzheimer's & Dementia: Translational Research & Clinical Interventions* 2017; **3**(3): 367–84.

17. World Health Organization. *Commission on Social Determinants of Health: Final Report* [Internet]. Geneva, World Health Organization, 2008 [cited 2020 Feb 29]. Available from www.who.int/social_determinants/thecommission/finalreport/en

18. World Health Organization. *World Report on Ageing and Health* [Internet]. Geneva, World Health Organization, 2015 [cited 2020 Feb 29]. Available from www.who.int/life-course/publications/2015-ageing-report/en

19. Shah A, Oommen G, Wuntakal B. Cross-cultural aspects of dementia. *Psychiatry* 2005; **4**(2): 103–6.

20. O'Connor ML, McFadden SH. A terror management perspective on young adults' ageism and attitudes toward dementia. *Educational Gerontology* 2012 Sep 1; **38**(9): 627–43.

21. Kivipelto M, Ngandu T, Laatikainen T, Winblad B, Soininen H, Tuomilehto J. Risk score for the prediction of dementia risk in 20 years among middle aged people: A longitudinal, population-based study. *Lancet Neurology* 2006 Sep 1; **5**(9): 735–41.

22. Debette S, Seshadri S, Beiser A, Au R, Himali JJ, Palumbo C, et al. Midlife vascular risk factor exposure accelerates structural brain aging and cognitive decline. *Neurology* [Internet]. 2011 [cited 2020 Mar 1]; **77**(5). Available from https://n.neurology.org/content/77/5/461

23. Mayer F, Di Pucchio A, Lacorte E, Bacigalupo I, Marzolini F, Ferrante G, et al. An estimate of attributable cases of Alzheimer disease and vascular dementia due to modifiable risk factors: The impact of primary prevention in Europe and in Italy. *Dementia and Geriatric Cognitive Disorders Extra* 2018 Feb 21; **8**(1): 60–71.

24. Cadar D, Lassale C, Davies H, Llewellyn DJ, Batty GD, Steptoe A. Individual and area-based socioeconomic factors associated with dementia incidence in England: Evidence from a 12-year follow-up in the English longitudinal study of ageing. *JAMA Psychiatry* 2018 Jul 1; **75**(7): 723–32.

25. Fratiglioni L, Paillard-Borg S, Winblad B. An active and socially integrated lifestyle in late life might protect against dementia. *Lancet Neurology* 2004 Jun 1; **3**(6): 343–53.

26. Power MC, Adar SD, Yanosky JD, Weuve J. Exposure to air pollution as a potential contributor to cognitive function, cognitive decline, brain imaging, and dementia: A systematic review of epidemiologic research. *NeuroToxicology* 2016 Sep 1; **56**: 235–53.

27. Cooper C, Lodwick R, Walters K, Raine R, Manthorpe J, Iliffe S, et al. Inequalities in receipt of mental and physical healthcare in people with dementia in the UK. *Age & Ageing* 2017 May 1; **46**(3): 393–400.

28. Cloos P. Is there a pathological way of ageing? Questioning 'Alzheimer's disease'. *Medicine Anthropology Theory* 2017; **4**(2): 60–9.

29. Chen C, Zissimopoulos JM. Racial and ethnic differences in trends in dementia prevalence and risk factors in the United States. *Alzheimer's & Dementia: Translational Research & Clinical Interventions* 2018 Oct 5; **4**: 510–20.

30. Anderson NB, Bulatao RA, Cohen B, National Research Council (US) Panel on Race. *Ethnic Differences in Dementia and Alzheimer's Disease* [Internet]. Washington, DC, National Academies Press, 2004 [cited 2020 Mar 2]. Available from www.ncbi.nlm.nih.gov/books/NBK25535

31. Lorenz K, Freddolino PP, Comas-Herrera A, Knapp M, Damant J. Technology-based tools and services for people with dementia and carers: Mapping technology onto the dementia care pathway. *Dementia* 2019; **18**(2): 725–74.

32. Delavande A, Hurd MD, Martorell P, Langa KM. Dementia and out-of-pocket spending on health care services. *Alzheimer's and Dementia* 2013; **9**(1): 19–29.

33. Kelley AS, McGarry K, Gorges R, et al. The burden of health care costs for patients with dementia in the last 5 years of life. *Annals of Internal Medicine* 2015; **163**(10): 729–36.

34. Kaufman JE, Gallo W, Fahs MC. The contribution of dementia to the disparity in family wealth between black and non-black Americans. *Ageing and Society* 2020; **40**(2): 306–27.

35. Charlesworth A, Johnson P. *Securing the Future: Funding Health and Social Care to the 2030s.* London, Institute for Fiscal Studies, 2018.

36. Baxter K. Self-funders and social care: Findings from a scoping review. *Research Policy and Planning* 2016; 179–93.

37. Lum T, Shi C, Wong G, Wong K. COVID-19 and long-term care policy for older people in Hong Kong. *Journal of Aging & Social Policy* 2020; 1–7.

38. World Health Organization. *World Report on Ageing and Health.* Geneva, World Health Organization, 2015.

39. Wittenberg R, Knapp M, Hu B, et al. The costs of dementia in England. *International Journal of Geriatric Psychiatry* 2019; **34**: 1095–1103.

40. Wübker A, Zwakhalen SM, Challis D, Suhonen R, Karlsson S, Zabalegui A, Soto M, Sas K, Sauerland D. Costs of care for people with dementia just before and after nursing home placement: Primary data from eight European countries. *European Journal of Health Economics* 2015; **16**(7): 689–707.

41. World Health Organization. *Global Action Plan on the Public Health Response to Dementia 2017–2025.* Geneva, World Health Organization, 2017.

42. Livingston G, Manela M, O'Keeffe A, Rapaport P, Cooper C, Knapp M, et al. Clinical effectiveness of START (STrAtegies for RelaTives) psychological intervention for family carers and the effects on cost of care for people with dementia: Six year follow-up of a randomised controlled trial. *British Journal of Psychiatry* 2019; **216**(1): 35–42.

43. Skinner M, Lorentzen H, Tingvold L, Sortland O, Andfossen N, Iegermalm M. Volunteers and informal caregivers' contributions and collaboration with formal caregivers in Norwegian long-term care. *Journal of Aging and Social Policy* 2020; 1–26.

44. Sharac J, McCrone P, Clement S, Thornicroft G. The economic impact of mental health stigma and discrimination: A systematic review. *Epidemiologia e Psichiatria Sociale* 2010; **19**(3): 223–32.

45. World Health Organization. *Dementia: A Public Health Priority.* Geneva, World Health Organization, 2017.

46. Netten A, Jones K, Knapp M, Fernandez JL, Challis, D, Glendinnig C, et al. Personalisation through individual budgets: Does it work and for whom? *British Journal of Social Work* 2012; **42**(8): 1556–73.

47. Hatton C, Waters J. *Older People and Personal Budgets: A Re-analysis of Data from the National Personal Budget Survey.* London, Lancaster University and In Control, 2012.

48. George KM, Lutsey PL, Kucharska-Newton A, Palta P, Heiss G, Osypuk T, Folsom AR Life course individual and neighborhood socioeconomic status and risk of dementia in the Atherosclerosis Risk in Communities Neurocognitive Study (ARIC-NCS). *American Journal of Epidemiology* 2020 Oct; **189** (10): 1134–42. doi.org/10.1093/aje/kwaa072

49. Livingston G, Sommerlad A, Orgeta V, Costafreda SG, Huntley J, Ames D, et al. Dementia prevention, intervention, and care. *Lancet* 2017; **390**: 2673–2734.

50. Hyde C, Peters J, Bond M, Rogers G, Hoyle M, Anderson R, et al. Evolution of the evidence on the effectiveness and cost-effectiveness of acetylcholinesterase inhibitors and memantine for Alzheimer's disease: Systematic review and economic model. *Age and Ageing* 2013; **42**: 14–20.

51. Knapp M, King D, Romeo R, Adams J, Baldwin A, Ballard C, et al. Cost-effectiveness of donepezil and memantine in moderate to severe Alzheimer's disease (the DOMINO-AD trial). *International Journal of Geriatric Psychiatry* 2017; **32**(12): 1205–16.

52. Howard R, McShane R, Lindesay J, Ritchie C, Baldwin A, Barber R, et al. Nursing home placement in the Donepezil and Memantine in Moderate to Severe Alzheimer's Disease (DOMINO-AD) trial: Secondary and post-hoc analyses. *Lancet Neurology* 2015; **14**: 1171–81.

53. Pestieau P, Ponthiere G. Long term care insurance puzzle. CORE: Discussion Paper 2010/23, 2010.

54. Brown J, Finkelstein A. Insuring long-term care in the United States. *Journal of Economic Perspectives* 2011; **25**: 119–42.

55. Courbage C, Roudaut N. Empirical evidence on long term care insurance purchase in France. *Geneva Papers on Risk and Insurance* 2008; **33**: 645–58.

56. Finkelstein A, McGarry K. Multiple dimensions of private information: Evidence from the long-term care insurance market. *American Economic Review* 2006; **96**: 938–58.

57. Muir T. *Measuring Social Protection for Long-Term care: OECD Health Working Papers No. 93*. Paris, OECD Publishing, 2017. http://dx.doi.org/10.1787/a411500a-en.

58. Drèze JH, Pestieau P, Schokkaert E. Arrow's theorem of the deductible and long-term care insurance. *Economics Letters* 2016; **148**: 103–5.

59. Basu R. Willingness-to-pay to prevent Alzheimer's disease: A contingent valuation approach. *International Journal of Health Care Finance and Economics* 2013; **13**: 233–45.

60. Neumann P, Cohen J, Hammitt J, Concannon T, Auerbach H, Fang C, Kent D. Willingness-to-pay for predictive tests with no immediate treatment applications: A survey of US residents. *Health Economics* 2012; **21**: 238–51.

61. Nocera S, Bonato D, Telser H. The contingency of contingent valuation: How much are people willing to pay against Alzheimer's disease? *International Journal of Health Care Finance and Economics* 2002; **2**: 219–40.

62. Nieboer A, Koolman X, Stolk E. Preferences for long-term care services: Willingness to pay estimates derived from a discrete choice experiment. *Social Science & Medicine* 2010; **70**: 1317–25.

63. Negrin MA, Pinilla J, Leon CJ. Willingness to pay for alternative policies for patients with Alzheimer's disease. *Health Economics, Policy and Law* 2008; **3**: 257–75.

64. Gerves-Pinquie C, Bellanger M, Ankri J. Willingness to pay for informal care in France: The value of funding support interventions for caregivers. *Health Economics Review* 2014; 4.

65. König M, Wettstein A. Caring for relatives with dementia: Willingness-to-pay for a reduction in caregiver's burden. *Expert Review of Pharmacoeconomics and Outcomes Research* 2002; **2**: 535–47.

66. Costa-Font J. 'Institutionalization aversion' and the willingness to pay for home health care. *Journal of Housing Economics* 2017; **38**: 62–9.

67. Wong G, Knapp M. Should we move dementia research funding from a cure to its care? *Expert Review of Neurotherapeutics* 2020. doi: 10.1080/14737175.2020.1735364

68. Mukadam N, Anderson R, Knapp M, Wittenberg R, Karagiannidou M, Costafreda SG, et al. Effective interventions for potentially modifiable risk factors for late-onset dementia: A costs and cost-effective modelling study. *Lancet Healthy Longevity* 2020; **1**: e13–e20.

Index

Printed in the United States
by Baker & Taylor Publisher Services